Michael

Michael

VENTRICULAR
Electrocardiography

VENTRICULAR
Electrocardiography

J. WILLIS HURST, M.D.*

Candler Professor of Medicine (Cardiology)
Emory University School of Medicine
Atlanta, Georgia

*Professor and Chairman, Department of Medicine,
Emory University School of Medicine, Atlanta, Georgia, 1957-1986.

J. B. Lippincott Company • Philadelphia

Gower Medical Publishing • New York • London

Distributed in USA and Canada by:
J.B. Lippincott Company
East Washington Square
Philadelphia, PA 19105
USA

Distributed in Southeast Asia, Hong Kong, India,
and Pakistan by:
Harper and Row (Asia) Pte Ltd.
37 Jalan Pemimpin 02–01
Singapore 2057

Distributed in UK and Continental Europe by:
Harper and Row Ltd.
Middlesex House
34–42 Cleveland Street
London W1P 5FB
UK

Distributed in Japan by:
Igaku Shoin Ltd.
Tokyo International
P.O. Box 5063
Tokyo
Japan

Distributed in Australia and New Zealand by:
Harper and Row (Australia) Pty Ltd.
P.O. Box 226
Artarmon, N.S.W. 2064
Australia

Library of Congress Cataloging–in–Publication Data
Hurst, J. Willis (John Willis), 1920-
    Ventricular Electrocardiography/ J. Willis Hurst.
        p.   cm.
    ISBN 0–397–44615–2
    1. Electrocardiography. 2. Heart--Ventricles--Disease-
-Diagnosis.   I. Title.
    [DNLM: 1. Electrocardiography. 2. Heart Diseases-
-diagnosis.   WG   140   H966v]
RC683.5.E5H84   1990
616.1'207543--dc20
DNLM/DLC
for Library of Congress   90–2939
                                                      CIP

British Library Cataloguing in Publication Data
Hurst, J. Willis (John Willis), *1920-*
        Ventricular Electrocardiography/ J. Willis Hurst.
        1. Man. Heart. Diagnosis. Electrocardiography
        I. Title
        616.1207547--dc20

        ISBN 0–397–44615–2

Editor: Erik L. Goldman
Copy Editor: Kenneth Lane
Designers: Lori Thorn, Nava Anav
Illustrators: Susan Tilberry
            Laura Pardi Duprey
            Wendy Jackelow
            Virginia Schoonover-Carr
Art Director: Jill Feltham
Illustration Director: Laura Pardi Duprey

10   9   8   7   6   5   4   3   2   1

Printed in Hong Kong

*T*HIS BOOK IS DEDICATED TO ROBERT PRESTON GRANT (1915 TO 1966),* A CREATIVE GENIUS AND EXCELLENT TEACHER, FOR HIS CONTRIBUTION TO THE FIELD OF VECTOR ELECTROCARDIOGRAPHY AND TO HIS ASSOCIATE, E. HARVEY ESTES, JR.,** WHO HELPED CLARIFY AND TEACH THE CONCEPTS TO A COUNTLESS NUMBER OF PHYSICIANS.

*Dr. Grant was Instructor in Medicine and Assistant Professor of Medicine and Physiology at Emory University, Atlanta, Georgia, from 1947 to 1950. He joined the National Institutes of Health in 1950 where he held several important positions. He became Director of the National Heart (now the Heart, Lung and Blood) Institute in 1966. He remained in that position until his untimely death in August 1966.

**Dr. Estes worked intimately with Dr. Grant when he was at Emory. He later joined the Department of Medicine at Duke University, Durham, North Carolina, where he became Professor of Medicine. In 1966, he became Professor and Chairman of the Department of Community and Family Medicine, a position he held until 1985. He is currently Professor of Medicine and Community and Family Medicine.

PREFACE

This book represents an effort to rekindle interest in the important and exciting subject of ventricular electrocadiography.

There has been a decline in the interest of physicians in learning and teaching ventricular electrocardiography. This has occurred despite the fact that the machines used for the purpose have been simplified, the recording process requires very little time, and more electrocardiograms are recorded today than at any time in history. There are many reasons for this waning of interest. Some of these are as follows:

- Physiology of the heart, including electrocardiography is taught less in modern medical schools than it was in the past. Molecular biology is taught beautifully in the modern curriculum of basic science departments, but the integrated physiology that is needed and used by clinicians is emphasized less now than in former decades. House staff programs may not include electrocardiography, and cardiology fellowship programs may not include in depth discussions of ventricular electrocardiography.
- There is a tendency on the part of students, house officers, fellows, indeed all of us, to memorize medical "facts" rather than understand them. The basic principles of electrocardiography are not stressed by all teachers, and often, they are not learned by beginners. It is difficult to memorize the infinite number of possible electrocardiographic abnormalities. This being true, many individuals who interpret electrocardiograms do not have the educational "building blocks" required to increase their knowledge of the subject. They interpret increasing numbers of electrocardiograms, but their skill at interpretation does not improve. The old adage is correct: Practice does not make perfect - - it is perfect practice that makes perfect.
- The correlation of cardiologic data is not emphasized adequately in medical schools or house-staff training. Accordingly, many physicians, even those who work in cardiac catheterization or echocardiographic laboratories, may not correlate the results of such procedures with the clinical data which includes the information gleaned from careful analysis of the electrocardiogram. They therefore miss a great learning opportunity.
- Though it is grossly inadequate, computer software for electrocardiography is being used more and more frequently. There is no computer program that can routinely identify all electrocardiographic abnormalities with precision, but because an interpretation is spelled out by an expensive machine, it is assumed to be accurate. Worse still, is the fact that the early learner assumes that he or she does not need to learn basic principles because the computer can interpret the tracing. Consequently, the computer acts as an obstacle to learning. This is not to say that the computer could not become a great teaching tool; what I am saying is

that it has not, thus far, been developed as such. Then, too, the identification of abnormalities alone, sometimes done precisely by computers, is not electrocardiography. As I view it, there are three steps involved in electrocardiography: the conversion of electrocardiographic deflections to vectors; the creation of an electrical differential diagnosis to explain each abnormal vector; and finally, the development of a clinical differential diagnosis that could explain the electrical abnormalities. The diagnostic clues found in the history, physical examination, and chest x-ray should then be used to support or deny the diagnostic possibilities considered from the analysis of the electrocardiogram.

- I believe that most medical educators will admit that during the last few years there has been a steady decline in the level of skill in history taking, physical examination, electrocardiographic interpretation and interpretation of the chest x-ray film. The lack of interest in these techniques on the part of the younger student is partly due to the old and routine nature of these methods; new techniques such as echocardiography, magnetic resonance imaging, nuclear cardiology, cardiac catheterization, and coronary arteriography are inviting competitors, and because training and study time is limited, the early learner spends most of his/her time observing and learning these new techniques. He or she may not understand that a decision to use a new technologic procedure for examining a patient should be made after a thorough and accurate analysis of the medical data gleaned from more routine techniques. Obviously, when low technology is used poorly, it is highly likely that high technology will also be used poorly.

This book does not deal with arrhythmia, because early learners are exposed to arrhythmias in the coronary care unit, the operating room, in intensive care units, and in other monitored units. Accordingly, the average medical trainee today knows more about arrhythmias than did his or her counterpart two decades ago.

Legend holds that Sir Thomas Lewis believed, after he investigated cardiac arrhythmia using the electrocardiograph machine, that the electrocardiogram had little else to offer. Dr. Frank Wilson and many others began to emphasize the value of the ventricular electrocardiogram, and for a while, this aspect of electrocardiography dominated the field. Then, as monitoring systems were developed, the interest in arrhythmias was again emphasized, and the ventricular electrocardiogram was de-emphasized. This is the major reason why I have written this book: I believe that the interest in ventricular electrocardiography needs resuscitation.

In summary, ventricular electrocardiography should be emphasized once again as a basic diagnostic tool. It should not be discarded in the teaching arena. As long as we order electrocardiograms on our patients, we should struggle to improve our ability to interpret them, and to use the information they provide in the integrative thought process that leads to a cardiac diagnosis.

MY OWN INTEREST

My own interest in electrocardiography began in 1948, when, as a fellow with Dr. Paul White at the Massachusetts General Hospital in Boston, I was expected to "read" the electrocardiograms from the cardiology service. Dr. Conger Williams was trying to determine which of several chest lead systems was the best. Was it CR, CL, CF, or the new unipolar chest lead (CV) described by Wilson? Later, Dr. Emanuel Goldberger visited the hospital and discussed his augmented extremity leads (aVR, aVL and aVF).

During the early months of 1949, I became interested in Robert Grant's approach to electrocardiography. He could simply inspect an electrocardiogram and determine the directions and magnitudes of the electrical forces of the heart. I wrote to Dr. Grant, who was working at Emory University, to send me as much information as he could about his new method. He did. He sent me a copy of the manuscript of his small book, which was later printed privately by Emory University. What an exciting document! I later joined the Emory faculty and was influenced greatly by Bob Grant. The Grant and Estes book, Spatial Vector Electrocardiography, was published in 1951(1). I published, with Dr. Grant looking over my shoulder, along with Dr. Grattan Woodson, an Atlas of Vector Electrocardiography in 1952(2).

Later, in 1957, I, along with Russell Wallace (a medical student at the time), investigated the method by total body mapping. Deflections from the extremity leads were recorded, and V leads were used to record the deflections from numerous electrode positions on the anterior surface of the chest. The recordings were organized by pasting small lead markers on the chest surface at the point from which each of the deflections was recorded. A chest roentgenogram was then made, and the electrocardiographic deflections were pasted on the chest film at the site of the lead markers, identifying the spot from which the electrocardiogram was recorded. The transitional pathways for the QRS complex and T waves were identified on the chest x ray film by locating the electrocardiograms in which the QRS complex and T waves were resultantly zero. The transitional pathways of the QRS complex and T waves divided the chest into positive and negative sides. The body maps used then were primitive compared to current, simplified techniques, but they were adequate to convince me that Grant's method was sufficiently accurate to be used as a clinicial tool. Consequently, I have applied Grant's method to thousands of electrocardiograms for nearly 40 years. Being a clinician, I have also tried to correlate the electrocardiographic abnormalities identified by this method with other clinical data. Grant's views, which were based on Einthoven's and Wilson's research, appear to be worth preserving.

HOW DOES THIS BOOK DIFFER FROM OTHERS?

Although the principles of interpretation described by Grant in the late 1940's are used in this book, certain new data have been woven into the text. For example, Robert Anderson and Anton Becker have continued their work on the anatomy of the heart and conduction system. Drs. D. Durrer, H.J.J. Wellens, and others have clarified the depolarization process in the atria and ventricles. Many of the concepts of Rosenbaum regarding the conduction system have also been included. The technique of vectorcardiography ran its course, but taught us a great deal. Now, total body mapping of the electrical forces is teaching us, and the techniques of magnetic resonance imaging, echocardiography, nuclear cardiography, cardiac catheterization and coronary arteriography have been added. This book differs from others in that the results of many of these techniques are utilized in a concerted effort to understand the ventricular electrocardiogram.

A DISCLAIMER

I do not claim that the vector method of interpretation is perfect. In fact, I claim that it is not, and I will later enumerate the faults of the system. I also remind the reader of this fact at the beginning of chapters 3 through 13. On the other hand, the reader should know that there is no perfect system of electrocardiographic interpretation. Facts are available to support many of the concepts discussed here, but there are instances when the explanation goes beyond the facts because it seems logical to do so. At times, the concepts are like the wind blowing on the leaves of a tree. One cannot see the wind but, by studying the movement of the leaves, one can draw a conclusion about its direction and force. The vector method appeals to me because it incorporates many basic principles, faulty as they are, into the method of interpretation. A system that uses imperfect basic principles is better than a system that uses no basic principles at all—a bad skeleton is better than no skeleton. I am not against the memorization of a number of electrocardiographic patterns, but anyone interested in learning appreciates that one's memory can be expanded when the items being memorized are correlated with something else. So, I contend, why not relate electrocardiographic patterns to vectors which, in turn, relate to certain basic principles? The figures in this book are designed to teach. At times they do not depict the absolute facts because the truth is either unknown or so complex that it is not teachable. Whenever this occurs I have labeled the figure as hypothetical or imaginary. I have also pointed out the flaws in the system as vigorously as I can.

COMMENTS

THE ELECTROCARDIOGRAMS

SOURCE OF THE ELECTROCARDIOGRAMS

Most of the electrocardiograms presented in this book came from the electrocardiographic laboratory of Emory University Hospital and Emory Clinic. A few came from the electrocardiographic laboratories of Henrietta Egleston Hospital for Children, and a small number came from Grady Memorial Hospital. All of these facilities are parts of, or affiliated with, the Woodruff Health Sciences Center of Emory University in Atlanta, Georgia. A few of the electrocardiograms were obtained from other facilities and are used with appropriate permission. When electrocardiograms were taken from previously published sources, permission to use them was obtained from the publishers and authors, and the original sources are cited in the Figure Credits section of each chapter.

REPRODUCTION OF ELECTROCARDIGRAMS

All of the electrocardiograms reproduced in this book were redrawn by Susan Tilberry of Gower Medical Publishing. This approach is necessary in order to present the reader with aesthetically pleasing electrocardiograms. This method permits the removal of smudges and scratches, and makes it possible to show the fine detail of the background grid; this cannot be accomplished with the usual photographic technique. I carefully checked the final rendition against the original electrocardiogram. Susan is a genius—her diagrams are virtually perfect.

CALIBRATION OF ELECTROCARDIOGRAMS

Each electrocardiogram was properly standardized (calibrated); the stylus was adjusted so that it moved 1 cm. The calibration signal is not shown, in order to conserve space.

MEASUREMENT OF INTERVALS

A computer readout was available for almost all of the electrocardiograms presented here. In many instances, the computer "read" the PR intervals, QRS-complex durations, and QT intervals longer than I did by visual inspection. My visual measurements are recorded in the legends of the electrocardiograms presented here because the normal and abnormal intervals established previously were obtained by visual inspection of the deflection. Even so, you, the reader, may obtain a different measurement than mine. The difference in measurements may be explained as follows: I had the opportunity to study many complexes in all of the leads before arriving at a measurement, whereas the reader can study only one electrocardiographic deflection in the figures shown here.

CORRELATION OF OTHER DATA WITH ELECTROCARDIOGRAPHIC ABNORMALITIES

It is valuable to correlate electrocardiographic abnormalities with the age, sex, and symptoms of patients, and with the results of cardiac catheterization, coronary arteriography, and echocardiography. Whereas every effort was made to do this as accurately as possible, it could not be accomplished to perfection because this was a retroactive study. For example, it was not always possible to locate an electrocardiogram that was recorded from a given patient on the same day on which the coronary arteriogram was made. In fact, at times, several months and even years may separate the two dates. A prospective study would be needed to be certain that all of the data were collected at the appropriate time so that more precise correlations could be made.

THE DIAGRAMS

SOURCE OF THE DIAGRAMS

I developed rough sketches for all of the original diagrams in this book. The three artists redrew my rough sketches in order to make them presentable and printable. Susan Tilbery redrew the diagrams associated with each electrocardiogram. Virginia Schoonover-Carr developed additional rough sketches for the diagrams in the first six chapters of the book. Laura Duprey completed the rough sketches of the first six chapters, and supervised the artwork for the entire book.

I checked and double-checked the diagrams for accuracy. Despite every effort to avoid errors, I suspect that minor errors will become evident as I relax from the intense effort of "producing" and switch to the casual effort of "just looking."

DETERMINING THE DIRECTION OF VECTORS

The direction of the vectors was determined by the method of Grant. I used many electrocardiographic complexes in 12 leads to determine the direction of the vectors. The reader is shown one deflection in each lead and therefore, must make his or her calculation from a single complex in each lead. This may, at times, account for minor differences between the readers's calculation of the direction of a vector and my own.

WHEN THE DIRECTIONS OF THE VECTORS ARE DIFFICULT TO DETERMINE

When the Grant method is used, it is possible to identify the frontal plane projection of a vector within an error range of about 5° of the actual direction of the vector, and to identify the anterior or posterior direction of the vector within an error range of about ±15°. It is surprising that the direction of the vectors representing the electrical forces can be computed with acceptable accuracy when one considers that the amplitudes and areas of the complexes were made by simple inspection of the electrocardiographic complexes.

There are times, when viewing electrocardiograms, that it is difficult or impossible to determine the directions of the vectors. These situations are highlighted below.

Already alluded to is the fact that the reader of this book has only one complex for each lead to make his or her computations, whereas I could study many complexes in each lead to make my calculation. It should be recalled that minor changes may occur because of inspiration and expiration; these changes cannot be identified from inspecting a single complex from each lead.

At times, all of the precordial leads record resultantly negative or positive deflections. When this occurs, it is not possible to determine the exact number of degrees to which a vector is directed anteriorly or posteriorly, unless additional deflections are recorded from the appropriate precordial lead sites. When this occurs, and no additional recordings are obtained, the transitional pathway is drawn on the chest at a reasonable location and a statement is made in the legend of the diagrams that it is just that—an estimate.

There are times, even when there are negative and positive deflections noted in the precordial leads, that the vectors illustrating the electrical forces cannot be drawn to fit the actual deflections seen in the precordial leads. This failure to fit can often be explained as follows:

The precordial lead electrodes are nearer the heart than the extremity lead electrodes. Because of this they are influenced to record larger deflections than the electrodes placed at a greater distance from the heart. This makes it impossible to use the area or amplitude of a precordial deflection to determine that the vector is parallel with the lead axis that exhibits the largest deflection, and forces one to use the resultantly smallest deflection to determine that the vector is perpendicular to the lead axis exhibiting the smallest resultant deflection. This minimizes the error, but does not eliminate it, and the transitional pathway may be miscalculated to a small degree. This is especially true in children, and in adults with thin chests.

The same diagram is used to represent all chests throughout the book. It is a "generic" replica of the chest. It must be remembered that the precordial electrode sites are determined by using anatomic guidelines, and that shape of the chest alters the relationship of some of the electrodes sites to the others. For example, the electrode sites V2, V3, and V4 are located almost one above the other in tall individuals, but almost side by side in broad-chested persons. This difference can alter where one preceives the transitional pathway to be on the chest. The fact that only one diagram is used throughout the book to represent the shape of the chest will obviously lead to errors in that a diagram may be constructed in which the deflections that are predicted from the diagram do not match those in the actual tracing. As a rule, in such a case, there are several deflections which actually fit the predicted deflections, and the anterior or posterior direction of the vector can be calculated from these deflections. The remaining actual deflections in the other leads may not fit the predicted deflections in the diagram. This lack of a fit is usually because the remaining leads record from near the transitional pathway of a vector, and a small difference in electrode location may change a deflection from negative (inverted) to positive (upright). This problem is especially likely in children. It is illustrated and discussed in many diagrams in Chapter 11.

Body surface mapping of the electrical fields reveals that the transitional pathway for each vector undulates. Accordingly, the transitional pathway of a vector may actually curve above or below a precordial electrode site whereas the transitional pathway as calculated from the electrocardiographic deflections from the usual precordial electrode sites is viewed as non-undulating. This accounts for many of the situations in which the deflections seen in the electrocardiogram are different from the deflections that would be predicted.

Each part of the diagram is used to depict a three-dimensional concept. For example, the rim of the arrowhead is the same color as the transitional pathway for a vector, and the base of the arrowhead is the same color as the zero potential plane for the vector. In addition to these artistic efforts to lead the reader to visualize in three dimension, I have drawn the electrode positions for V6 a little higher than electrode position for V5, and electrode position V5 is a little higher than electrode position V4. Because of this the predicted deflections, which are based on the direction of the vectors in the diagrams, may not match the actual deflections. There is a poor "fit". As a rule, the deflections that do not fit will be recorded by the electrodes that are located near the transitional pathway.

In an effort to show the transitional pathway in three dimensions, I permitted the artist to show a thick transitional pathway. This makes it more difficult to diagram the pathway coursing between two precordial electrode positions. Actually, the transitional pathway is a fine line. This also explains why some of the actual deflections do not "fit" the predicted deflections.

ACKNOWLEDGEMENTS

I wish to thank the masters of the past for their interest in solving the mysteries of animal electricity. I thank Dr. Robert Grant for his contribution to electrocardiography and his influence on me. I thank Dr. Harvey Estes of Duke University for reviewing the first six chapters of the book. Dr. Estes is an expert in vector electrocardiography who, more than anyone, worked side by side with Dr. Grant. I must add, however, that any errors found in the document are mine and not his.

I thank some of my associates at the Emory University School of Medicine, Emory University Hospital, and Emory Clinic. These include Dr. Wayne Alexander, Dr. Robert Schlant, Dr. Steve Clements, Dr. Paul Walter, Dr. Woodfin Cobbs, Dr. Paul Robinson, Dr. Spencer King, Dr. John Douglas, Dr. Nick Lembo, Dr. Robert Franch, and Dr. Jerre Lutz. Together, they have supplied me with many of the electrocardiograms appearing in this text. Dr. Charles Brown, a cardiology fellow at Emory, and Dr. Mark Hanson, Chief Resident in Medicine at the Emory University Hospital, were also helpful in supplying me with electrocardiograms, and challenged me at every turn. I thank Dr. William Weintraub for identifying the electrocardiograms of patients who had cardiac catheterization and coronary arteriography; Dr. Gordon DuPuey for supplying me with the electrocardiograms of patients who had thallium scans and other nuclear tests; and Dr. Roderic Pettigrew, who supplied the magnetic resonance images of the heart.

I thank Mary Cotton and Carol Miller for their expert typing and organizational abilities.

It is my hope that the reader will understand the complex problem of trying to depict a three dimensional structure on a flat, two dimensional surface. The artists who were responsible for the illustrations deserve special praise for accomplishing this feat. This book could not have been written without their help. I thank Virginia Schoonover-Carr, of Atlanta, for her ability to take my crude drawings and convert them into works of art. I met with her early in the development of the book for one to two hours almost every week for several months, in order to guide this portion of the project. She developed the sketches for almost all of the illustrations for the first six chapter of the book. I thank Susan Tilberry, of Washington, D.C., for creating the illustrations for the last seven chapters of the book. She magnified and redrew all of the electrocardiograms in the book, in an effort to present the reader with aesthetically pleasing figures. I thank Laura Duprey, and Wendy Jackelow of New York City, for completing the illustrations in the first six chapters. I thank Laura for supervising the artwork for the entire book. I carefully checked the accuracy of the reproductions and illustrations. I thank Nava Anav for her skillful design work.

I thank Kenneth Lane for his excellent contributions as a copy editor and Erik Goldman for his effort as Development Editor. They are skilled professionals.

I thank Abe Krieger and Bill Gabello, of Gower Medical Publications, for their willingness to proceed with this book when the market is replete with books on electrocardiography and interest in the subject is at a low ebb.

Finally, my wife Nelie, who supports my every effort and has made our house a home while I made our home a library. She was the major force in rearing our three sons. No accomplishment of mine would have been possible without her. So, as I pause to smell a few roses, I am blessed that I have her hand to hold.

J. Willis Hurst, M.D.
Candler Professor of Medicine(Cardiology)
Emory University School of Medicine
Atlanta, Georgia

CONTENTS

PART

The Electrical Forces of the Heart

ONE

ELECTRICITY AND THE CREATION OF ELECTROCARDIOGRAPHY

Louis N. Katz and Herman K. Hellerstein wrote a scholarly discussion on the evolution of our knowledge of electrocardiography and published it in *Circulation of the Blood: Men and Ideas* edited by Fishman and Richards (1).* Interested readers will be spellbound to discover how early observers gradually began to understand that lightning, lodestone, amber (when rubbed), and the torpedo fish had something in common—electricity!

Apparently, the torpedo fish was the subject of great interest. Bancraft, in 1676, suggested that the strange fish was capable of delivering a shock of electricity (2). John Walsh (3), John Hunter (4), and Henry Cavendish (5) supported Bancraft's contention. Accordingly, it was gradually accepted that certain animals generated electrical current.

Luigi Galvani (1737–1798) can be acclaimed as the scientist who proved that electrical stimulation of the crural nerves of a frog would make the frog's leg muscles contract. In his own account (6,7) of this important experiment, he wrote:

The course of the work has progressed in the following way. I dissected a frog and prepared it. Having in mind other things, I placed the frog on the same table as an electrical machine...so that the animal was completely separated from and removed at a considerable distance from the machine's conductor. When one of my assistants by chance lightly applied the point of a scalpel to the inner crural nerves...suddenly all the muscles of the limbs were seen so to contract that they appeared to have fallen into violent tonic convulsions. Another assistant who was present when we were performing electrical experiments thought he observed that this phenomenon occurred when a spark was discharged from the conductor of the electrical machine. Marvelling at this, he immediately brought the unusual phenomenon to my attention when I was completely engrossed and contemplating other things. Hereupon I became extremely enthusiastic and eager to repeat the experiment so as to clarify the obscure phenomenon and make it known. I myself, therefore, applied the point of the scalpel first to one then to the other crural nerve, while at the same time some one of the assistants produced a spark; the phenomenon repeated itself in precisely the same manner as before. Violent contractions were induced in the individual muscles of the limbs and the prepared animal reacted just as though it were seized with tetanus at the very moment when the sparks were discharged.

Galvani and Volta had their differences, but each stimulated the other to extensive experimentation (9). Galvani discovered, in an experiment in which no metal was used, that when the nerve of one frog was placed on the injured muscle of another frog, the muscles of the first frog would contract (8).

As time passed, many workers pursued the mysteries of animal electricity, including the great Emil Du Bois-Reymond

(9). The next giant step was taken by Kolliker and Muller (10), who placed the nerve portion of a nerve–leg preparation of one frog on the beating heart of another frog. The frog's leg contracted each time the heart contracted.

These investigators soon recognized that a measuring device was needed. Dr. Du Bois-Reymond invented the rheotome, which interrupted the current in such a fashion that the heart's own current could be recorded with a galvanometer (11). Marchand in 1877 (12) and Engelmann in 1878 (13) were among the first to record the electrocardiogram from the surface of the heart of a lower animal.

The search for improved measuring devices continued until the mercury capillary electrometer was invented by Gabriel Lippmann in 1875 (14). Augustus Waller (Fig. 1.1), who was destined to play a major role in the events that followed, wrote the following passage about the device (15):

The instrument is, in fact, an exceedingly delicate electrical manometer; a rise of electrical pressure on the mercury side or a fall of electrical pressure on the sulphuric acid side, causes the mercury to move towards the point of the capillary; a fall of electrical pressure on the mercury side or a rise on the sulphuric acid side, causes the mercury to recede from the point of the capillary. The instrument accordingly is an indicator of "potential" or "pressure"; not of "current." Its delicacy is such that it will react to as little as 1/40,000 volt. It offers, moreover, the following advantages: the indications are practically instantaneous, free of lost time, and of after-oscillation; the resistance in the circuit is immaterial; unpolarisable electrodes may for most purposes be dispensed with.

Although Marey recorded the first electrocardiogram using the mercury capillary electrometer in 1876 (16), Waller was the first to record the electrocardiogram of a human heart (17). Waller, who was born in Paris, later moved to London, where he became Director of the Physiological Laboratory at the University of London. Sir Thomas Lewis (Fig. 1.2) wrote the following statement about his contribution (17):

Waller was the first to show that currents set up in the beating of the human heart can be recorded; he was the first to obtain a human electrocardiogram.

The search for an improved measuring device continued. Willem Einthoven of Leiden, who had heard Waller lecture in May of 1887 and witnessed the recording of an electrocardiogram, improved upon Ader's galvanometer (18) so that it could record the electrical current of the intact human heart. In Einthoven's words (19):

The string galvanometer is essentially composed of a thin silver-coated quartz filament (about 3μ thick): which is stretched like a string, in a strong magnetic field. When an

*I thank Dr. Hellerstein, Dr. Fishman and the Oxford University Press for permitting me to abstract certain parts of the chapter on electrocardiography¹.

electric current is conducted through this quartz filament, the filament reveals a movement which can be observed and photographed by means of considerable magnification; this movement is similar to the movements of the mercury contained in the capillary-electrometer. It is possible to regulate the sensitivity of the galvanometer very accurately within broad limits by tightening or loosening the string.

Einthoven (Fig. 1.3A) and his string galvanometer (Fig. 1.3B) soon gained international recognition. Einthoven labeled the waves of the electrocardiogram as P, Q, R, S, and T. Legend holds that he chose the letters from the center of the alphabet because he did not know what the waves meant, or whether other waves preceding the P wave and following the T wave would be discovered as the instrumentation improved (Fig. 1.3C). In fact, the U wave was added later.

Sir Thomas Lewis of London (Fig. 1.2) extended the work of Einthoven. His pioneering work formed the basis for much of our current knowledge and influenced many clinicians throughout the world (20).

The brilliant work of Frank Wilson (Fig. 1.4) and his associates dominated the field for many decades. He developed a new lead system that permitted accurate recordings from new body positions, including the precordial sites (see Chapter 4). He emphasized the ventricular electrocardiogram and developed many new concepts (21-33), which will be taken up in later discussions.

As modern technology developed in the 1940s, the bulky machine designed by Einthoven was replaced by a more modern, portable, photographic electrocardiograph machine. Finally, the direct-writing machine was invented, and although it did not record with the precision of the photographic machine, its practicality soon made it the most frequently used instrument. Oscilloscopic recordings, or vectorcardiograms, were used during the 1950s and for a decade or so afterward. They were the most accurate of all recordings but they never gained widespread acceptance by clinicians, and as a practical tool, vectorcardiography did not survive. The machine and lead system used today are discussed in Chapter 4. Computer interpretation of electrocardiograms is now commonplace. The software varies with the manufacturer and, regrettably, none of the programs is accurate.

Robert P. Grant (Fig. 1.5) was a creative genius. While working at Emory University in Atlanta, he built on the work of Einthoven, Lewis, and Wilson, and developed a way to apply vector concepts to the interpretation of a 12-lead electrocardiogram. The results of his investigations were published, with the collaboration of Harvey Estes, in *Spatial Vector Electrocardiography* (34). This book, as well as the *Atlas of Spatial Vector Electrocardiography* by J. Willis Hurst and Grattan Woodson, could not have been written without the basic contribution of Robert Grant (35).

FIGURE 1.1
Augustus D. Waller (1856-1922). Using a mercury capillary electrometer, he was the first to record a human electrocardiogram (15, 17). (Photograph provided by and reproduced with permission of The National Library of Medicine, Bethesda, Maryland.)

FIGURE 1.2
Sir Thomas Lewis (1881-1945). Lewis extended the work of Einthoven. His pioneering work, for the most part related to understanding cardiac arrhythmias, influenced clinical practice throughout the world. (Photograph provided by and reproduced with permission of The National Library of Medicine, Bethesda, Maryland.)

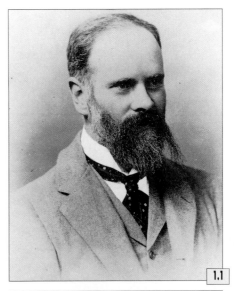

1.1

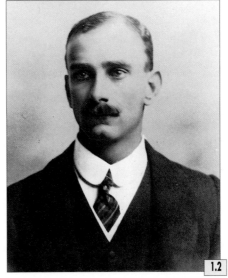

1.2

FIGURE 1.3

A. Willem Einthoven (1860-1927). This Dutch physiologist improved Ader's galvanometer so that it would record the electrical current of the human heart (18,19). Einthoven's instrument introduced the field of electrocardiography. (Photograph provided by and reproduced with permission of The National Library of Medicine, Bethesda, Maryland.)
B. Einthoven's string galvanometer, Leyden model. (Original source unknown; see Figure Credits.)
C. Evolution of the electrocardiogram from the electrometer. The upper record was made using the capillary electrometer, the middle record is a "corrected curve," and the lower record was made using Einthoven's string galvanometer. (See Figure Credits.)

FIGURE 1.4

Frank Norman Wilson (1890-1952). Wilson and his associates dominated the field of electrocardiography for many decades. His research effort was directed toward understanding the ventricular electrocardiogram as well as arrhythmias. (Photograph provided by and reproduced with permission of The National Library of Medicine, Bethesda, Maryland.)

FIGURE 1.5

Robert Purves Grant (1915-1966). While working at Emory University, Grant developed the concept of vector electrocardiography, which enabled the observer to characterize the electrical forces responsible for the electrocardiogram. His concepts, based mainly on the work of Wilson, form the basis for this book. (Photograph provided by and reproduced with permission of The National Library of Medicine, Bethesda, Maryland.)

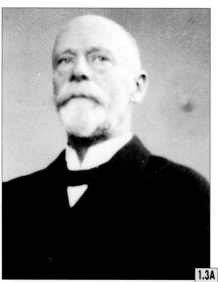

1.3A

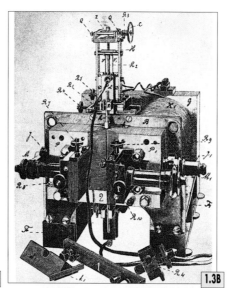

1.3B

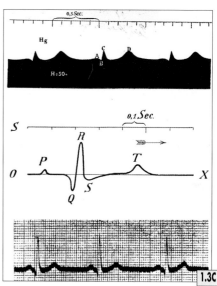

1.3C

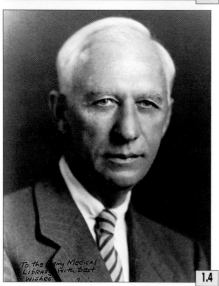

1.4

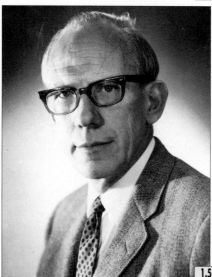

1.5

REFERENCES

1. Katz LN, Hellerstein HK: Electrocardiography, in Fishman AP, Richards DW (eds): *Circulation of the Blood: Men and Ideas*. New York, Oxford University Press, 1964, p 265.
2. Fleming JA: Electricity, in *Encyclopedia Britannica* Cambridge, England, New York, Cambridge University Press, ed 11, Vol 9, 1910, p 179.
3. Walsh J: Of torpedoes found on the coast of England. *Philos Trans R Soc Lond (Biol)* 1773-75;64:464.
4. Hunter J: Anatomical observations on the torpedo. *Philos Trans R Soc Lond (Biol)* 1773;63:481.
5. Cavendish H: An account of some attempts to imitate the effects of the torpedo by electricity. *Philos Trans R Soc Lond (Biol)* 1776;66:196.
6. Galvani L: De viribus electricitatis in motu musculari commentarius. *De Bononiensi Scientarium et Artium Instituto atque Academia Commentarii* 1791;7:363-418.
7. Cohen IB: Introduction, in Galvani L: *Commentary on the Effects of Electricity on Muscular Motion*, M G Foley (trans). Norwalk, CT, Brundy Library, 1954.
8. Galvani L: *Dell'uso e dell'Attivita dell'Arco Conduttore nelle Contrazioni die Muscoli*. Bologna, Tommaso d'Aquino, 1794.
9. Du Bois-Reymond E: *Untersuchungen über Thierische Elektricitat*. Berlin, Reimer, 1848-60, Vols 1 and 2.
10. Kolliker A, Muller H: Zweiter Bericht über die im Jahr 1854/55 in der physiologischen Anstalt der Universität Wurzburg angestellten Versuche. VII. Nachweis der negativen Schwankung des Muskelstroms am naturlich sich contrahirender Muskel. *Verh Phys-Med Ges Wurzb* 1856; 6:528.
11. Hoff HE, Geddes LA: The rheotome and its pre-history: A study in the historical interrelation of electrophysiology and electromechanics. *Bull Hist Med* 1957;31:327.
12. Marchman R: Beitrage zur Kenntniss der Reizwelle und Contractionswelle des Herzmuskels. *Pflügers Arch* 1877; 15:511.
13. Engelmann TW: Über das Verhalten des thatigen Herzens. *Pflügers Arch* 1878;17:68.
14. Lippmann G: Relations entre les phenomenes électriques et capillaires. *Ann Chir (Phys.) (Ser. 5)* 1875;5:494.
15. Waller AD: *An Introduction to Human Physiology*, ed 2. New York, Longmans Green, 1893.
16. Marey EJ: Des variations électriques des muscles et du coeur en particulier, étudiées au moyen de l'electromètre de M. Lippmann. *C R Acad Sci (Paris)* 1876;82:975.
17. Lewis T: Comments in obituary notice of A. D. Waller. *Br Med J* 1922;1:458.
18. Ader C: Sur un nouvel appareil enregistreur pour cables sousmarins. *C R Acad Sci (Paris)* 1897;124:1440.
19. Einthoven W: The galvanometric registration of the human electrocardiogram, likewise a review of the use of the capillary-electrometer in physiology. In Willius FA, Keys E (eds): *Cardiac Classics*, Willius FW (trans). St Louis, CV Mosby, 1941.
20. Lewis T, Rothschild MA: The excitatory process in the dog's heart. Part II. The ventricles. *Philos Trans R Soc Lond (Biol)* 1915;206:181.
21. Wilson FN: A case in which the vagus influenced the form of the ventricular complex of the electrocardiogram. *Arch Intern Med* 1915;16:1008.
22. Wilson FN: The distribution of the potential differences produced by the heart beat within the body and at its surface. *Am Heart J* 1930;5:599.
23. Wilson FN, Bryant JM, Johnston FD: On the possibility of constructing an Einthoven triangle for a given subject. *Am Heart J* 1949;37:493.
24. Wilson FN, Johnston FD: The vectorcardiogram. *Am Heart J* 1938;16:14.
25. Wilson FN, Johnston FD, Barker PS: The use of the cathode ray oscillograph in the study of the monocardiogram. *J Clin Invest* 1937;16:664.
26. Wilson FN, Herrmann GR: Bundle branch block and arborization block. *Arch Intern Med* 1920;26:153.
27. Wilson FN, Johnston FD, Hill IGW: The interpretation of the galvanometric curves obtained when one electrode is distant from the heart and the other near or in contact with the ventricular surface. Part II. Observations on the mammalian heart. *Am Heart J* 1934;10:176.
28. Wilson FN, Johnston FD, Rosenbaum FF, et al: On Einthoven's triangle, the theory of unipolar electrocardiographic leads, and the interpretation of the precordial electrocardiogram. *Am Heart J* 1946;32:277.
29. Wilson FN, Macleod AG, Barker PS: The interpretation of the initial deflection of the ventricular complex of the electrocardiogram. *Am Heart J* 1931;6:637.
30. Wilson FN, Macleod AG, Barker PS: The potential variations produced by the heart at the apices of Einthoven's triangle. *Am Heart J* 1931;7:207.
31. Wilson FN, Macleod AG, Barker PS: *The Distribution of the Currents of Action and of Injury Displayed by Heart Muscle and Other Excitable Tissues*. Ann Arbor, University of Michigan Press, 1933.
32. Wilson FN, Macleod AG, Barker PS, et al: The determination and the significance of the areas of the ventricular deflections of the electrocardiogram. *Am Heart J* 1934;10:45.
33. Wilson FN, Macleod AG, Barker PS, et al: The electrocardiogram in myocardial infarction with particular reference to the initial deflections of the ventricular complex. in Johnston FD, Lepeschkin E (eds): *Selected Papers, F N Wilson*. Ann Arbor, MI, Edwards, 1954.
34. Grant RP, Estes EH: *Spatial Vector Electrocardiography*, Philadelphia, New York, Toronto, The Blakiston Company, 1951.
    Hurst JW, Woodson GC: *Atlas of Spatial Vector*
35. *Electrocardiography*. New York, Toronto, The Blakiston Company, 1952.

FIGURE CREDITS

Figure 1.3B From Katz LN, Hellerstein HK Electrocardiography. *In Fishman AP, Richards DW (eds): Circulation of the Blood: Men and Ideas*. New York, Oxford University Press, 1964, p 294, 295.

Figure 1.3C The upper and middle portions of this figure are from Einthoven W: Die galvanometrische Registrirung des menschlichen Elektrokardiogramms, zugleich eine Beurtheilung der Anwendung des Capillar-Elektrometers in der Physiologie. *Archiv fur die Gesammte Psysiologie des Menshen und der Thiere*, 99:473, 1903. The exact source for the lower portion of this figure is unknown because it was not shown in the original figure published in 1903. It did appear in Fishman AP, Richards DW (eds): *Circulation of the Blood: Men and Ideas*. New York, Oxford University Press, 1964, p 295.

CHAPTER TWO

THE BLACK BOX AND THE ARROW

A *black box* is often used to signify an enigma (Fig.2.1). The black box discussed here is one that represents a special puzzle: a small arrow is located in the center of the box and suspended from the top of the box in such a manner that it can rotate through 360° in any direction (Fig. 2.2A).

Let us suppose that you spin the arrow (Fig. 2.2B) and close the front panel of the box before the arrow stops spinning. Can you determine the direction of the arrow after it stops spinning without opening the black box? The answer, of course, is no.

The black box, however, is accompanied by a device that may help us determine the direction of the arrow without opening the box (Fig. 2.3). The device will register a plus (+) sign when the arrow points toward it and a negative (–) sign when the arrow points away from it. It will register zero (0) when the arrow is located precisely perpendicular to it. Furthermore, it will register its largest plus (+) sign when the arrow is pointing directly toward the device and its largest negative (–) sign when the arrow is pointing directly away from it. Now, can you determine the direction of the arrow without looking inside the black box? The answer is yes. Now play the game. Spin the arrow and close the front panel of the box. Explore the outside of the box with the device. Plus (+) signs, negative (–) signs, and zeros (0) are identified with the device and recorded on the surface of the black box (Fig. 2.4A). You can deduce the direction of the arrow from the distribution of the signs on the surface of the box (Fig. 2.4B). Now open the front panel of the black box and observe the direction of the arrow to check your deduction (Fig. 2.4C).

THE PROBLEM OF THE HUMAN THORAX AND THE ELECTRICAL FORCES OF THE HEART

Let us now assume that the black box is analogous to the human thorax. The arrow is symbolic of an electrical force generated by the heart, and the simple measuring device is an electrocardiograph machine.

The problem facing the clinician is analogous to the one facing the individual trying to solve the *black box* puzzle (Figs. 2.1 and 2.2); how to measure and interpret the electrical forces generated in the heart by studying the electrical activity on the surface of the body (Fig. 2.5). If we assume that the electrical forces of the heart can be represented as arrows, we can then analyze these forces in terms of their direction and size.

FIGURE 2.1
A black box is often used to signify an enigma.

FIGURE 2.2
A. Arrow located in the center of a black box. **B.** Arrow suspended from the top of the box so it can rotate through 360° in any direction. Suppose you spin the arrow and close the front panel of the box before the arrow stops spinning. Can you determine the direction of the arrow after it stops spinning?

FIGURE 2.3
A. Measuring device used to determine direction of the arrow. **B.** A positive (+) signal is registered by the measuring device when the arrow points toward it. **C.** A negative (–) signal is registered by the device when the arrow points away from it. **D.** A zero (0) signal is registered by the device when the arrow is perpendicular to it.

The measuring device will register its largest positive signal when the arrow is pointing directly toward it, and its largest negative signal when the arrow is pointing directly away from it. The measuring device will register its smallest signal when the arrow is perpendicular to it.

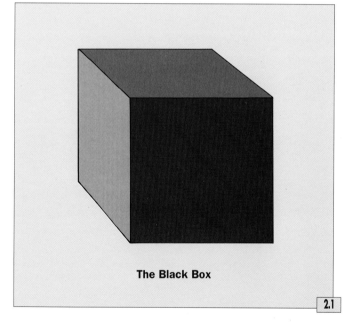

The Black Box

2.1

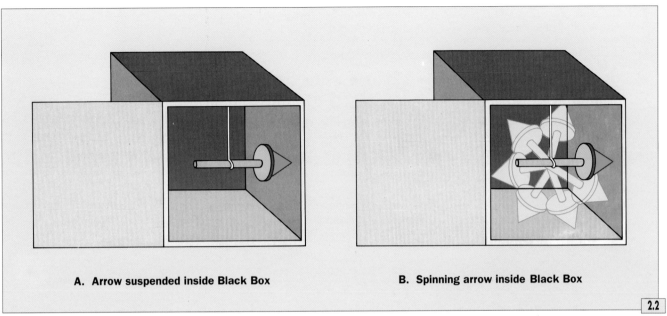

A. Arrow suspended inside Black Box

B. Spinning arrow inside Black Box

2.2

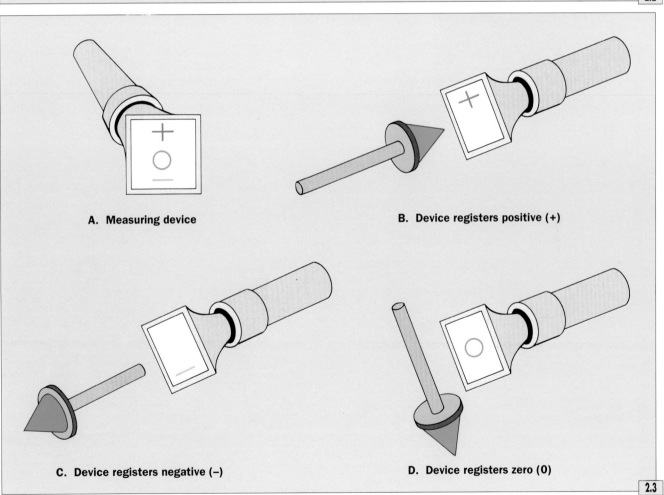

A. Measuring device

B. Device registers positive (+)

C. Device registers negative (−)

D. Device registers zero (0)

2.3

FIGURE 2.4
A. When the external surface of the black box is explored in an orderly manner using the device, it is possible to identify areas on the box where positive signs (+) will be found, negative signs (–) will be found, and zeros (0) will be found. **B.** By studying the positive (+), negative (–), and zero (0) signs on the surface of the box, it is possible to determine that the arrow should be directed as shown. **C.** Opening the

front panel of the box reveals that the direction of the arrow was correctly determined using the principles described in Figure 2.3.

FIGURE 2.5
A. Note the location of the heart within the thorax. The faint outline of the black box is shown to remind the reader that the problem facing the clinician in electrocardiography is similar to the puzzle of the black box. The sampling sites are

shown as electrodes located on the right arm, left arm, and leg. **B.** The electrocardiograph machine. Note the faint outline of the measuring device described in Fig. 2.3. It is shown here to emphasize that the electrocardiograph machine is capable of determining if an electrical force is positive (+), negative (–), or zero (0). The deflections shown on the paper to the right of the electrocardiograph machine are characteristic of the human electrocardiogram.

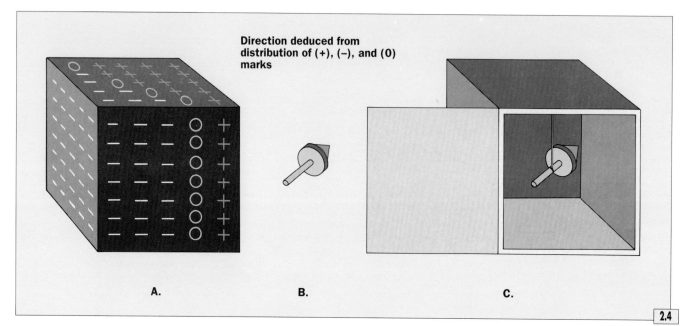

Direction deduced from distribution of (+), (–), and (0) marks

A.   B.   C.

2.4

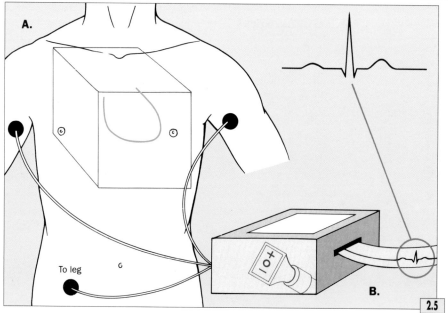

A.

To leg

B.

2.5

CHAPTER THREE

The Hypothetical Myocardial Cell

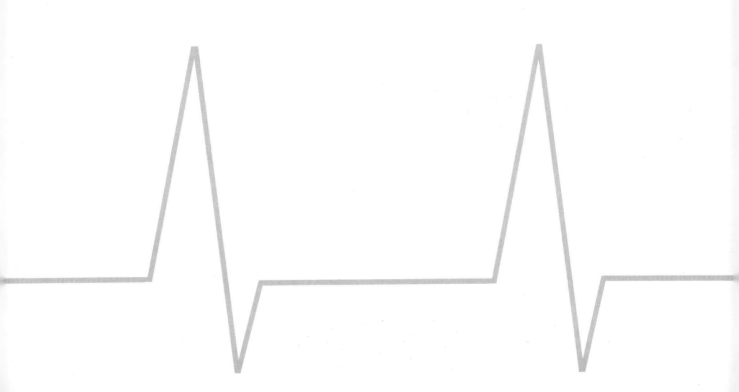

Single cells generate electricity sufficient to be recorded by a very sensitive measuring device. Suppose, for teaching purposes, that the cell and the measuring device could be depicted as in Figure. 3.1A. The inside of the cell, which is shown as a three-dimensional structure, is lined with negative (–) electrical charges, while the outside is covered with an equal number of positive (+) electrical charges. A flow of electricity is produced when ions move across the cell membrane. This flow of electricity is from negative to positive, and it produces *electrical forces*, which can be visualized as *vectors* and represented as *arrows*. The measuring device is designed so that it will write an upward deflection when the arrow representing an electrical force points toward its positive pole, and a downward line when the arrow points toward its negative pole (Fig. 3.2).

A SAGITTAL VIEW OF A HYPOTHETICAL CELL

A sagittal view of a hypothetical cell is shown in Figure 3.1B. Several different views of the cell are shown in Figures 3.3 and 3.4, because it is metabolically active and periodically loses and regains its electrical charges.

THE DEPOLARIZATION PROCESS

The *resting cell*, referred to as a polarized cell, is shown in Figure 3.3A. There is no flow of electrical current across the cell wall because each negative charge is balanced by a positive charge. Accordingly, no electrical forces are recorded by the machine.

When the resting cell is stimulated on its right side (Fig. 3.3B), the cell membrane begins the process of losing its electrical charges. The loss of charge takes place in an orderly manner, and the first charges lost are those at the location of the stimulus. The loss of charges can be visualized more vividly if a small arrow is used to represent the relationship of each negative (–) charge to each positive (+) charge on the cell membrane. We must assume that a finite period of time elapses between the loss of one electrical charge and another, and that the measuring device writes an upward line when the electrical force is dominated by arrows that are directed to the left (toward the positive pole).

As a few arrows are removed on the right side of the cell, the arrows located on the left side of the cell dominate the electrical field. This diagram (Fig. 3.3B) represents *early depolarization*. The process of depolarization proceeds from right to left, producing electrical forces represented by arrows directed from right to left. This results in an upward deflection because the arrows are directed toward the positive pole of the measuring device.

Figure 3.3C depicts the depolarization process as it is imagined to be at the halfway point. The measuring device is influ-

enced by all of the arrows on the left side of the cell. The influence on the measuring device is maximum, and the device cannot record a taller line.

Figure 3.3D shows the continuing depolarization of the cell. The process is about three-quarters complete. The sum of the directions of the arrows produces a positive deflection, but one that is less positive than when depolarization was at the halfway mark.

Figure 3.3E illustrates the completion of the depolarization process. This state is sometimes referred to as the *excited state*. There are no negative (–) charges inside the cell and no positive (+) charges on the surface of the cell. The measuring device is now recording zero (0) because there is no flow of electricity across the cell membrane.

THE REPOLARIZATION PROCESS

The cell in our discussion is metabolically active and programmed to rebuild the electrical charges it has lost. So, after a time delay, the cell membrane begins to restore its charges. It begins to rebuild its charges at the exact spot where it initially lost them. Let us imagine that the time needed for recovery of the charge at each spot on the membrane is the same. When this is true, the spot where the stimulus initiated depolarization will recover its charge first, and the spot at which the charge was lost last will recover its charge last. The time interval between losing and rebuilding the charge will be the same for all parts of the membrane. The repolarization process is depicted in Figure 3.4A through D.

Figure 3.4A depicts the cell actively rebuilding its charges, initially on the right side because it initially lost them there. The amount of time that elapses between the loss and the rebuilding of charge is the same for all parts of the cell membrane. Note that the electrical forces, represented by arrows, now point away from the positive pole of the measuring device and toward its negative pole. This is recorded as a downward deflection.

Figure 3.4B shows the repolarization process at the halfway point. Note that the (repolarization) process itself moves from right to left, but that the measuring device records it as a downward deflection because the electrical forces (represented as arrows) are directed from left to right, away from the positive pole.

Figure 3.4C depicts the repolarization process nearing completion.

Figure 3.4D shows the complete restoration of the electrical charges within and outside the cell membrane. The last area to regain its charges is the spot where the charges were lost last. The cell is now repolarized. It is resting and waiting for another stimulus on its membrane to initiate depolarization once again. Note that in this hypothetical cell, the *depolariza-*

Note: George Burch and Travis Winsor wrote A Primer of Electrocardiography in 1945 (1). The book was very popular and was reprinted many times. The authors simplified the basic concepts created by Wilson, Ashman, and others so that clinicians could grasp and use them. I have drawn heavily on their text and have modified their illustrations with the permission of Dr. Winsor and the publisher (Lea & Febiger) (1).

As stated in several places in this book, the model presented here is a clinically useful approximation of the real situation within the heart. At times, the explanation moves beyond the known evidence. When this occurs, every effort has been made to extend the facts in a logical manner.

tion process takes place from right to left. This produces electrical forces, represented by arrows, that are directed from right to left. The response of the measuring device is to write an upward deflection. The *repolarization* process also takes place from right to left, but because the electrical forces, represented as arrows, are directed from left to right, away from the positive pole of the measuring device, it draws a deflection in a downward direction.

FACTORS INFLUENCING THE DEPOLARIZATION AND REPOLARIZATION PROCESS OF THE HYPOTHETICAL CELL

The diagrams shown in Figures 3.3 and 3.4 depict the depolarization and repolarization processes taking place across the membrane of a hypothetical cell in a simple and orderly manner. At this juncture, the question can be asked: what might alter the orderliness of the depolarization and repolarization of the hypothetical cell? The *direction* of depolarization can be altered by stimulating the cell at a spot other than that illustrated in Figure 3.3B. This, of course, would also alter the *direction* of the repolarization process. A portion of the cell membrane could also be *altered by some intrinsic or extrinsic force* such as temperature, pressure, or intrinsic disease. One can also conceive of conditions that would influence repolarization but would not alter depolarization. Figure 3.5 illustrates how cooling one side of the cell could alter the sequence of repolarization without significantly altering depolarization.

Figure 3.5A shows a hypothetical cell that has been *cooled* on its right side. The measuring device records a straight line, indicating a resting cell that is generating zero (0) electrical forces.

Figure 3.5B shows the cell being stimulated on the right side. The direction of the wave of depolarization is again from right to left, as shown in Figure 3.3, but because of the cooling, the upstroke produced by the measuring device is more sluggish than that shown in Figure 3.3. Accordingly, the measuring device will again record an upward deflection, but one that is slightly more slanted than that shown in Figure 3.3.

Figure 3.5C shows complete depolarization of the cell. The cell is now in an excited state. Cooling of the right side of the cell did not change the direction of the depolarization process, but did slow the initial part of it, as shown by the ascending limb of the deflection wave. It is more slanted than the descending limb, which registers the depolarization of the non-cooled side of the cell.

Figure 3.5D illustrates the early phase of the repolarization process. The coolest part (on the right) is not able to restore its electrical charges as quickly as the uncooled portion of the cell (on the left). Accordingly, the recovery process begins on the left, and proceeds from left to right. Note carefully that

this creates electrical forces, represented as arrows, that are directed from right to left. Therefore, as the recovery process moves, it influences the measuring device to write an upright deflection.

Figure 3.5D shows the recovery process at its halfway mark.

Figure 3.5E depicts the completion of the repolarization process. Note that the measuring device records an upright deflection for both depolarization and repolarization. The latter process is slower than the former, and therefore produces a deflection that is longer than, but not as tall as, that produced by depolarization. The number of charges lost and regained is the same, and the area under the depolarization curve is the same as that under the repolarization curve.

THE HYPOTHETICAL CELL IN THREE DIMENSIONS

Figures 3.1B through 3.5 have depicted a sagittal view of a hypothetical cell. Obviously, this is a great oversimplification of the true condition. Even a single cell is not flat, but has a spatial configuration. This being true, the depolarization and repolarization processes might be directed upward or downward, to the right or left, or from front to back. The heart, which is made up of millions of cells, produces electrical forces that are propagated over the entire surface of the body. The recording device (electrocardiograph machine) and its sampling system (lead system) are used to identify the electrical signals that reach the body surface. The clinician's initial objective is to identify the direction, magnitude, and sense of the electrical forces that are generated by the heart. These electrical forces may be directed upward or downward, to the right or left, or from front to back. This should lead the reader to recall the puzzle of the black box (see Fig. 2.1).

THE ORIGIN OF CELLULAR ELECTRICITY

The origin of animal and plant cellular electricity has intrigued scientists for generations (2). Denis Noble's *The Initiation of the Heartbeat* summarizes our current knowledge as it relates to cardiac cells (3). The following passage from his book is reproduced with permission of the publisher and author (3):

> The species of ions that carry most of the current flow across cardiac cell membranes are sodium (Na^+), calcium (Ca^{2+}), potassium (K^+), and chloride (Cl^-). In each case, the intracellular concentrations are very different from the extracellular concentrations. The sodium and potassium concentration gradients run in opposite directions and are maintained by the Na^+–K^+ exchange pump that accumulates K^+ inside the cell and keeps the intracellular concentration of Na^+ low. The Na^+–K^+ exchange pump is important in all excitable cells since the resting potential is primarily

determined by the K^+ concentration gradient and sodium ions are usually responsible for the depolarization phase of the action potential. So far as cardiac muscle is concerned, we may note three important properties of the pump that will be relevant to the interpretation of both normal and pathological behaviour:

1. The pumping rate is steeply dependent on the extracellular K^+ concentration below a certain level. At low K^+ concentrations, therefore, the Na^+ concentration gradient will be K^+-dependent. Moreover, since the Ca^{2+} gradient is dependent on the Na^+ gradient, the calcium gradient may also be K^+-dependent. Variations in plasma K^+ are common, and sometimes severe in certain cardiac diseases, particularly those associated with renal malfunction. It is conceivable that some of the cardiac disturbances in these cases are secondarily produced by hypokalaemia (low-plasma K^+). The level of plasma K^+ has a large effect on the electrical activity of the heart, though it is likely that most of this effect is attributable to changes in K^+ conductance rather than to changes in ionic pumping over physiological ranges of plasma K^+ (2mM to 5mM).

2. The cardiac glycosides, digitalis and ouabain, are specific blockers of the Na^+–K^+ pump. Digitalis (usually as digoxin) is widely used in clinical practice to treat heart-failure. It is still not clear whether or how its restorative action on a failing heart is related to its action on the Na^+ pump, though it is possible, once again, that the secondary dependence of the calcium gradient on sodium pumping may be involved.

3. In most excitable cells, it has been found that the pump moves more sodium ions than potassium ions. It tends therefore to carry net positive charge from the inside of the cell and so hyperpolarizes it, i.e. the activity of the pump may contribute directly to the negative intracellular potential. Isenberg and Trautwein (4) have shown that cardiac glycosides reduce the outward current in Purkinje fibres.

The existence of the Na^+–K^+ pump has been established for a long time. It is only relatively recently that the existence of the Ca^{2+} pumps has been demonstrated. Two mechanisms appear to exist. The first is a direct outward Ca^{2+} pump involving the use of energy from ATP. The second is an outward movement dependent primarily on the Na^+ concentration gradient and appears to derive its energy from this gradient. It is therefore secondarily dependent on the Na^+–K^+ pump. The evidence for these pumps in a variety of tissues has been reviewed recently by Baker (5). In the case of excitable cells, the Na^+-dependent Ca^{2+} pump appears to be the most important and it has been clearly demonstrated in cardiac muscle (see Refs. 6–9).

Unlike the Na^+–K^+ pump, the Na^+–Ca^{2+} pump is not blocked by cardiac glycosides. The dependence on exter-

nal sodium ions is very specific. The very similar ion Li^+, which is accepted by the Na^+ conductance mechanism in excitable cells, will not substitute for sodium ions in the pump mechanism.

In the case of calcium ions, there is a further factor to be taken into account that determines the concentration gradients, and which is also very important in relation to the role of calcium ions in the initiation of contraction. Unlike the monovalent cations Na^+ and K^+, which are largely free, the majority of intracellular Ca^{2+} is in a bound or sequestered form. Part of this binding may be attributable to Ca^{2+} binding sites on intracellular proteins but the great majority is attributable to Ca^{2+} uptake by internal membranous organelles such as mitochondria or the sarcoplasmic reticulum. Since the fraction of Ca^{2+} bound in this way is very large, minor variations in uptake may have a large effect on the intracellular calcium concentration. This may be particularly important in cardiac muscle since the uptake and release mechanisms are probably controlled by drugs like adrenaline that are important in the natural control of cardiac function. They may also be affected by the cardiac glycosides. Finally, there is some evidence that chloride ions may be actively transported into cardiac cells (10). The estimated intracellular chloride concentration is somewhat larger than would be expected if chloride ions moved purely passively across the membrane.

Figure 3.6 summarizes the ion pumps in cardiac cells and gives typical values of the various ion concentrations. These values may now be used to estimate the electrochemical gradients acting on the various ion species.

ACTION POTENTIAL OF THE HUMAN VENTRICULAR MYOCYTE

The electrical activity of individual cells can be measured using specialized techniques. Although there is a difference in the action potential produced by atrial cells, conduction tissue cells, and ventricular myocytes, I have chosen to illustrate the last of these (Fig. 3.7) and refer the reader to other sources for a more detailed discussion of the subject. The ionic exchange across the cell membrane is shown for each phase of the action potential curve.

ELECTRICAL-MECHANICAL MYOCARDIAL COUPLING AND RELAXATION

An electrical stimulus sets in motion a series of cellular actions that culminate in contraction and relaxation of the myocardial cell. Whereas the precise sequence of events is not known, a great deal of information is available on the subject. Our current knowledge about the subject is shown in Figures 3.8 and 3.9.

FIGURE 3.1
A hypothetical cell. It should be visualized as being spherical. **A.** The reader should imagine that the inside of the cell is lined with negative electrical charges and the outside is covered with positive electrical charges. In this illustration, the positive and negative charges are balanced throughout the cell. Therefore, no electrical forces are produced. **B.** A sagittal view of the hypothetical cell, showing that the inside of the cell is electrically negative while the outside is electrically positive. Small hypothetical arrows project through the cell membrane. They are used to demonstrate how the electrical forces are balanced. These balanced forces will not influence the measuring device in any way. This is so because the addition of the electrical forces represented by all of the arrows throughout the cell produces a sum that is zero.

FIGURE 3.2
The measuring device writes an upward deflection when the arrow, representing an electrical force, points toward its positive pole. It writes a downward deflection when the arrow points away from its positive pole.

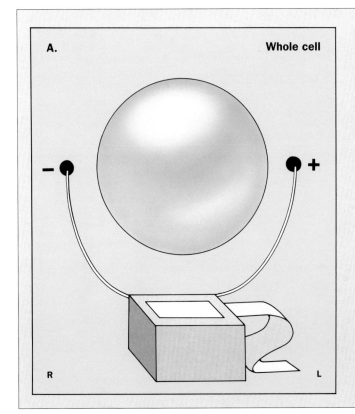

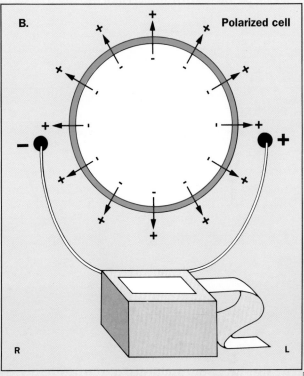

3.1

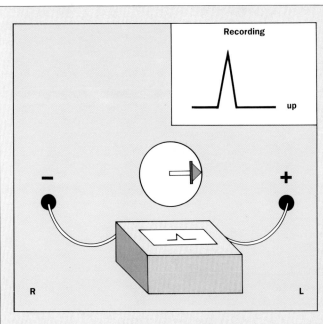

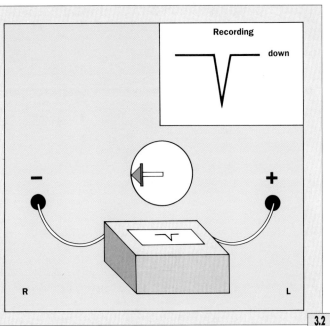

3.2

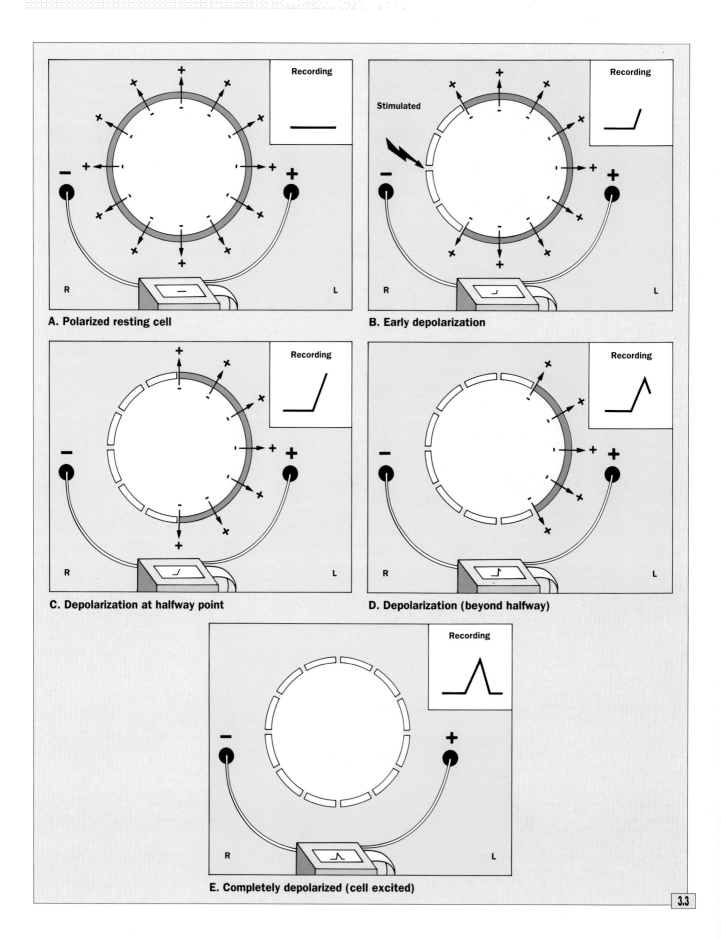

A. Polarized resting cell

B. Early depolarization

C. Depolarization at halfway point

D. Depolarization (beyond halfway)

E. Completely depolarized (cell excited)

Recording

FIGURE 3.3

A. The hypothetical cell is shown in the **polarized state**. The cell is said to be **resting**. This implies that the electrical charges inside and outside are arranged in such a manner that no electrical force can be recorded. Accordingly, the measuring device will record a straight line. (see the left side of the illustration). **B.** The cell is stimulated on the right side, causing the cell membrane to lose its charges on the right side, and permitting the electrical charges on the left side of the cell to gain dominance. The depolarization process spreads from right to left, toward the positive pole of the measuring device, producing an upright deflection on the recording paper. **C.** The depolarization of the cell has reached the halfway point. The upward deflection has reached its maximum height. **D.** The depolarization process is about three-quarters complete. The sum of the electrical forces is smaller than when depolarization was at the halfway mark. The forces still produce a line that is above the baseline on the recording paper. **E.** The depolarization is completed and the deflection returns to the baseline. The cell is said to be in the **excited** state.

FIGURE 3.4

A. The repolarization process (the rebuilding of electrical charges) begins in the area of the hypothetical cell where the depolarization process (the loss of electrical charges) began. Note that the repolarization spreads from right to left but that it produces electrical forces directed from left to right. These forces are directed away from the positive pole of the measuring device. **B.** This figure shows the repolarization process at the halfway point. The deflection it produces on the recording paper cannot become more negative (downward). **C.** This figure shows the repolarization process nearing completion. The sum of the arrows is negative, but less so than when repolarization was at the halfway point. **D.** The repolarization process is complete. All charges have been restored and the cell has returned to the resting state.

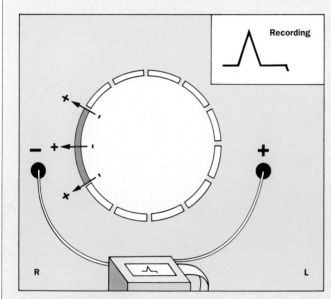

A. Early repolarization

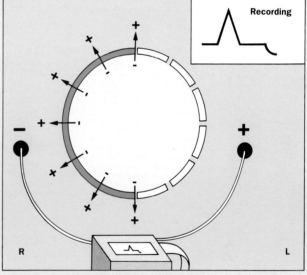

B. Repolarization at halfway point

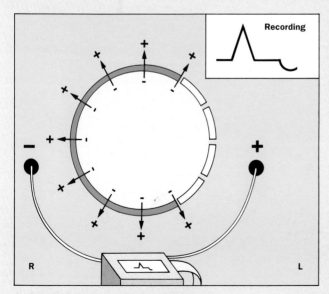

C. Repolarization nearing completion

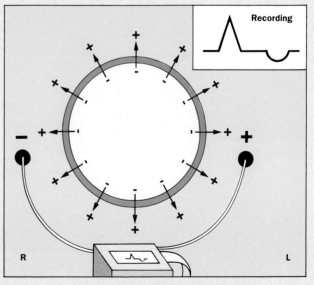

D. Repolarization complete (begins resting state)

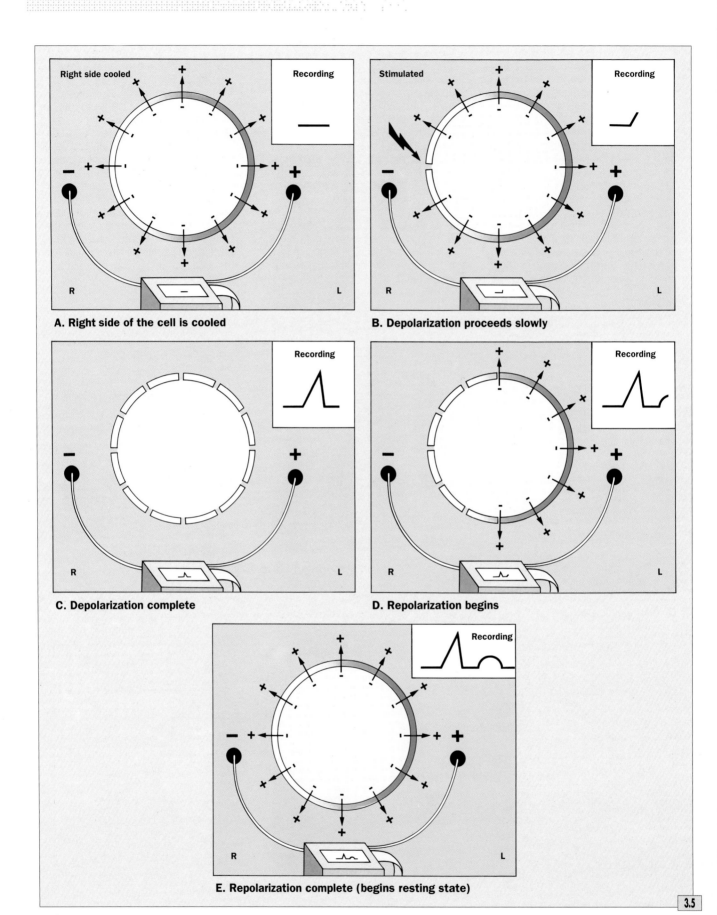

A. Right side of the cell is cooled

B. Depolarization proceeds slowly

C. Depolarization complete

D. Repolarization begins

E. Repolarization complete (begins resting state)

FIGURE 3.5

A. The hypothetical cell has been cooled on the right side. The electrical charges are arranged to show that the cell is resting and no electrical force is generated. This registers a straight line on the recording paper. **B.** The cell is stimulated on the right side. Because the right side of the cell is cooled, it loses its electrical charges more slowly that it did in Figure 3.3B. Depolarization proceeds from right to left, as it did in Figure 3.3, producing a positive (upright) line on the recording paper. Note, however, that the ascending limb of the deflection is slanted a little more than it was in Figure 3.3C because depolarization occurs more slowly in the cooled portion of the cell. **C.** The depolarization process is complete. The cell is now in the excited state. The cooling of the right side of the cell did not alter the direction of electrical discharge but it did prolong the ascending limb of the deflection. The descending limb, which represents the uncooled portion of the cell, appears just as it did in Figure 3.3E. **D.** Repolarization begins on the left side of the cell; as a result of the cooling, it is delayed on the right side. The recovery process proceeds from left to right, creating arrows that are directed from right to left. The arrows are directed toward the positive pole of the measur-ing device and, because of this, generate a positive (upright) deflection on the recording paper. The repolarization process shown here is at the halfway point. **E.** This figure illustrates the completion of repolarization The deflection created by the repolarization process lasts longer but is not as tall as that created by the depolarization process.

FIGURE 3.6

Ion movements across the cell membrane due to pumps. The typical ion concentration within and outside the cell is shown to the reader's left. (Reproduced with permission; see Figure Credits.)

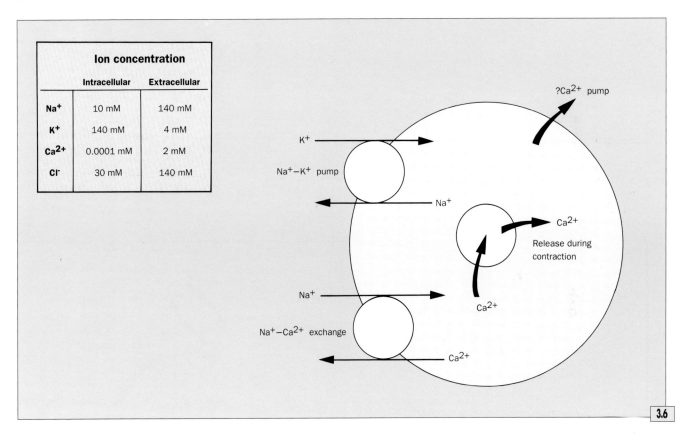

Ion concentration		
	Intracellular	**Extracellular**
Na$^+$	10 mM	140 mM
K$^+$	140 mM	4 mM
Ca^{2+}	0.0001 mM	2 mM
Cl$^-$	30 mM	140 mM

3.6

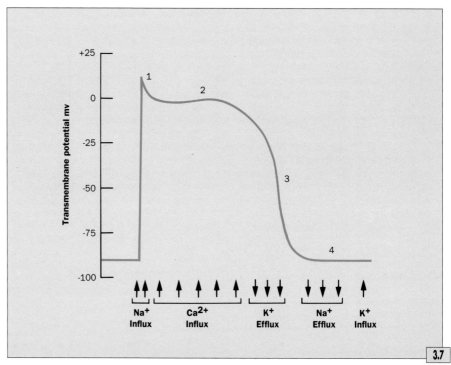

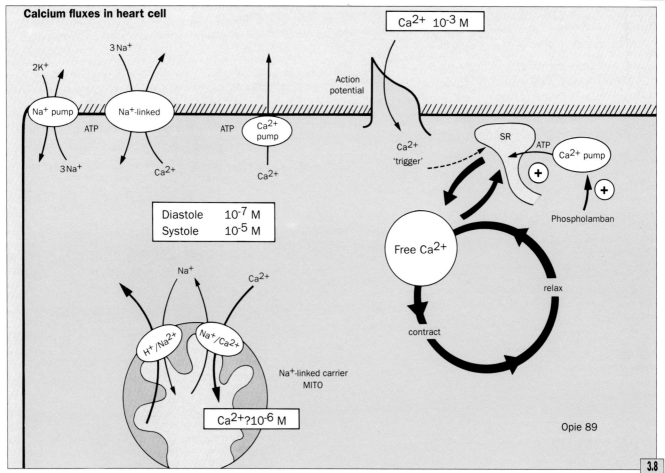

FIGURE 3.7

Schematic diagram showing the action potential of human ventricular myocardium together with probable electrolyte movements. The initial phase 0 spike and overshoot are related to a sudden influx of Na^+. This is followed by a slower, maintained influx of Ca^{2+} during the plateau phase 2. The phase of Ca^{2+} efflux is not well defined for human ventricular myocardium, but it presumably occurs during phase 4. (Reproduced with permission; see Figure Credits.)

FIGURE 3.8

Calcium fluxes in the myocardium. Most of the free Ca^{2+} that is responsible for contraction is released from the sarcoplasmic reticulum. Mitochondria could act as a "buffer" against excessive changes in the free cytosolic calcium concentration. SR = sarcoplasmic reticulum; MITO = mitochondria. (Reproduced with permission from Opie, L.H.; see Figure Credits.)

FIGURE 3.9

Schematic diagram of the events that produce (**A**) myocardial excitation-contraction coupling and (**B**) myocardial relaxation. With depolarization of the cardiac cell membranes (sarcolemma and transverse T system), the Na^+ channels open, followed by the Ca^{2+} channels. The initial transsarcolemmal influx of Ca^{2+} triggers the release of Ca^{2+} from the sarcoplasmic reticulum (SR). Ca^{2+} in higher concentrations then binds to troponin C; this produces conformational changes in whole troponin (troponin I-tropon in C-troponin T complex) that relieves a troponin I interaction with actin. Tropomyosin can then roll back into the grooves of the F-actin superhelix, allowing the interaction of actin and myosin to produce contraction. The transsarcolemmal Ca^{2+} current has both a faster and a slower component. The former may trigger the release of Ca^{2+} from the SR, whereas the slow component may cause the SR to accumulate calcium. Ca^{2+} influx may also occur via the Na^+–Ca^{2+} exchange mechanism. Relaxation is initiated by an unknown stimulus that produces the active uptake of Ca^{2+} by the SR Ca^{2+} ATPase, which is under the control of phospholamban. The resulting lower concentration of cytoplasmic Ca^{2+} produces decreased Ca^{2+} binding to troponin C, and relaxation. During relaxation, Ca^{2+} efflux may occur both by Ca^{2+} ATPase and by a Na^+–Ca^{2+} exchange mechanism. (Reproduced with permission; see Figure Credits.)

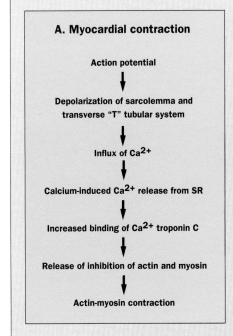
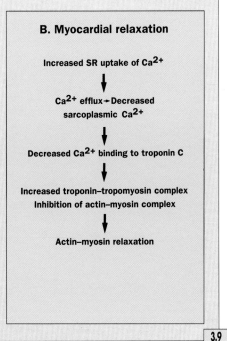

3.9

REFERENCES

1. Burch G, Winsor T: *A Primer of Electrocardiography.* Philadelphia, Lea & Febiger, 1945.
2. Fishman AP, Richards DW (eds): *Circulation of the Blood: Men and Ideas.* New York, Oxford University Press, 1964.
3. Noble D: *The Initiation of the Heartbeat*, ed 2. Oxford, Clarendon Press, 1979, pp 10–13.
4. Isenberg G, Trautwein W: The effect of dihydro-ouabain and lithium ions on the outward current in cardiac Purkinje fibres. Evidence for electrogenicity of active transport. *Pflugers Arch* 1974;350:41.
5. Baker PF: Transport and metabolism of calcium ions in nerve. *Prog Biophys* 1972;24:177.
6. Luttgau HC, Niedergerke R: The antagonism between calcium and sodium ions on the frog's heart. *J Physiol Lond* 1958;143:486.
7. Niedergerke R: Movements of Ca^+ in beating ventricles of the frog. *J Physiol Lond* 1963;167:551.
8. Reuter H, Seitz N: The dependence of calcium efflux from cardiac muscle on temperature and external ion composition. *J Physiol Lond* 1968;195:451.
9. Glitsch HL, Reuter H, Scholz H: The effect of internal sodium concentration on calcium fluxes in isolated guinea-pig auricles. *J Physiol Lond* 1970;209:25.
10. Vaughan-Jones RD: Intracellular chloride activity of quiescent cardiac Purkinje fibres. *J Physiol Lond* 1977;272:32.
11. Schlant RC, Sonnenblick EH: Normal physiology of the cardiovascular system. In Hurst JW (ed); *The Heart*, 7th ed, McGraw-Hill, New York, 1990, pp 36–39.

FIGURE CREDITS

Figure 3.6 Reprinted from Noble D: *The Initiation of the Heartbeat.* (2nd ed., 1979) Oxford University Press, 1979, p 12.

Figure 3.7 From Schlant RC, Sonnenblick EH: Normal physiology of the cardiovascular system. In Hurst JW (ed): *The Heart*, 7th ed. New York, McGraw-Hill, 1990, p 36.

Figure 3.8 From Opie LH: *The Heart.* New York, Grune & Stratton, 1984, p 89. Legend modified by Schlant RC, Sonnenblick EH: Normal physiology of the cardiovascular system. In Hurst JW (ed): *The Heart*, 7th ed, New York, McGraw-Hill, 1990, p 37.

Figure 3.9 From Schlant RC, Sonnenblick EH: Normal physiology of the cardiovascular system. In Hurst JW (ed): *The Heart*, 7th ed, New York, McGraw-Hill, 1990, p 37.

*T*HE ELECTRICAL FORCES OF THE HEART AND THEIR MEASUREMENT

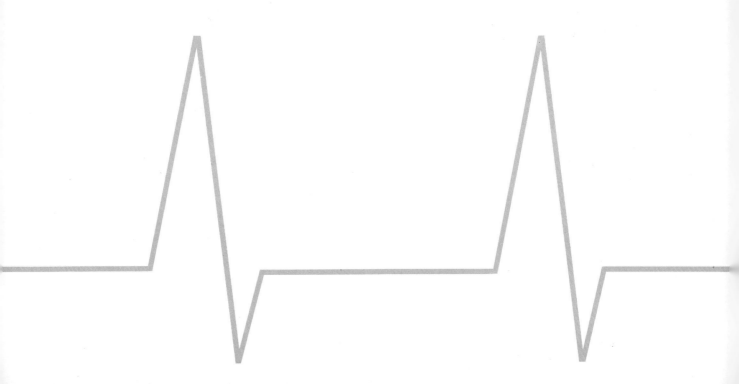

THE ELECTRICAL FORCES OF THE HEART

Let us assume that the heart generates only three electrical forces (Fig. 4.1). An inquisitive observer will ask, "what determines the characteristics of the vectors (arrows) that are used to represent the three electrical forces?"

There are five major factors that determine the characteristics of the vectors (arrows) that represent the electrical forces of the heart. They are: (a) the location of the heart in the thorax; (b) the transmission of the electrical forces of the heart to the body surface; (c) the exact location and anatomic features of the atria and ventricles; (d) the unique anatomy of the conduction system; and (e) the sensitivity of the measuring device (the electrocardiograph machine).

THE LOCATION OF THE HEART IN THE THORAX

Austin Flint, of auscultation fame, published a beautiful drawing of the heart (Fig. 4.2) in 1859 (1). Note that the heart is nearer to the anterior portion of the chest wall than it is to the lateral or posterior portions.

THE TRANSMISSION OF THE ELECTRICAL FORCES OF THE HEART TO THE BODY SURFACE

The electrical forces generated by the heart are transmitted through the tissues of the body to the skin. Whenever an electrocardiogram is recorded from the right wrist, the deflection has the same size and shape as when it is recorded from the right upper arm (Fig. 4.3A, left). Similarly, when the electrocardiogram is recorded from an electrode placed on the right ankle, the deflection has the same size and shape as when it is recorded from an electrode on the right knee (Fig. 4.3A, right). This suggests that the tissue of the legs and arms transmits electrical forces to the skin without great difficulty. It also indicates, as will be discussed later, that any portion of the legs or arms is "electrically" equidistant from the origin of the electrical forces generated by the heart. As Dr. Estes has pointed out, the extremities are like wires attached to the trunk, and a connection made at any point along the wire will produce the same recording. The lower extremities represent an upside down, Y-shaped wire*.

When an electrocardiogram is recorded from an electrode placed on the back of the thorax, the waves will be smaller than in an electrocardiogram recorded from an electrode on the front of the thorax (Fig. 4.3B). This occurs because the sampling electrode placed on the front is nearer the electrical field generated by the heart than when it is placed on the back. In addition to this, the lung tissue, which is sparse anteriorly as compared to posterolaterally, impedes the transmission of the electrical field to a greater degree posteriorly than anteriorly. The precordial deflection will also be larger than the deflections recorded from the extremities (Fig. 4.3A). The size of the electrical forces recorded from the body surface decreases considerably when the sampling electrode is moved from the anterior portion of the chest toward the extremities, but after about 10 cm, the electrodes have to be moved greater and greater distances before there

is a change in the magnitude of the recorded electrical forces (Fig. 4.4). The point is that recordings made beyond 10 cm are made in a region where the isopotential lines have become so "thinned out"* that distance is relatively unimportant; therefore, the surface points can be considered to be equidistant.

THE PRECISE LOCATION AND ANATOMIC FEATURES OF THE ATRIA AND VENTRICLES

The names of the four chambers of the heart—the right atrium, left atrium, right ventricle, and left ventricle—prevent us from perceiving the precise location of these structures in the thorax. The right atrium is in reality located to the right and slightly anterior to the left atrium. The left atrium is a posterior structure and is actually located in a central position within the chest. The right ventricle is located to the right and is predominantly an anterior structure, while the left ventricle rests on the left leaf of the diaphragm in a left lateral and slightly anterior position. The anatomic position of the cardiac structures is shown in Figures 4.5, 4.6, and 4.7. The reader should recall that the heart is located more vertically in tall, thin individuals and more horizontally in broad chested, obese individuals.

In addition to their location, the size, thickness and integrity of the walls of the four cardiac chambers are major determinants of the electrical field created by the heart. The heart of a normal newborn exhibits a right and left ventricle of equal wall thickness, whereas the left ventricle of a one-year-old child and an adult has a thicker wall than the right ventricle. These normal anatomic conditions influence the characteristics of the heart's electrical field. A large right or left atrium may be associated with large, deformed P waves in the electrocardiogram. A hypertrophied right ventricle may produce large rightward and anteriorly directed electrical forces, whereas a hypertrophied left ventricle may produce large leftward and slightly posteriorly directed electrical forces. Damage to the left ventricle, as with myocardial infarction, may also alter the electrical field. All of these conditions will be discussed later. The objective of the current discussion is to emphasize that the location of the chambers of the heart and the anatomical status of the muscle influence the characteristics of the heart's electrical field and its distribution.

THE CARDIAC CONDUCTION SYSTEM

The cardiac impulse is a self-perpetuating process that begins in the *sinoatrial node (SA node)*. The SA node is normally "beating" a certain number of times each minute, and periodically leaks electrical potential, causing the neighboring cells to depolarize. This node is located at the junction of the superior vena cava, the right atrium, and right atrial appendage.

Anton Becker, one of the modern authorities on the conduction system of the heart (2-5), does not believe that there is any specialized conduction tissue within the atria. However, he maintains that there are preferential electrical pathways

---

Note: As stated in several places in this book, the model presented here is a clinically useful approximation of the real situation within the heart. At times, the explanation moves beyond the known evidence. When this occurs, every effort has been made to extend the facts in a logical manner.
* Personal communication with Harvey Estes, M.D.

(Figure 4.3 continued.)
shape of the electrocardiographic deflections are the same. This simple experiment shows that electrically speaking, the ankles are no further away from the heart (the origin of electrical activity) than the knees, and the wrists are no further away than the upper arms. **B.** The electrocardiographic deflections were recorded from the front of the chest and the back of the thorax. The deflection recorded from the front of the chest is larger than that recorded from the back. This difference occurs because an electrode placed on the front of the chest is nearer the heart than one on the back or on the extremities.

FIGURE 4.4
The influence of distance on the size of the electrocardiographic deflections. When electrodes are placed near the heart (central circle on the front of the chest), the size of the deflections is influenced considerably by their near-ness to the origin of electrical activity. For electrodes placed in the middle circle, the size of the deflections is influenced less by their proximity to the heart than when they are placed in the central circle. The size of the deflections recorded by electrodes placed on the body in the outer circle will be influenced very little by the distance from the heart. When electrodes are placed within the outer circle, they are considered to be electrically equidistant from the origin of electrical activity.

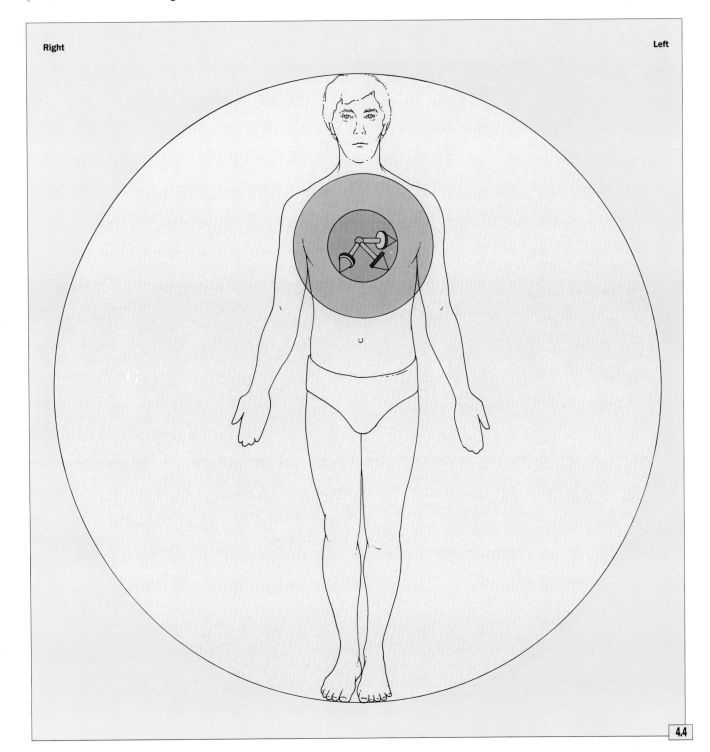

Right   Left

FIGURE 4.5

The gross anatomy of the heart (frontal view). In order to understand electrocardiography it is necessary to know cardiac anatomy. The technique of magnetic resonance imaging (MRI) can be used to show the frontal view, transverse view (see Fig. 4.6), and left lateral view (see Fig. 4.7) of the heart. They are the same views that must be kept in mind as one analyzes the electrical forces of the heart. (Image of Dr. Mark Lowell; provided by Dr. Roderic I. Pettigrew and the Radiology Department of Emory University Hospital).

FIGURE 4.6

The gross anatomy of the heart (transverse view). **A.** Magnetic resonance image (transverse view) showing the left and right ventricles. (Image of Dr. Mark Lowell; provided by Dr. Roderic I. Pettigrew and the Radiology Department of the Emory University Hospital.) **B.** Magnetic resonance image (transverse view) showing the left atrium, right atrium, right ventricle, and left ventricle. (Image of Dr. Mark Lowell; provided by Dr. Roderic I. Pettigrew and the Radiology Department of the Emory University Hospital.)

FIGURE 4.7

The gross anatomy of the heart (magnetic resonance image of left lateral view). (Image of Dr. Mark Lowell; provided by Dr. Roderic I. Pettigrew and the Radiology Department of Emory University Hospital.

FIGURE 4.8

Diagram showing the three internodal pathways: Anterior (A), middle (M), and posterior (P). Bachmann's bundle (BB) contains the major interatrial pathway and the first portion of the anterior internodal pathway. RV = right ventricle; LV = left ventricle; Ao = aorta; SN = sinus

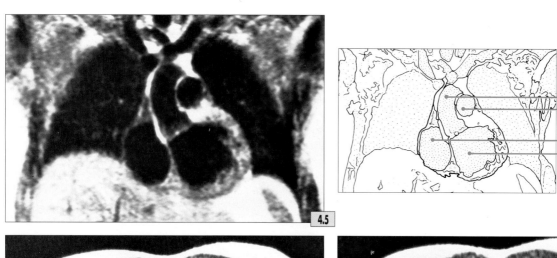

4.5

Aorta
Pulmonary Artery

Right Atrium
Left Ventricle

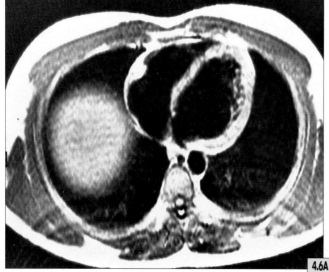

4.6A

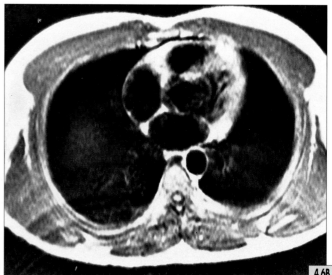

4.6B

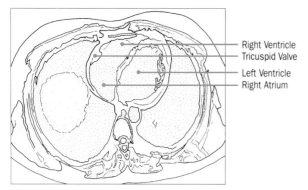

Right Ventricle
Tricuspid Valve

Left Ventricle
Right Atrium

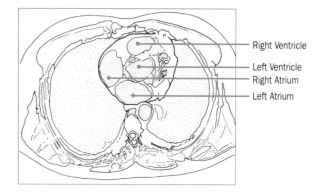

Right Ventricle

Left Ventricle
Right Atrium

Left Atrium

(Figure 4.8 continued.)
node; AVN=AV node. (Reproduced with permission; see Figure Credits.)

FIGURE 4.9

Depolarization of the atria. **A.** Mean vector representing depolarization of the right atrium. This vector is referred to as P1. **B.** Mean vector representing depolarization of the left atrium. This vector is referred to as P2. **C.** Mean vector representing depolarization of both atria. This vector is referred to as Pm.

FIGURE 4.10

Tawara's view of the left bundle branch. This diagram is taken from the monograph by Tawara (1906) (10), which established and elucidated the signifi-

cance of the atrioventricular conduction axis. It shows the fanlike arrangement of the left bundle branch. The clinical value of the so-called concept of hemiblocks should not be extended to presume that the left bundle branch is arranged anatomically in bifascicular fashion. As shown here, it is arranged as a fan, and if it divides at all, it forms three rather than two divisions.

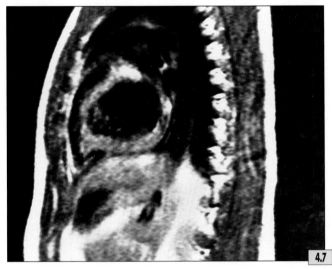

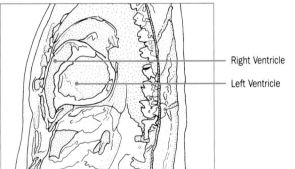

Right Ventricle

Left Ventricle

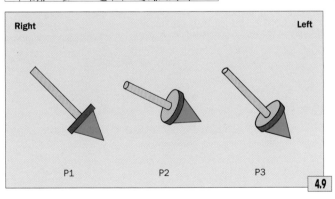

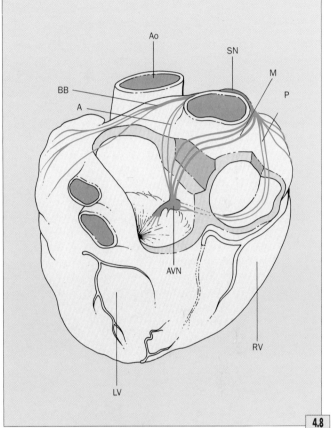

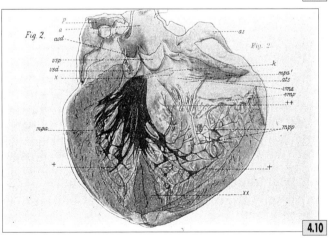

FIGURE 4.11

The left bundle branch provides an early twig to the left upper portion of the interventricular septum. The left bundle divides to form two branches although Tawara called it tripartite. The major divisions are the anterior-superior and the posterior-inferior divisions. The arrows indicate the direction of depolarization of the myocytes that results from the electrical stimulus transmitted by the conduction system.

FIGURE 4.12

The mean direction of a vector representing the wave of depolarization of the ventricles of a normal adult is toward the left, inferiorly, and slightly posteriorly.

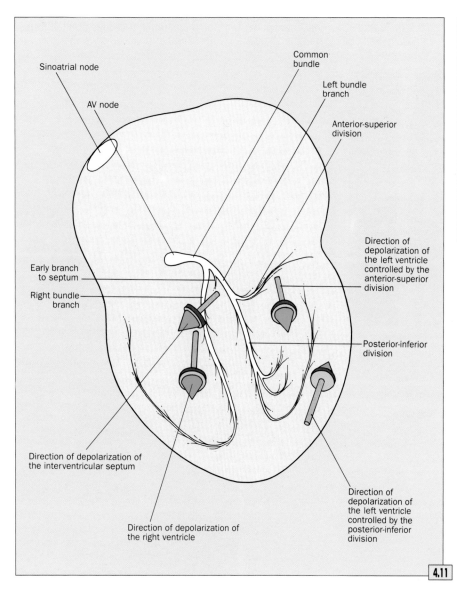

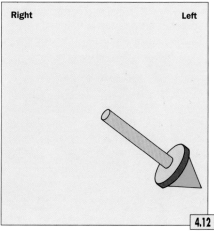

THE MEASUREMENT OF THE ELECTRICAL FORCES OF THE HEART

As discussed earlier, in deference to simplicity, let us assume that the heart generates only three electrical forces (Fig. 4.1). Later in the book we will deal with the *infinite* number of electrical forces actually generated by the heart. The three electrical forces do not occur simultaneously; Force 1 occurs a brief moment before Force 2, and Force 2 occurs a brief moment before Force 3. Force 1 is produced by depolarization of the interventricular septum; Force 2 is due to depolarization of the endocardial layers of the right and left ventricles; and Force 3 is due to the depolarization of the thicker, superior portion of the left ventricle. Clinicians can identify the important characteristics of the electrical forces by studying the distribution of electrical fields on the body surface (arms, legs, and thorax).

At this point the reader should review the puzzle of the black box discussed in Chapter 2. Note, too, that a simple measuring device was also discussed in Chapter 2. That device could detect whether an arrow, representing an electrical force, was directed toward it by recording a positive (+) response, or away from it by recording a negative (–) response. The device could also detect whether an arrow representing an electrical force was perpendicular to it by recording a zero (0) response. This simple device, which was used to record the distribution of the positive and negative signs from the surface of the black box, can be viewed as an analogue of an electrocardiograph machine (Fig. 2.3).

THE MACHINE

The evolution of our knowledge of the electricity produced by the heart and its measurement was discussed in Chapter 1 (12). The capillary manometer was replaced by Einthoven's bulky galvanometer. Einthoven's machine was replaced by a portable electronic and photographic machine that recorded from one or two sampling sites at a time. This machine was replaced by the portable electronic, direct-writing machine, which also recorded from one or two sampling sites at a time. The latter machine was replaced by the modern portable, electronic, direct-writing machine, which records from 12 sampling sites simultaneously (Fig. 4.13). The direct-writing machine does not record with the precision of the photographic machine, but the practical value of an immediate readout of waves and deflections overrides the value of a more precise but more time-consuming photographic recording.

THE ELECTROCARDIOGRAPHIC PAPER

A sample of the paper used for electrocardiography is shown in Figure 4.14A. The stylus of the electrocardiograph machine moves upward to record a positive deflection and downward to record a negative deflection (Fig. 4.14B). Each small, 1-mm square represents 0.04 second along the horizontal axis and 0.1 mv along the vertical axis. Five of the small squares, or one large square, represents 0.2 second on the horizontal axis and 0.5 mv along the vertical axis. The machine is then standardized (calibrated) so that 1 mv of electrical force will record a visible signal of 10 mm (two large squares) on the paper (Fig. 4.14C). This reference figure is called the standard. The paper speed is preset to a uniform 25 mm per second.

SAMPLING SITES AND LEAD AXES

Back in the time of Waller and Einthoven, in order to record an electrocardiogram, it was necessary for subjects to place their hands and feet into buckets of saline. The wires of the capillary electrometer or galvanometer were connected to the outer bucket of a double-bucket apparatus. The subjects' extremities were immersed in saline-soaked cotton held within the inner bucket (which was actually a porous pot), and each wire was attached to the outer bucket, which contained zinc sulfate. Sir Thomas Lewis published the photograph shown in Figure 4.15 in the fourth edition of his book *Clinical Electrocardiography,* published in 1928 (13).

Improvements gradually took place, and today it is quite easy to "hook up" the patient to a modern electrocardiograph machine. The wires connecting the machine and the skin surface are called *leads.* They are attached to the skin by electrodes and electrode paste. This paste, which is capable of transmitting electricity, is placed between the skin and electrode in order to insure that the electricity that reaches the skin has good contact with the electrode.

A *lead axis* for a *bipolar extremity lead* can best be visualized by considering the Bayley triaxial reference system (see later discussion). A bipolar lead axis passes from one extremity electrode, through the center of the heart, which represents the origin of electrical activity, to another extremity electrode. A *lead axis* for a *unipolar extremity lead* passes from the extremity electrode, through the center of the heart, to the opposite side of the body (see later discussion). The hexaxial reference display system is used to represent the bipolar and unipolar extremity lead axes. The lead axes for the *six unipolar chest leads* pass from the chest electrodes through the center of the heart, to the opposite chest wall. As will be discussed later, electrodes attached to the extremities are, from an electrical viewpoint, equidistant from the origin of electrical activity in the center of the heart. This is not the case with electrodes attached to the anterior chest wall—they are not equidistant from the origin of electrical activity. Einthoven's lead system (14), Bayley's triaxial reference lead system (15), Wilson's unipolar chest leads (16), and Goldberger's augmented unipolar extremity leads will all be discussed later (17).

Once the electrical energy from a lead is introduced into the machine, it is translated into a positive or negative movement of the recording stylus. An upward movement occurs when electrical forces are directed toward the electrode attached to the positive pole of the machine, and a downward movement occurs when the forces are directed away from the positive pole electrode (Fig. 4.14B). The stylus does not move at all when there are no electrical forces being generated by the heart, or when the electrical forces are perpendicular to the lead axis being used.

It would be possible to characterize the distribution of the electrical fields generated by the heart by placing the electrode of a lead on every centimeter of the skin of the thorax, just as we studied the distribution of electrical charges on the surface of the black box shown in Figure 2.4. This, of course, would be so time consuming that it would be impossible to utilize the system in any practical way (see the discussion of *precordial mapping* at the end of this chapter). Accordingly, a system has gradually evolved whereby a minimum of sampling sites (electrode positions) can be used to represent the thousands of potential sampling sites on the thorax. We should not forget, however, that the small numbers of sampling sites routinely used may not always reveal an accurate picture of the true events just as a Gallup Poll does not always reveal an accurate estimate of the true feelings of a population interested in a political election.

LEAD SYSTEMS

EINTHOVEN BIPLOAR EXTREMITY LEADS:The first electrocardiographic lead system was designed by Einthoven (14). He was undoubtedly influenced by the fact that he could only use the extremities as sampling sites since only they could be placed in buckets of saline. Einthoven connected the negative pole of his galvanometer to the right arm and the positive pole to the left arm, and labeled this as lead I. For lead II, he connected the negative pole of the galvanometer to the right arm and the positive pole to the left leg. He then connected the negative pole of the galvanometer to the left arm and the positive pole to the left leg, labeling this as lead III. Figure 4.16A shows Einthoven's system.

Einthoven broke the sequence of measuring around the periphery of the electrical field when he reversed the polarity of lead II. Had the same sequence been maintained, he would have connected the negative pole of the galvanometer to the left leg and the positive pole to the right arm to create lead II. The sum of the deflections recorded on each lead would have equaled zero (the deflections on leads I + II + III = 0). As Einthoven designed the system, however, the deflection recorded on lead I, plus the deflection recorded on lead III, plus the deflection recorded on a *reversed* lead II equaled zero (the deflection on I + (-II) + III = 0, or I + III = II). This equation is known as Einthoven's law and, as will be discussed later, can be used to determine if the electrode positions have been accidentally switched. Legend holds that Einthoven preferred to see upright deflections. Such would not occur in the majority of adults had he attached the negative pole of the galvanometer to the left leg and its positive pole to the right arm, so he reversed the polarity of lead II.

One should note that Einthoven's leads I, II, and III are bipolar leads. In other words, lead I is influenced by the electrical potential of both the left and right arm. The recording one sees on the paper represents the difference between the electrical potential recorded at the two electrode sites. Lead II records the difference in electrical potential recorded from the right arm and left leg, and lead III records the difference between the left arm and left leg. Einthoven's leads form a triangle that is often called an equilateral triangle. *This designation does not imply that it is an anatomic equilateral triangle:* obviously, the distance between the center of the chest and a leg is greater than the distance between the center of the chest and an arm. The term equilateral is used here to suggest that Einthoven's leads form an *electrically equilateral triangle*. At this point, the reader should review Figures 4.3 and 4.4. They show that the electrical potential recorded at the ankle is no different from that recorded at the knee, and that the potential recorded at the wrist is no different from that recorded higher on the arm. This being true, one can assume that electrodes connected to the extremities are electrically equidistant from the origin of the electrical force in the center of the heart and thorax, and that the sampling sites (electrode positions) located on the extremities are electrically equidistant from each other. This understanding led Einthoven to create his equilateral triangle.

Burger's investigations proved that Einthoven's hypothesis was not accurate (18). He found that one extremity might be influenced more than another by the electrical field originating in the center of the heart and thorax. For practical purposes however this variance does not matter, and Einthoven's views regarding this matter will be used throughout this book.

The bipolar and unipolar extremity leads are sometimes called frontal plane leads because their lead axes are influenced by electrical forces that are directed up or down and to the left or right, but not by electrical forces that are directed only anteriorly or posteriorly.

BAYLEY'S TRIAXIAL REFERENCE SYSTEM: Robert Bayley accepted Einthoven's equilateral triangle which displayed the extremity bipolar lead system, and he used it as the basis for designing a simpler display system (15). He also accepted that the influence of an electrical force on the leads of Einthoven's triangle could be represented by projecting the magnitude of the force onto the lead axes. Bayley created a simpler display by moving the leads of Einthoven's equilateral triangle so that they all passed through the origin of electrical activity located at the center of the triangle (the center of the heart and thorax.) The orientations of the lead axes themselves were not changed (Fig. 4.16B). The influence of an electrical force, represented as an arrow, that is perpendicular to Einthoven's lead axis I is shown in Figure 4.17A. The projection of the electrical force is smallest on lead I and equal in size on leads II and III (the magnitude of the deflection on lead I + the magnitude of the deflection on lead III = the magnitude of the deflection on lead II). The arrow representing the electrical force points inferiorly because it points relatively toward the positive poles of lead axes II and III. An electrical force, represented as an arrow, projects the same quantity on the lead axes of this new display system as it projects on the lead axes of the Einthoven triangle. The new display system is called the triaxial reference system of Bayley.

In order to measure and communicate the direction of electrical forces in the frontal plane, the right side of Bayley's diagram was designated as 0° (this is the patient's left side), the inferior vertical position was designated as +90°, the left side of the diagram was designated as ± 180° (this is the patient's right side), and the upper part of the diagram was designated as -90° (Fig. 4.17B). The electrical force represented as a vector as shown in Figure 4.17B, is directed at +90°.

BIPOLAR CHEST LEADS: The extremity leads used in electrocardiography are called bipolar leads because each lead uses two electrodes. The electrocardiograph machine measures the difference in the electrical potential between the two electrode sites. As electrodes were developed and improved, and buckets of saline were no longer used for contact with the patient's skin, it became possible to place one of the electrodes of a bipolar lead on the precordium and the other on one of the extremities. The precordial (chest) electrode was connected to the positive pole of the galvanometer and the extremity electrode was connected to the negative pole. The electrocardiograph machine measures the difference in electrical potential between the two sites. Accordingly, such a lead was called a bipolar chest lead. In the beginning, only one precordial electrode site was used, and it was labeled CF, CL, or CR, with the letter C signifying chest and F, L, or R signifying foot, left arm, or right arm, respectively (Fig. 4.18). Later, six precordial electrode positions were designated, as shown in Figure 4.19. Still later, the seventh precordial lead position (3R) was defined. The precordial electrode positions are:

1. Fourth right intercostal space adjacent to the sternum.
2. Fourth left intercostal space adjacent to the sternum.
3. Halfway between electrode positions 2 and 4.
4. Fifth intercostal space to the left in the midclavicular line.
5. Anterior axillary line on the left, at the same level as electrode position 4.
6. Midaxillary line on the left, at the same level as electrode positions 4 and 5.

7. The 3R electrode is placed in same position as 3, but located on the right side of the thorax rather than the left.

The six precordial electrode positions were originally established because it was believed that electrode positions 1, 2, and sometimes 3 recorded the electrical forces generated by the right ventricle; electrode positions 3 or 4 recorded the electrical forces generated by the interventricular septum; and electrode positions 5, 6 and sometimes 4 recorded the electrical forces generated by the left ventricle. While this concept has some merit, it is not accurate. All precordial electrode positions are influenced by the electrical forces from all parts of the heart. Electrode positions 1, 2, and 3 are influenced by the right ventricle more than positions 4, 5, and 6, but the electrocardiographic recordings made from positions 1, 2, and 3 reveal left ventricular electrical forces to a greater extent than they do right ventricular electrical forces. Electrode positions 5 and 6 are influenced predominantly by the left ventricle, but the right ventricle also influences the recording made from these positions. A recording from electrode positions 3 or 4 is not from the septum, but represents one of the numerous positions on the chest where the electrical field shifts from negative to positive (see the later discussion of the transitional pathway in this chapter). Also, it must be remembered that when a bipolar chest lead is used, the electrocardiogram represents the difference between the potentials recorded at the chest and the extremity electrode positions.

UNIPOLAR LEADS: Frank Wilson (16), more than anyone, realized the need to record the electrical potential from the body surface using a lead axis that would record the true electrical potential at the electrode site. Such a lead should be better than a bipolar lead because a bipolar lead records the difference in electrical potential between two different sites. Wilson's unique contribution was the realization that if one connects the three extremity electrode lead wires together, according to Einthoven's law, the electrical potential at the point of their common connection should always record a zero potential (Fig. 4.20). This common point was called the *central terminal*. Wilson then connected the central terminal to the negative pole of the electrocardiograph machine and called it the *indifferent electrode*. He connected the positive pole of the machine to a wire which was connected to the *exploring electrode*. Wilson added resistances to the wires from each extremity in order to equalize the effects of varying skin resistances, and then amplified the resulting signal. He performed many carefully designed experiments to determine whether the indifferent electrode recorded a zero potential, and whether it was in fact an indifferent electrode. He discovered that it recorded an almost, but not true, zero potential. He concluded, however, that for practical purposes the exploring electrode could be considered to be a true unipolar lead, largely uninfluenced by the electrical potential recorded by the indifferent electrode.

UNIPOLAR CHEST LEADS: Wilson recommended that the unipolar lead be used to explore the surface of the chest. The electrode positions discussed earlier and shown in Figure 4.19 were used, and the leads themselves were designated as V leads because V is the symbol for electrical potential. Accordingly, the seven precordial V leads were born and called V1, V2, V3, V4, V5, V6, and V3R (Fig. 4.21A). The precordial V lead axes are shown in Figures 4.21B and 4.21C. The magnitude of the deflections from each precordial lead was adequate for analysis because the electrode positions were near the heart.

As pointed out by Grant, the V leads are used to identify and measure the extent to which the heart's electrical forces are directed anteriorly or posteriorly. Lead V6 is influenced by forces that are directed predominantly to the left or right and parallel with the frontal plane; it is almost a frontal plane lead. This is why a deflection recorded by lead V6 is often similar to the deflection recorded by lead I.

For many years, clinicians compared the deflections recorded by V leads with those recorded by the CR, CL, and CF leads, in an effort to determine which system yielded the best clinical information (Fig. 4.22). It was eventually concluded that the V lead system was superior to the others.

It would be advantageous to use different chest electrode positions than those currently in use. For example, the electrode positions shown in Figure 4.23 could be used. The old system has, however, been deeply ingrained by years of usage, and a new system is unacceptable. This point is made here to reinforce the previous statement of the clinician's challenge: to determine the characteristics of the electrical forces of the heart by placing electrodes on the surface of the body. A limited number of sampling sites (electrode positions) are used because it is impractical to record from every centimeter of the skin surface. Although other, better sampling sites (electrode positions) might be used, it is unlikely that the current seven precordial electrode positions will be changed. There are times, however, when additional electrode sites are needed, and it is important for the clinician to be able to determine where to place the electrode on the chest in order to clarify the characteristics of the electrical forces. For example, lead V3R, which is not used routinely in adults as it is in children, is often useful in those adults who have had an inferior infarction to determine whether the right ventricle is also involved. Other electrode positions may be needed, the location being determined on an individual basis (see the discussion later in this chapter).

UNIPOLAR EXTREMITY LEADS: When Wilson placed the exploring electrode of the lead system he designed on each of the extremities, he discovered that the magnitude of the electrical forces at those sites was too small to be used in association with the deflections recorded by the bipolar extremity leads. In other words, a mathematical relationship between the unipolar extremity leads and the bipolar extremity leads could not be established without amplifying the magnitude of the electrical inputs to the unipolar lead system. However, World War II, of necessity, drained off the electronic technology of the United States so that amplifying systems could not be mass produced. Therefore, it was necessary to develop another way of augmenting the magnitude of the Wilson unipolar extremity leads.

Emanuel Goldberger (17) discovered that the magnitude of the deflection recorded from a specific electrode site using a Wilson unipolar extremity lead could be *augmented* if the extremity-to-central terminal electrode was disconnected when the exploring electrode was placed on that extremity (17). As a result, leads aVR, aVL, and aVF were born (Fig. 4.24).

Figure 4.25 shows two deflections. One was recorded with a Wilson V lead from the left leg and the other with an augmented lead (aVF) attached to the left leg. Note that the contours of the two deflections are identical but the size of the deflection recorded with the V lead is slightly smaller than that recorded by lead aVF.

The lead axes of the unipolar lead system bisect the angles of Einthoven's bipolar lead axis display system and those of Bayley's triaxial system. The resulting display of lead axes is called the hexaxial lead axis display system (Fig. 4.16C).

The unipolar extremity leads, like the bipolar extremity leads, are called frontal plane leads because they are influenced by electrical forces that are directed upward and downward or to the right or left; they are not influenced by electrical forces that are directed precisely anteriorly or posteriorly.

SUMMARY: The leads used in modern electrocardiography are Einthoven's bipolar extremity leads (Bayley's triaxial reference system), Goldberger's augmented Wilson unipolar extremity leads; and Wilson's six unipolar chest leads. A seventh chest electrode position (V3R) is used in children and in some adults when needed. Other chest electrode positions are occasionally used when the clinician determines that the usual chest leads are inadequate to characterize the electrical forces of the heart.

FIGURE 4.13
A modern direct-writing electrocardiograph machine. The machine records all 12 leads simultaneously. The recordings of three leads are displayed one above the other so that leads I, II, and III can be viewed on the first segment of the paper. These are followed by the recordings of aVR, aVL, and aVF; V1, V2, and V3; and V4, V5, and V6. The electrodes are small suction cups, and the electrode paste assures excellent skin contact. Not only is this an efficient system, but it permits the study of simultaneously recorded leads, which assists in the effort to diagram more accurate

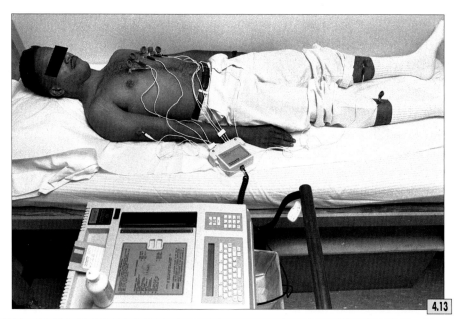

4.13

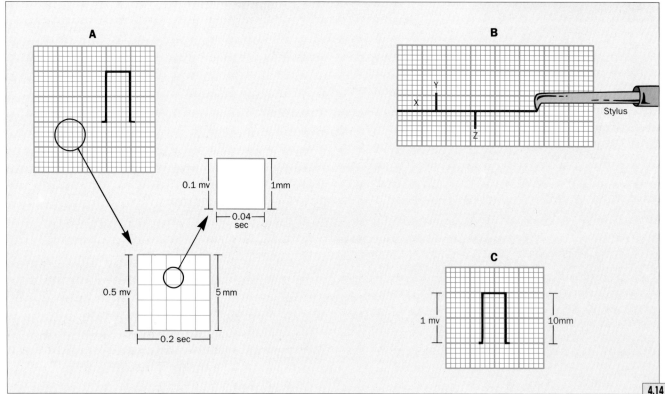

4.14

(Figure 4.13 continued.)
vectors. I thank The Marquette Electronics Company for their permission to use this photograph.

FIGURE 4.14
The electrocardiograph paper and stylus. **A.** Electrocardiograph paper. **B.** Electrocardiograph paper and writing stylus. The stylus registers a positive deflection by writing upward (y) and a negative deflection by writing downward (z). The baseline is labeled X. **C.** The machine is standardized (calibrated) by adjusting the stylus so that it moves upward 10 mm to represent 1mV.

FIGURE 4.15
During the Waller and Einthoven era, contact between the electrocardiograph machine and the subject was accomplished by placing the extremities of the subject in buckets of saline. The need to use this type of contact between the patient and the machine prevented the development of chest leads. (Reproduced with permission; see Figure Credits.)

FIGURE 4.16
A. Einthoven's equilateral triangle. Note that lead I is created by attaching the negative pole of the galvanometer to the right arm and the positive pole of the galvanometer to the left arm. Lead II is created by attaching the negative pole of the galvanometer to the right arm and the positive pole of the galvanometer to the left or right leg. Lead III is created by attaching the negative pole of the galvanometer to the left arm and the positive pole of the galvanometer to the left or right leg. (A fourth wire is used as a ground wire.) **B.** Bayley triaxial lead system. **C.** Hexaxial lead system. Note that the unipolar extremily lead axes bisect the angles of Einthoven's equilateral triangle (see complete discussion later in chapter).

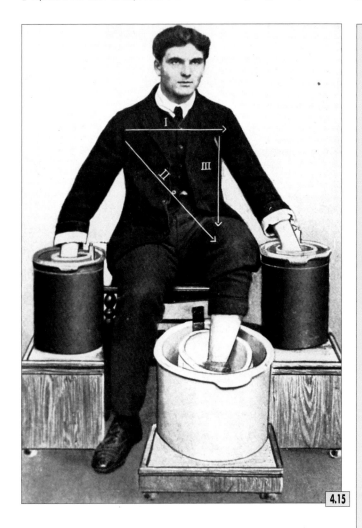

4.15

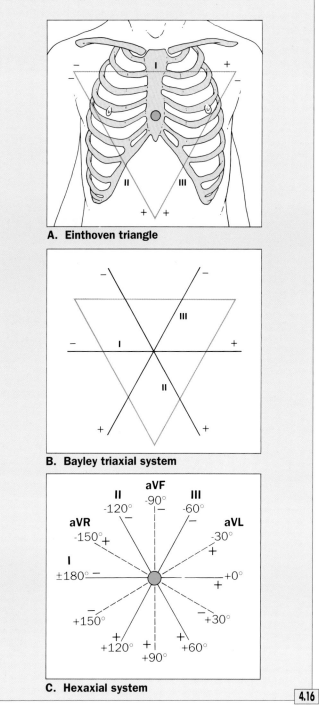

A. Einthoven triangle

B. Bayley triaxial system

C. Hexaxial system

4.16

FIGURE 4.17
A. Bayley's triaxial reference system. Einthoven's lead axes are moved over to pass through the center of electrical activity. Note that the vector will project the same quantity on the transposed axes as it does on the Einthoven axes. The curved arrows illustrate how the lead axes are translated from the Einthoven system to the Bayley system. In the example shown, the dotted lines represent the projection of the vector onto lead axis II. **B.** The display system used to communicate the direction of an electrical force represented by a vector. The right horizontal position in the figure is labeled as zero (this is the patient's left side), the inferior vertical position is labeled +90°, the superior vertical position is labeled -90°, and the left horizontal position is labeled ± 180° (this is the patient's right side). The vector shown here is directed at +90°.

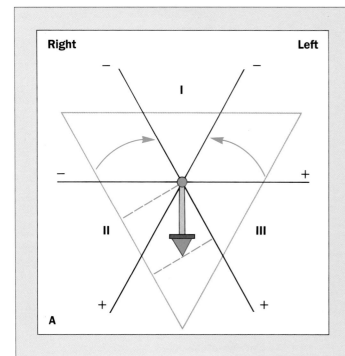

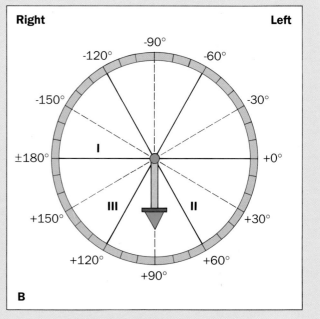

4.17

4.18

FIGURE 4.18
A bipolar chest lead. A bipolar chest lead is produced when the negative pole of the galvanometer is attached to an electrode placed on an extremity (left or right leg, or left or right arm) and the positive pole is attached to an electrode placed on the chest. The bipolar lead shown here is called a CF lead (C = chest and F = foot).

FIGURE 4.19
The seven precordial chest lead positions. **1.** Fourth right intercostal space adjacent to the sternum. **2.** Fourth left intercostal space adjacent to the sternum. **3.** Halfway between positions 2 and 4. **4.** Fifth intercostal space to the left in the midclavicular line. **5.** Anterior axillary line on the left at the same horizontal level as position 4. **6.** Midaxillary line on the left, at the same horizontal level as electrode positions 4 and 5. **7.** The 3r position is located in the same position as 3 but on the patient's right side.

FIGURE 4.20
Wilson's unipolar lead. Wilson connected the wires from the left arm, right arm, and leg electrodes to a common point. This point is called a *central terminal.* The central terminal is then connected to the negative pole of the electrocardiograph machine and is called an *indifferent electrode.* The *exploring electrode* is connected to the positive pole of the machine. Resistances are added to the wires from each extremity in order to equalize the effect of varying skin resistances. The exploring electrode is considered to be a unipolar lead because it records the true electrical potential at the electrode site. This is possible because a unipolar lead measures the difference in electrical potential between the central terminal and the exploring electrode. The electrical potential recorded by the central terminal is almost zero so the potential measured by the exploring electrode is a true potential. When a Wilson unipolar lead is used as an extremity lead, it is necessary to amplify the size of the deflections.

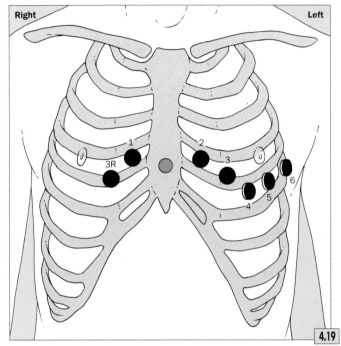

4.19

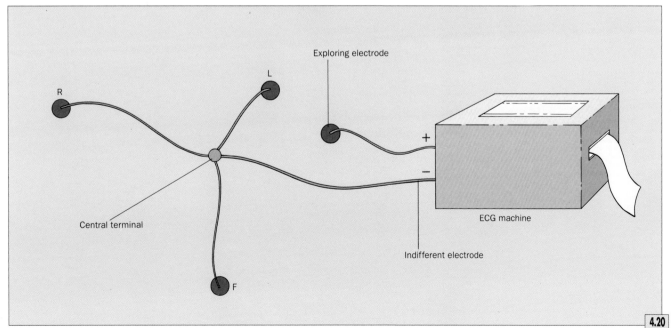

Exploring electrode

Central terminal

ECG machine

Indifferent electrode

4.20

FIGURE 4.21
Unipolar chest lead axes. **A.** When
unipolar chest leads are used,
they are identified as V1, V2, V3, V4,
V5, V6, and V3R. **B.** A frontal plane
view of the precordial lead axes.
C. A transverse view of the precordial
V lead axes.

FIGURE 4.22
The precordial deflections at all six
precordial electrode positions using
CR, CL, CF, and V leads. The
deflections recorded on leads I, II,
and III are shown at the bottom of the
illustration. Note the influence
of the extremity leads on the
precordial deflections as compared
to the deflections recorded with the

unipolar V lead system. (Reproduced
with permission; see Figure
Credits.)

FIGURE 4.23
An example of a different precordial
lead system. Other precordial lead systems could be developed, but it is
unlikely they would replace the conventional system now in use.

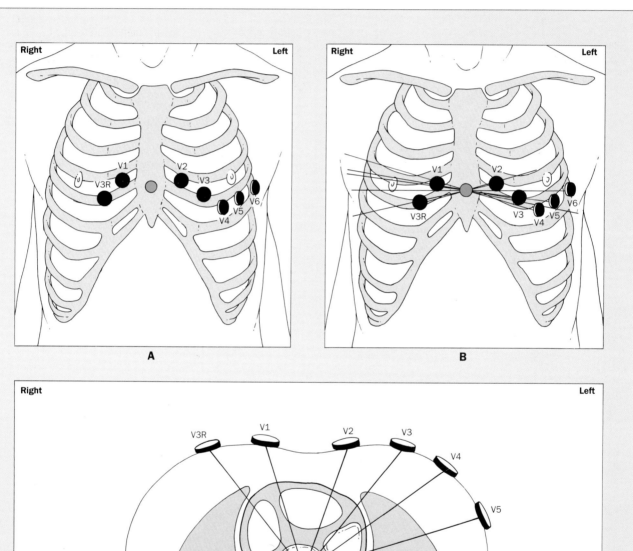

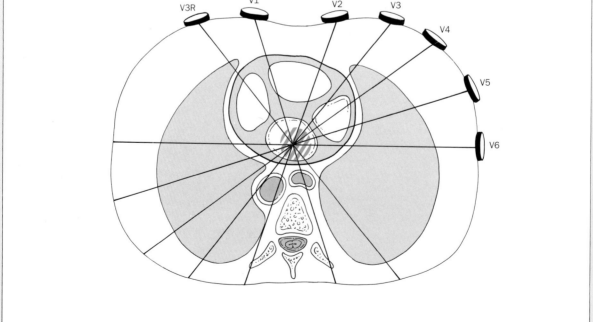

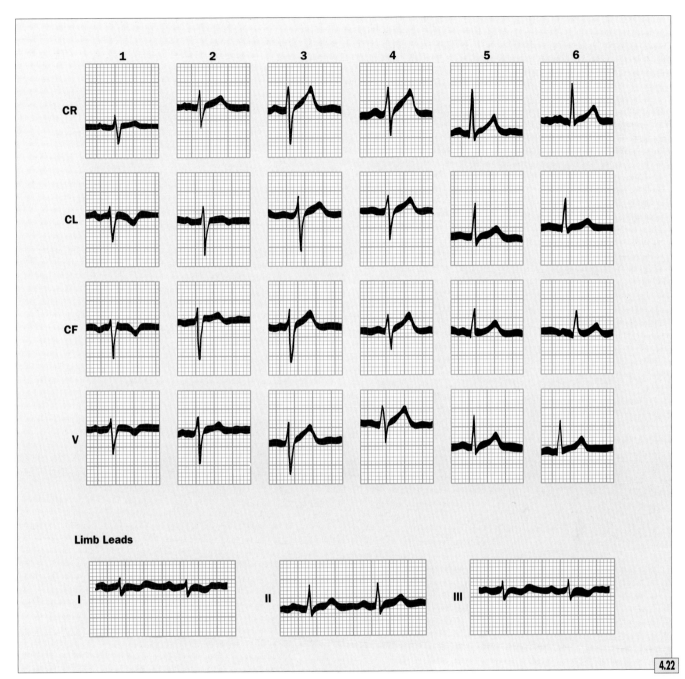

4.22

Limb Leads

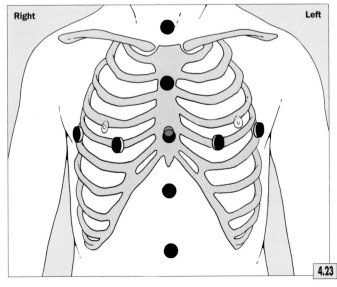

4.23

FIGURE 4.24

Goldberger's lead system. **A.** Lead aVR is created by placing an electrode on the left arm (L) and leg (F), and connecting the two electrodes by wires to a central terminal. A connection to the right arm (R) is omitted. The central terminal is connected to the negative pole of the electrocardiograph machine. The positive pole of the electrocardiograph machine is attached to a wire and electrode that is placed on the right arm. **B.** Lead aVL is created by placing electrodes on the right arm (R) and leg (F), and connecting the two electrodes by wires to a central terminal. A connection to the left arm (L) is omitted. The central terminal is connected to the negative pole of the electrocardiograph machine. The positive pole is attached to a wire leading to the electrode placed on the left arm. **C.** Lead aVF is created by placing electrodes on the right arm (R) and left arm (L), and connecting the electrodes by wires to a central terminal. A connection to the leg (F) is omitted. The central terminal is connected to the negative pole of the electrocardiograph machine, with the positive pole attached to a wire and electrode that is placed on the leg.

FIGURE 4.25

Comparison of the deflection produced by VF with the deflection produced by aVF. **A.** Electrocardiogram recorded by using Wilson's unipolar lead (VF). **B.** Electrocardiogram recorded by using Goldberger's augmented unipolar extremity lead (aVF). Note that the deflection in A is not as large as the deflection in B. The shape of the two deflections however, is about the same.

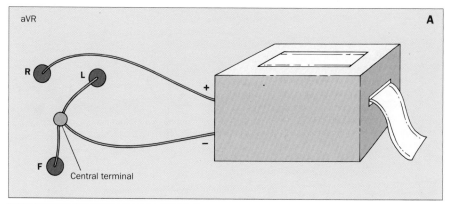

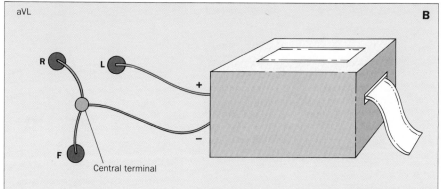

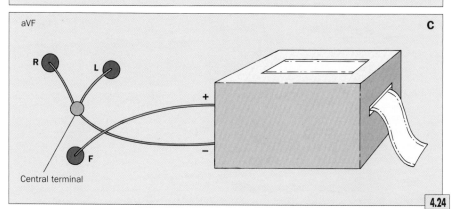

4.24

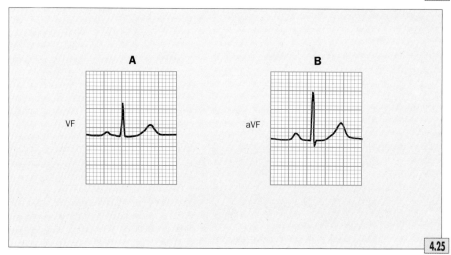

4.25

THE ELECTRICAL FORCES OF THE HEART REPRESENTED AS VECTORS

The electrical forces of the heart can be represented as vectors (19). This being true, it is necessary to discuss the characteristics of a vector. A vector, represented as an arrow, has three characteristics: direction, magnitude, and sense. The direction (or inclination) of the arrow indicates the *orientation* of the vector in space; the length of the arrow represents the *magnitude* of the vector; and the location of the arrowhead is used to designate the direction (or *sense*) of the flow of electrical energy from its origin (Fig. 4.26).

THE PROJECTION OF ELECTRICAL FORCES (REPRESENTED AS VECTORS) ON TO THE LEAD AXES

The projection of electrical forces (represented as vectors) onto the lead axes used in electrocardiography must be carefully considered (19-21). This concept can be illustrated by the use of a screen, pencil, and light source (Fig. 4.27) (20). Suppose a pencil (which represents an electrical force) is placed in front of a screen (which represents a lead axis), and imagine that a light source is arranged so that the pencil casts a shadow on the screen. The shadow cast will be largest when the pencil is precisely parallel with the screen, and will be smallest when it is precisely perpendicular. Similarly, the magnitude, direction, and sense of the electrical forces of the heart, represented as vectors, can be visualized by identifying the projection of the vectors onto the lead axes.

THE FRONTAL PLANE PROJECTION OF ELECTRICAL FORCES: The projection of electrical forces, represented as vectors, onto the axes of the extremity leads can be used to determine the magnitude, direction, and sense of the electrical forces as viewed in the frontal plane. Suppose an electrical force, represented as a vector, is directed to the left, as shown in Figure 4.28A. The extremity leads are used to identify the frontal plane projection of the vector. The display of the hexaxial axis lead system is shown superimposed on the vector in Figure 4.28B. Observations such as those illustrated in Figure 4.28 lead to formulation of the following rule: *whenever an electrical force, represented as a vector, is parallel with a frontal plane lead axis, it will project its largest "shadow" onto that axis, and the electrocardiograph machine will write its largest deflection on that lead. Whenever an electrical force, represented as a vector, is perpendicular to a frontal plane lead axis, it will project its smallest shadow" onto that axis, and the machine will write its smallest deflection on that lead. The positivity or negativity of the deflection is determined by identifying whether the vector is directed toward or away from the electrode that is attached to the positive pole of the electrocardiograph machine* (19). When the force is directed toward the positive pole, it produces an upright deflection, and when it is directed away from the positive pole, it produces a negative deflection. Part C of Figure 4.28 shows the deflections that would be recorded on the electrocardiograph paper.

The frontal plane projection of a cardiac vector onto the axes of the hexaxial lead system is *always performed as the first step* in determining the magnitude, spatial direction, and sense of an electrical force represented as a vector (19).

THE SPATIAL ORIENTATION OF ELECTRICAL FORCES: The projection of the electrical forces of the heart, represented as vectors, onto the precordial lead axes can be used to determine their anterior or posterior direction, and their sense. As emphasized

subsequently, the magnitude of an electrical force cannot be accurately determined because the chest lead electrodes are not electrically equidistant from the heart.

Suppose an electrical force, represented as a vector, is directed to the left and inferiorly, as shown in Figure 4.29A. Imagine that this force is directed posteriorly because the zero potential plane is oriented in such a way that the transitional pathway passes between electrode positions V3 and V4. Figure 4.29B shows the hexaxial lead system superimposed on the spatially oriented vector shown in Figure 4.29A. Figure 4.29C shows how the extremity lead axes would be influenced by the vector.

Figure 4.29D illustrates the type of deflection that would be recorded at positions V1, V2, V3, V4, V5, and V6. Note that the electrical field divides the thorax into two halves; negative charges will be recorded from the right half and positive charges will be recorded from the left. When this occurs, leads V1 and V2 record negative deflections, lead V3 records a slightly negative deflection, and leads V4, V5, and V6 record positive deflections. One can see how a plane that is perpendicular to the arrow intersects the surface of the chest and divides the thorax into two halves. In this case the transitional pathway passes between leads V3 and V4; it is slightly negative but smallest in lead V3. The vector is directed about 35° posteriorly.

Observations such as those illustrated in Figure 4.29 lead to the formulation of the following rule: *whenever an electrical force, represented as a vector, is perpendicular to a precordial lead axis, it will project its smallest "shadow" on that axis and the electrocardiograph machine will write its smallest deflection on that lead.* A vector representing such an electrical force will be directed toward the area of the chest where the precordial electrodes record upright deflections. It is not possible to state, as was the case with the extremity leads, that whenever an electrical force represented as a vector is parallel to a precordial lead axis, it will project its largest "shadow" and therefore record its largest deflection on that lead axis. This is because some of the precordial electrode positions, especially V1, V2, V3, and V3R, are nearer the heart than the others and would record larger deflections; the precordial electrodes are not electrically equidistant from the heart. Therefore, to restate the situation, one can assume that when an electrical force is perpendicular to a precordial lead axis, the electrocardiograph machine will write its smallest deflection on that lead, but one cannot assume that an electrical force parallel to a precordial lead axis will produce its largest deflection on that lead (19).

SUMMARY: It is possible to determine the direction, magnitude, and sense of an electrical force represented as a vector by inspecting the deflections recorded on the extremity lead axes and the precordial lead axes. The process is divided into two steps. Step one is implemented initially to determine the frontal projection of a vector which has spatial orientation. Step two is used to determine the anterior and posterior direction of the vector.

•Step one: Determining the frontal plane direction of a vector.:

Identify the lead axis in the extremity lead that reveals the largest or smallest deflection on the electrocardiograph tracing; the vector will be relatively parallel with the axis of the lead in which the deflection is largest, and relatively perpendicular to the axis of the lead in which the deflection is smallest. Inspect all of the extremity leads and adjust the vector so that it "fits" the projection of the force on all of the extremity lead axes (Fig. 4.29A and B). With practice, it is possible to identify the frontal plane direction of the vector with an accuracy of 5°.

•Step two: Determining the anterior or posterior direction of a vector.:

Having identified the frontal plane projection of a vector, one should mentally redirect it anteriorly or posteriorly until it is perpendicular to the precordial lead axis that exhibits the smallest deflection. This is done by identifying the precordial electrode position that records the smallest deflection and then arranging the vector so that a plane perpendicular to it will, when extended to the surface of the chest, pass through this electrode position (Fig. 4.29A and D). This action will divide the thorax into an area where the precordial electrodes record upright deflections and an area where they record downward deflections. The vector will be directed relatively toward the area from which upright deflections are recorded. With practice, it is possible to identify the anterior or posterior direction of the vector with an accuracy of 10° to 15°.

FIGURE 4.26
An arrow is used to represent a vector. The three characteristics of a vector are (A) direction (inclination), (B) magnitude (size), and (C) sense (direction of the flow of energy from its origin). The arrowhead is used to indicate the sense of the electrical force.

FIGURE 4.27
The projection of the shadow of a pencil onto a screen is similar to the projection of an electrical force (represented by a vector) onto the lead axes. Note that when the pencil is perpendicular to the screen, it produces its smallest shadow, and when it is parallel with the screen, it produces its largest shadow. In this graphic metaphor, the screen is analogous to a lead axis and the pencil is analogous to an electrical force. (Adapted with permission; see Figure Credits.)

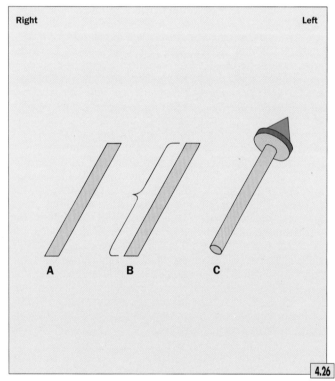

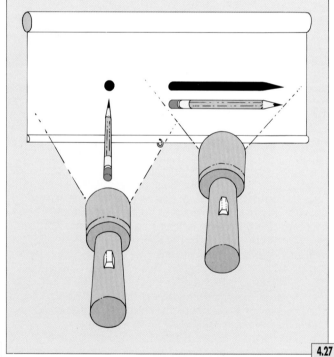

FIGURE 4.28
The extremity leads are used to determine the frontal plane projection of an electrical force (represented as a vector). **A.** The electrical force shown here is directed to the left. **B.** This figure illustrates how the vector shown in (A) will appear on the hexaxial lead system. Note that the vector is parallel to lead axis I, and will project its largest quantity onto lead axis I. The electrocardiograph machine writes an upright deflec-

tion because the electrical force represented as a vector is directed toward the positive pole of the machine. The vector is perpendicular to lead axis aVF, and will project its smallest quantity onto lead axis aVF. **C.** This figure illustrates the deflections the electrical force shown in (A) will produce in the extremity leads.

FIGURE 4.29
The spatial orientation of an electrical

force represented as a vector. **A.** This figure depicts an electrical force, represented as a vector, which is directed to the left, inferiorly, and posteriorly. **B.** This figure illustrates how the vector shown in (A) projects onto the lead axes of the hexaxial lead system. **C.** This figure shows the deflections that would be recorded on the extremity leads. **D.** This figure shows the deflections that would be recorded on the precordial lead axes.

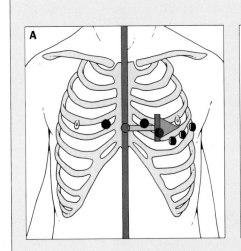 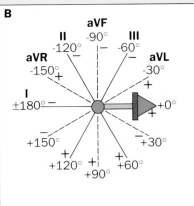 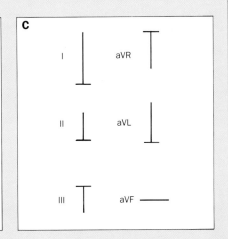

4.28

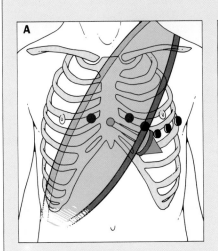 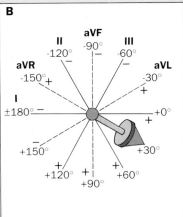 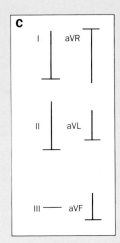 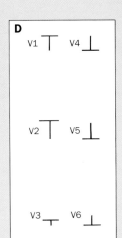

4.29

THE ART OF DIAGRAMMING VECTORS

Beginners may have some difficulty in visualizing the spatial orientation of the vectors that represent the electrical forces of the heart. The following points may assist them.

THE TILT OF THE ARROWHEAD

Arrows are used to represent vectors. The tilt of the arrowhead is used to indicate how far anteriorly or posteriorly a vector is directed. Figure 4.30 has been designed to illustrate how to visualize and diagram the arrowhead. The figure shows an arrow directed to the left, inferiorly and posteriorly. Note the plane perpendicular to the direction of the arrow. This plane extends in all directions to reach the surface of the chest, dividing the thorax into two areas. An exploring electrode will record a positive deflection from the left side of the chest and a negative deflection from the right side. An electrode will record zero potential when it records from the edge of the plane.

The plane that is perpendicular to the vector is called the *zero potential plane*. The line on the chest that is produced by extending the zero potential plane to the surface is called the *transitional pathway* (Fig. 4.30). A deflection recorded from the edge of the plane is called transitional because it is located between the negative and positive areas of the electrical field. *The base of the arrowhead is oriented so as to be parallel with the zero potential plane, and the rim of the arrowhead represents the transitional pathway.* In other words, the orientations of the base of the arrowhead and its rim are used to represent the zero potential plane and the transitional pathway, respectively.

THE FIRST AND SECOND GLANCE

Figure 4.31 illustrates the "first and second glance" approach to determining the direction of a vector. The reader should study the illustration and its legend. This is how the frontal plane direction of a vector can be adjusted to be within 5° of accuracy.

Figures 4.32A, B, and C illustrate the first and second glance approach to the anterior-posterior rotation of the vector. The reader should study the illustration and the legend. This is how the spatial direction of a vector can be adjusted to be within 10° to 15° of accuracy.

THE NEED FOR ADDITIONAL PRECORDIAL ELECTRODE POSITIONS

Suppose the precordial lead electrodes reveal only negative or positive deflections, and that no separation between negative and positive deflections can be identified. This rarely occurs when the frontal plane projection of the vector is located between 0° and +90°. It may occur, however, when the frontal plane direction of the vector is somewhere between 0° and -90°, or between +90° and ±180°. This is illustrated in Figure 4.33. Note in Figure 4.33A that it is impossible to compute the anterior or posterior direction of the vector because all of the precordial electrodes record negative deflections. In Figure 4.33B, an exploring electrode placed superior to position V2 records an isoelectric deflection, and having identified this, it is possible to determine that the vector is directed about 20° to 30° posteriorly. Note in Figure 4.33C that it is impossible to compute the anterior or posterior direction of the vector because all of the precordial electrodes record positive deflections. In Figure 4.33D, an exploring electrode

placed superior to position V2 records an isoelectric deflection. This makes it possible to determine that the vector is directed 20° to 30° anteriorly.

AREA VERSUS AMPLITUDE

The purpose of this short section is to point out an error that is commonly committed when the direction of a mean vector is computed. It was not necessary to consider this point when we were dealing with a single hypothetical electrical force represented by a single vector. However, when one is considering an entire electrocardiographic deflection produced by an infinite number of electrical forces generated in a sequential manner during a finite period, it is useful to treat them by adding them together to create a mean force that is represented as a mean vector. The beginner is likely to use the amplitute of an electrocardiographic deflection to determine the direction of a mean vector. This approach is incorrect. It is necessary to estimate the area enclosed within the lines of a deflection in order to determine the direction of a mean vector. This is illustrated in Figure 4.34. This concept holds for all elements of the electrocardiogram, such as the mean P wave, the first and second halves of the P wave, the QRS complex, the initial 0.04-second portion of the QRS complex, the terminal 0.04-second portion of the QRS complex, the ST segment deflection, and the T wave.

THREE ELECTRICAL FORCES

Thus far we have discussed a single electrical force represented as a vector. We have shown how a single vector would be projected on the extremity and precordial lead axes. As we work our way toward the analysis of the electrocardiogram itself, it is useful to study the projection of three vectors onto the lead axis system. This is illustrated in Figures 4.35A, B, and C. The three vectors labeled 1, 2, and 3 do not occur simultanteously. Vector 1 is generated at 0.01 to 0.02 second, vector 2 at 0.02 to 0.05 second, and vector 3 at 0.05 to 0.08 second.

The projections of these vectors on lead 1 is shown in Figure 4.35A. Their projections on the precordial leads V1 and V6 are shown in Figures 4.35B and C.

THE COMPLETE ELECTROCARDIOGRAM

Initially, a single vector was used to illustrate an electrical force of the heart. Then, three vectors were used to illustrate three electrical forces of the heart. These simple hypothetical illustrations were used because it is easier to visualize them and to use them to teach a number of basic principles that must be understood in order to understand, analyze and interpret the more complex deflections and the significance of the different waves of the electrocardiogram.

A complete electrocardiogram is generated by an infinite number of electrical forces. Some of these occur simultaneously, while others are generated at one point in time only to be followed by others which are followed by still others until the electrical cycle is complete. These electrical forces, acting in sequence, create the P loop, the QRS loop, and the ST-T loop. These loops are projected on to the lead axes to create the deflections seen in the electrocardiogram. It is then possible to determine the mean P vector, mean QRS vector, mean initial 0.04-second QRS vector, mean terminal 0.04-second QRS vector, QRS loop, mean ST vector, and mean T vector. All of these will be discussed in Chapter 5.

FIGURE 4.30
The importance of the base and rim of the arrowhead. **A.** A vector directed to the left, inferiorly, and posteriorly. **B.** The vector is shown inside the thorax in an effort to demonstrate the meaning of the parts of the arrowhead. The plane that is perpendicular to the vector extends to intersect the surface of the body. This plane is colored light blue and is called the *zero potential plane.* It divides the chest into areas of electrical negativity and positivity. The pathway on the surface of the chest produced by the edge of the zero potential plane is colored dark gray. It is called the *transitional pathway* because it is located between the negative and positive areas of the chest. A tracing recorded from the transitional pathway will register a zero deflection, and one recorded from the left lower side will register a positive deflection. An electrocardiogram recorded from the right upper side of the chest will record a negative deflection.

The base of the arrowhead identifies the inclination of the zero potential plane. It is colored light blue. The rim of the arrowhead represents the transitional pathway. In other words, the rim of the arrowhead, which is colored dark gray, is the displaced transitional pathway. Just as Bayley changed Einthoven's triangle to the triaxial system, the plane of the base of the arrowhead here represents the zero potential plane and the rim represents the transitional pathway

FIGURE 4.31
Refining the frontal plane direction of an electrical force (represented as a vector). **A.** "Electrocardiographic" deflections shown in the extremity leads. **B.** At first glance, the vector is drawn perpendicular to lead axis I because the smallest deflection is in lead I. **C.** On second glance, it is observed that the deflection, though small, is actually negative in lead I. Accordingly, the direction of the vector is adjusted to record a small negative quantity onto lead axis I.

FIGURE 4.32
Refining the spatial orientation of an electrical force represented as a vector. **A.** Suppose the "electrocardiogram" appears as shown here. **B.** The frontal plane projection of the electrical force represented as a vector is perpendicular to lead axis aVF, and records its small- est deflection on that axis. The largest deflection is in lead axis I, and the force records its largest deflection on that lead axis. Accordingly, the vector is drawn as shown. It is directed to the left because the electrical force producing it is directed toward the positive pole of the electrocardiograph machine. At first glance, the observer might notice that the electrical force records a negative deflection in lead axes V1 and V2, and a positive deflection in lead axes V4, V5, and V6. As a result of this first glance, the electrical force would be depicted as being posteriorly directed, so that the transitional pathway passes through lead axis V3. **C.** The second glance at the deflection shown in (A) reveals that there is, in reality, a small positive deflection in lead axis V3. This would require that the spatial orientation of the electrical force be modified slightly. The transitional pathway is adjusted so that lead axis V3 records a small positive deflection. At first glance, the electrical forces were shown to be directed 40° posteriorly. A second glance leads to a more accurate determination. The force is directed 35° rather than 40° posteriorly.

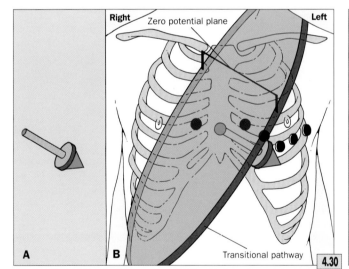

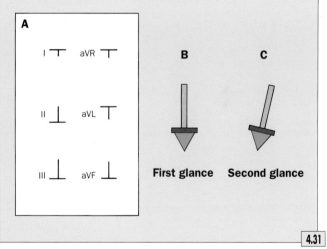

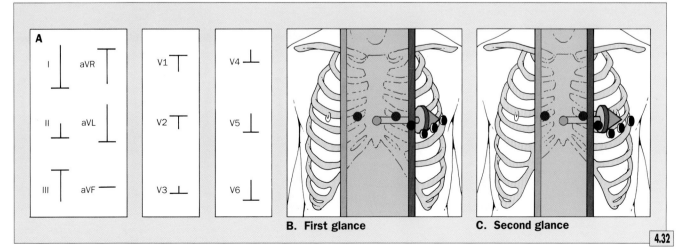

FIGURE 4.33

In certain cases, additional sampling sites are needed. **A.** This figure shows a vector directed far to the left. A negative deflection is recorded at six precordial electrode positions. **B.** It appears logical to explore the upper part of the chest with the exploring electrode in quest of a transitional deflection that is located between the negative and positive electrical fields. Such a deflection is found in this case a few centimeters above electrode position V2. **C.** This figure shows a vector directed far to the right. A positive deflection is recorded at all electrode positions. **D.** It appears logical to check for a transitional deflection between the positive and negative electrical fields. Such a deflection is found in this case a few centimeters above electrode position V2.

FIGURE 4.34

The area contained within an electrocardiographic deflection is used to calculate the direction of a mean vector. The figure illustrates this point. The sum of the positive area contained within the complex above the line, and the negative area contained within the complex below the line equals a negative quantity. The beginner is often misled by the height of the initial deflection, and makes an error by considering the total complex to be positive when it is, in fact, negative.

FIGURE 4.35

The shape of the QRS complex. **A.** This figure illustrates the fact that the heart generates more than one single force. The figure shows three vectors. Actually, the heart generates an infinite number of electrical forces that can be represented by vectors. In this illustration, Vector 1 is generated at 0.01 to 0.02 second, Vector 2 is generated at 0.02 to 0.05 second, and Vector 3 is generated at 0.05 to 0.08 second. The entire process is over at 0.08 second. This figure also shows how the three vectors would project onto the axis of lead I. **B.** This figure shows how the three vectors would project onto the lead axis of V1. **C.** The three vectors projected onto the lead axis of V6.

Prior to this figure, the illustrations have, for the most part, shown that the heart generates a simple electrical force represented as a single line in the electrocardiogram. This figure shows three electrical forces, represented as vectors, occurring in a time sequence, and thus explains the contour of an electrocardiographic deflection.

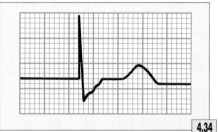

4.34

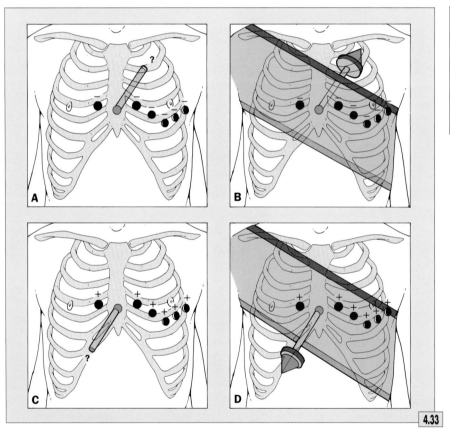

4.33

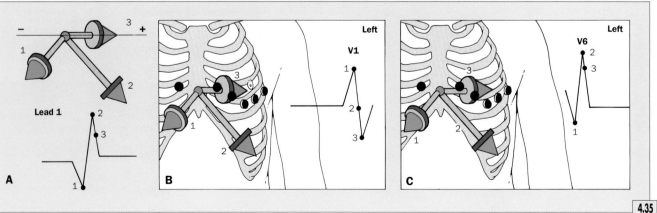

4.35

OTHER METHODS OF RECORDING

VECTORCARDIOGRAPHY

Vectorcardiography was popular in the 1960s (21). The oscilloscopic recording of electrical forces is more precise, but the technique did not produce sufficient additional information over conventional electrocardiographic recordings to replace the latter. Then, too, when electrocardiograms are interpreted using vector concepts, much of the information found in vectorcardiograms can be identified in linear electrocardiograms. A vectorcardiogram is shown in Figure 4.36 (21).

BODY-SURFACE MAPPING

Body-surface mapping utilizes numerous precordial electrode positions. The technology of body-surface mapping has improved to the degree that the application of the electrodes is relatively simple, but the technique has not added sufficient information to justify it as a replacement for the conventional method of electrocardiographic recording (22). As time passes, however, body-surface mapping may eventually come to replace conventional electrocardiographic techniques. An example of body-surface mapping published by Dr. L. E. Widman and his colleagues is shown in Figure 4.37.

An editorial on the current status of body-surface electrocardiographic mapping by Dr. David M. Mirvis is pertinent to this discussion (23). He constructed a table (Table 4.1) which compares body-surface mapping with conventional electrocardiography and vectorcardiography. The following passage is from the editorial and is reproduced with permission from the publisher and Dr. Mirvis (23):

> This brief review clearly supports the current clinical utility of body surface electrocardiographic mapping. However, widespread or even limited clinical implementation beyond the research laboratory has not occurred. Acceptance by cardiologists and, indeed, by "nonmapping" electrophysiologists has been limited.
>
> Several reasons for this disappointment may be identified. First, there is a general sense that electrocardiography—in all of its forms—has a limited role in cardiac diagnosis. The common notion is that other noninvasive procedures, such as echocardiography and radionuclide imaging, provide more useful clinical information.
>
> It is true that certain imaging techniques do provide better anatomic resolution than does electrocardiography. Electrocardiography as currently implemented, however, can be performed repeatedly in any office by personnel with little technical training in a totally non-invasive manner at a relatively low cost. In addition, identification of subjects at risk of sudden cardiac death—an electrophysiologic phenomenon—may best be approached by electrophysiologic rather than anatomic techniques.
>
> Second, there is a perception that body surface mapping entails prohibitive technical complexity. Problems generated by use of hundreds of torso electrodes and expensive and complex custom-designed computer systems have been largely obviated by development of accurate lead subsets that require as few as 24 electrodes and high-power but inexpensive microcomputer-based data acquisition systems. Turn-key systems similar to those widely marketed for routine electrocardiographic processing should be relatively simple to develop.
>
> A third major problem is the use of a new display format. The isopotential surface map does not at all resemble the scalar waveform. Diagnostic criteria are totally different and presently involve spatial rather than amplitude criteria. Many features are qualitative and not readily amenable to computerized interpretations. For such formats to become accepted by the general cardiologic public will require a major retraining that few may be willing to undertake, especially given the perception of limited value of the electrocardiogram. It may be—and it may be best that complex, surface mapping electrocardiography will become a specialized, hospital-based department similar to that for isotope imaging or invasive electrophysiologic procedures rather than a general technique to be applied routinely and a skill expected of all internists and cardiologists. Expanded use of numerical and statistical techniques will also facilitate automated, objective diagnoses.
>
> Thus, solutions—or at least approaches to solutions to many of the problems that hamper broader acceptance of surface mapping as a clinically valuable technique do exist. This is especially true of the technical complexities that plagued early applications. Once these and related issues are resolved, body surface electrocardiographic mapping should proceed to serve the cardiologic public with its demonstrated worth (23).

SIGNAL AVERAGING

Signal averaging is a technique for detecting electrical potentials occurring after the QRS complex. This electrical activity is not detected by the ordinary electrocardiograph machine. The after-potential correlates with ventricular arrhythmias. This technique will be discussed in Chapters 5 and 6 (24).

FIGURE 4.36

Normal electrocardiogram and vectorcardiogram from a 28-year-old male. The initial forces are almost directly anterior and do not produce Q waves in leads I, II or III. In this and subsequent examples, tracings of the QRS loop of the vectorcardiogram are seen to the right, each plane being identified as F (frontal), T (transverse), and S (left sagittal). The interruptions are spaced at 0.01-second intervals The horizontal plane, which is referred to as the transverse plane in this book, has been reoriented with the author's permission so that the viewer can imagine that he or she is viewing the transverse loop from a position at the feet of a patient in the supine position. (Reproduced with permission; see Figure Credits.)

FIGURE 4.37

Illustration of the advances that have been made in body-surface potential mapping (BSPM). This technique may well be used routinely in the future. The BSPM shown is of a 40-year-old normal Caucasian male. The recording was made from 180 electrodes placed on the anterior and posterior surfaces of the chest. A special vest is used for the recording. Vertically and on the viewer's right is the color scale for the six maps. A potential of 0 (zero) is displayed as black. Increasing positive potentials are on the upper scale, in this case up to 3,000 μV. Increasing negative potentials are on the lower side, in this case up to 3,000 μV. Increasing positive voltages would be shown by varying shades of yellow to orange to pink to lavender, and increasing negative voltages, by varying shades of green to blue (in this figure, increasing and decreasing voltages appear as different shades of gray). Each map is divided into four sections, with the clavicle located superiorly and the waist just above the navel, inferiorly. Vertical lines separate the maps into four sections. The three vertical lines, viewed from the viewer's left to right, are the sternum, left midaxillary line, and spine. The lateral margin on each side is the right midaxillary line. Therefore, the first two of the four sections are the anterior chest, and the next two are the posterior chest, or, in order from the viewer's left to right, the right anterior chest, left anterior chest, left posterior chest, and right posterior chest. This methodology allows the viewer to interpret the map as in a living subject, with the anterior chest facing the viewer. The illustration shows the electrical potential on the chest wall at 0.036 to 0.046 second of the QRS complex (see the marker in the center of the QRS wave in the lower portion of the illustration). (Reproduced with permission; see Figure Credits.)

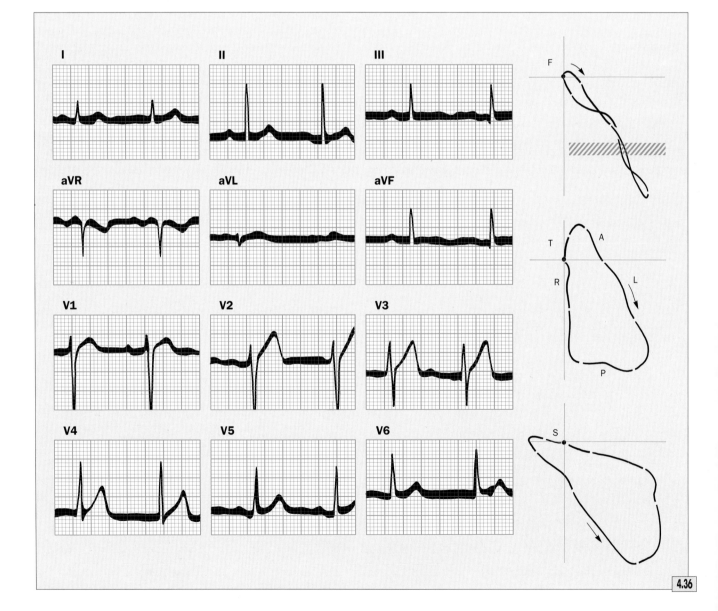

4.36

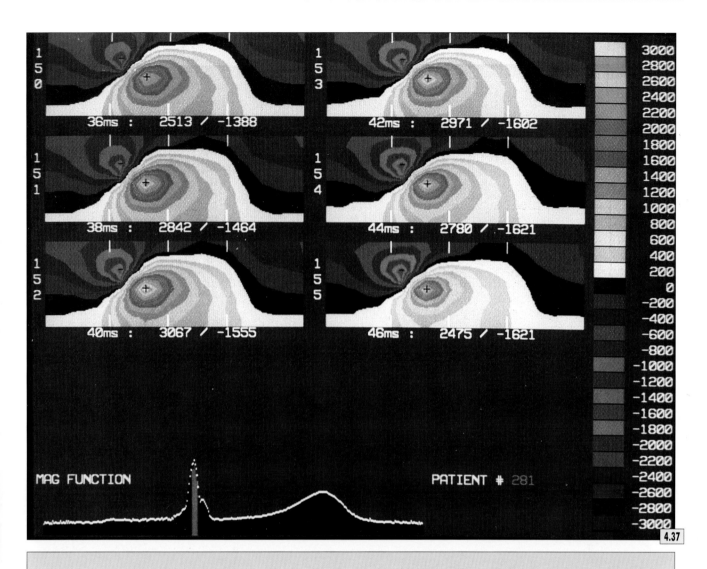

4.37

TABLE 4.1 COMPARISON OF BODY-SURFACE MAPPING AND OTHER ELECTROCARDIOGRAPHIC METHODS

BODY SURFACE MAPPING	STANDARD ELECTROCARDIOGRAPHY	VECTORCARDIOGRAPHY
1. Sensitive to regional cardiac events.	1. Limited sensitivity to regional cardiac events.	1. Not sensitive to regional cardiac events.
2. Widespread, direct torso sampling.	2. Limited precordial sampling; use of remote-field leads.	2. Conceptualizes all forces into three vectoral terms.
3. Emphasis on spatial features of cardiac direction field.	3. Emphasis on intensity of ECG forces.	3. Emphasis on intensity of forces.
4. Permits evaluation of cardiac equivaent generator models.	4. Does not permit model evaluation.	4. Assumes a fixed location, single dipole model.

Reproduced with permission from the American Heart Association and the author; see Figure Credits.

THE IMPERFECTIONS OF THE VECTOR METHOD OF ANALYSIS

I wish to emphasize the imperfections of the method of electrocardiographic interpretation described here. At the outset, however, it should be stated that there is no perfect method of electrocardiographic interpretation. I believe, despite its imperfections, that knowledge of the gross anatomy of the heart and thorax, the anatomy of the conduction system, the electromotive forces produced by the myocytes of the atria and ventricles, the propagation of electrical forces to the body surface, vector concepts, the characterization of electrical forces as vectors, normal cardiac vectors, and abnormal cardiac vectors will assist the clinician in the interpretation of electrocardiograms. Such a system is built on basic principles that, imperfect as they are, assist in understanding the cardiac condition responsible for a particular electrocardiographic abnormality, and makes the memorization of an infinite number of electrocardiographic patterns unnecessary. The vector method assists clinicians in interpreting electrocardiograms they have not seen (or memorized) before. It also enables clinicians to learn more electrocardiography as they correlate electrocardiographic abnormalities with the other clinical data they have collected from their patients.

Some imperfections of the method are that the electrical field is treated as if it originated from a single dipole, which is not correct; Einthoven's triangle is not an electrically perfect equilateral triangle, but is assumed to be so in this book. The central terminal is not electrically zero, and the augmented extremity leads are not perfect unipolar leads. The precordial electrodes are influenced by their nearness to the heart. The zero potential plane and transitional pathway are not straight, as shown in the illustrations, but are undulating and irregular. The direct writing electrographic machine does not inscribe a perfect recording.

In addition to the above, in an effort to teach, I have taken advantage of the known facts and used diagrams as graphic metaphors. An example of this is the hypothetical cell shown in Chapter 3. The depolarization and repolarization processes in this hypothetical cell and in the ventricles are largely based on theoretical considerations. The diagrams used to illustrate these and the phenomena discussed in subsequent chapters should be considered as graphic descriptions. I especially call attention to the use of the diagrams representing the chest. Whereas the same diagram is used throughout the book, the reader should recognize that a single diagram cannot represent the shapes of all chests. Consequently, I do not wish to imply that what is written here describes the situation as it exists in nature; I can say, as a clinician, that the method assists me in solving clinical problems. Perhaps as time passes, the imperfections will be eliminated.

REFERENCES

1. Flint A: *A Practical Treatise on the Diagnosis, Pathology, and Treatment of Diseases of the Heart.* Philadelphia, Blanchard and Lea, 1859, p 15.
2. Anderson RH, Ho SY, Becker AE: The clinical anatomy of the cardiac conduction system. In Rowland DJ (ed): *Recent Advances in Cardiology,* No. 9. Edinburgh, Churchill Livingstone, 1984.
3. Becker AE: Relation between structure and function of the sinus node. General comments. In Bonke FIM (ed): *The Sinus Node, Structure, Function and Clinical Relevance.* The Hague, Martinus Nijhoff, 1978, p 212.
4. Anderson RH, Ho SY, Smith A, Becker AE: The internodal atrial myocardium. *Anat Rec* 1981;201:75.
5. Becker AE: Personal letter, May 20, 1988.
6. Bachmann J: The inter-auricular time interval. *Am J Physiol* 1916;41:309.
7. James TN: The connecting pathways between the sinus node and the A-V node and between the right and the left atrium in the human heart. *Am Heart J* 1963;66:498.
8. Durrer D, Van Dam RT, Freud GE, et al: Total excitation of the isolated human heart. *Circulation* 1970;41:899.
9. Anderson RH, Becker AE, Brechenmacher C, et al: The human atrioventricular junctional area. *Eur J Cardiol* 1975;3:11.
10. Tawara S: Das reizleitungssystem des saugetierherzens. Jena, Gustav Fischer, 1906.
11. Lewis T, Rothschild MA: The excitatory process in the dog's heart. Part II. The ventricles. *Philos Trans R Soc Lond* (Biol) 1915;206:181.
12. Katz LN, Hellerstein HK: Electrocardiography. In Fishman AP, Richards DW (eds): *Circulation of the Blood: Men and Ideas.* New York, Oxford University Press, 1964, pp 265-351.
13. Lewis T: *Clinical Electrocardiography,* Ed 4. London, Shaw & Sons, 1928, p 6.
14. Einthoven W, Fahr G, de Waart A: On the direction and manifest size of the variations of potential in the human heart and on the influence of the position of the heart on the form of the electrocardiogram. HE Hoff, P Sekel (trans). *Am Heart J* 1950;40:163.
15. Bayley R: *Electrocardiographic Analysis,* Vol. 1, *Biophysical Principles.* New York, Paul Hoeber, 1958 p 41.
16. Wilson FN, Johnston FD, MacLeod AG, Barker PS: Electrocardiograms that represent potential variations of single electrode. *Am Heart J* 1934;9:477.
17. Goldberger E: Simple indifferent, electrocardiographic electrode of zero potential and a technique of obtaining augmented, unipolar, extremity leads. *Am Heart J* 1942; 23:483.
18. Burger HC, Van Milaan JB: Heart-vector and leads. *Br Heart J* 1946;8:157.
19. Grant RP, Estes EH Jr: *Spatial Vector Electrocardiography.* New York, Blakiston, 1951.
20. Hurst JW, Woodson GC Jr: *Atlas of Spatial Vector Electrocardiography.* New York, Blakiston, 1952.
21. Estes EH Jr: Electrocardiography and vectorcardiography. In Hurst JW, Logue RB (eds): *The Heart,* Ed 1 New York, McGraw-Hill, 1964, p 130.
22. Widman LE, Liebman J, Thomas C, et al: Electrocardiographic body surface potential maps of the QRS and T of normal young men. Qualitative description and selected quantification. *J Electrocardiol* 1988; 21:121.
23. Mirvis DM (editorial): Current status of body surface electrocardiographic mapping. *Circulation* 1987;75:684.
24. Winters SL, Stewart D, Gomes JA: Signal averaging of the surface QRS complex predicts inducibility of ventricular tachycardia in patients with syncope of unknown origin: A prospective study. *J Am Coll Cardiol* 1987;10:775.

FIGURE CREDITS

Table 4.1 From Mirvis DM: Current status of body surface electrocardiographic mapping (editorial). *Circulation* , 1987; 75:684.

Figure 4.2 Diagrams and legends from Flint A: *A Practical Treatise on the Diagnosis, Pathology, and Treatment of Diseases of the Heart.* Philadelphia, Blanchard and Lea, 1859, p 15. Book reprinted by The Cardiac Classics of Cardiology Library, Birmingham, Alabama.

Figure 4.8 Modified from James TN: The connecting pathways between the sinus node and the A-V node and between the right and the left atria in the human heart. *Am Heart J* 1963; 66:489.

Figure 4.15 From Lewis T: *Clinical Electrocardiography,* Ed 4. London, Shaw & Sons, 1928, p 6.

Figure 4.22 From Graybiel A, White PD: *Electrocardiography in Practice.* W.B. Saunders Company, Philadelphia, 1946, p 23.

Figure 4.27 From Hurst JW, Woodson GC Jr: *Atlas of Spatial Electrocardiography.* New York, Blakiston, 1952, p 18.

Figure 4.36 From Estes EH: Electrocardiography and vectorcardiography. In Hurst JW, Logue RB (eds): *The Heart,* Ed 1. New York, McGraw-Hill, 1966.

Figure 4.37 The figure and a portion of the text and legend are from Widman LE, Liebman J, Thomas C, et al: Electrocardiographic body surface potential maps of the QRS and T of normal young men. Qualitative description and selected quantifications. *J Electrocardiol* 1988; 21(2):121.

PART

Mechanisms Responsible for the Normal and Abnormal Electrocardiogram

TWO

CHAPTER FIVE

The Normal Ventricular Electrocardiogram

THE CLINICIAN'S USE OF THE ELECTROCARDIOGRAM

Clinicians are primarily concerned with the diagnosis of disease and the treatment and care of patients. They are the physicians on the firing line of medical decision-making and the delivery of patient care. Clinicians commonly use the electrocardiogram to assist them in the diagnosis of heart disease, and this book is herefore written for them.

THE CORRELATION OF DATA[1]

In order to screen individual patients for the presence of heart disease, clinicians utilize data collected from: (1) the medical history, (2) the physical examination, (3) the chest x-ray film, and (4) the electrocardiogram (1). Data collected by each of these methods of examination should be *correlated* with the data collected by the other three. Clinicians who learn to correlate data gathered by these four methods are able to diagnose their patients' problems with greater precision than clinicians who partition such data into separate mental compartments. Those who correlate such data can select the next diagnostic procedure, if needed, with greater precision, and can gradually learn more about the clinical significance of an abnormality they find.

THE COMPLETE CARDIAC DIAGNOSIS

Excellent clinicians will construct differential diagnoses for every abnormality they identify in the history, physical examination, chest x-ray film, and electrocardiogram of a given patient. The same diagnostic possibility may be considered to explain the abnormalities found by several of the methods of examination, and a diagnostic thread can be established (Table 5.1). When this skill is fully developed, the clinician can make use of small diagnostic clues that are of little predictive value individually, but are highly predictive if taken together. This approach permits the clinician to construct a more accurate appraisal of the patient.

A *complete cardiac diagnosis*(2)* is established when the clinician can identify the following five elements of a patient's problem: (1) the etiology, (2) altered anatomy, (3) physiologic derangement, (4) cardiac status, and (5) the prognosis for the patient(2). The correlation of data collected by the four methods of routine examination described earlier permits the clinician either to establish these five components or to state the patient's problem more precisely. If a complete cardiac diagnosis cannot be established, but the patient's problem has been stated as precisely as possible, the clinician must then judge whether the problem *should* be solved. If the decision is made to solve the problem, it is essential to create a differential diagnosis that encompasses all of the diagnostic possibilities. The clinician should then order the diagnostic procedure that yields a result having an acceptable predictive value; if this is not done, various procedures may be used improperly, and decision-making deteriorates.

THE PREVALENCE OF ELECTROCARDIOGRAPHIC ABNORMALITIES

The likelihood that an electrocardiogram will be abnormal in a given patient is predetermined by the type and severity of the patient's disease process. This limitation also applies to the history, physical examination, and chest x-ray film. The electrocardiogram may occasionally yield the only clue to the diagnosis, or it may yield a diagnostic clue that, when added to other clues, supports a particular diagnosis. There was a time in medical history when excellent physicians believed that 70 percent of the diagnostic information about a patient was detected in the patient's history, 20 percent was found on the physical examination, and 10 percent was obtained from laboratory testing (including the electrocardiogram and chest x-ray film). As stated above, the diagnostic method that yields the most information is predetermined by the patient's disease. For example, the history is obviously all-important if the patient has angina pectoris, because the other methods of routine examination may yield no abnormalities. The physical examination, on the other hand, may be the only method of routine examination that identifies the diastolic murmur of slight aortic valve regurgitation. Similarly, annular calcification of the mitral valve may be detected only on the chest x-ray film, and pre-excitation of the ventricles may be detected only on the electrocardiogram. To repeat, however, four, three, or two of the methods may uncover diagnostic clues suggesting the same abnormality. It is my view that during recent years, both major and minor electrocardiographic abnormalities have not been used advantageously for the purpose of reaching a diagnosis.

THE NORMAL RANGE

An analysis of the biologic phenomena exhibited by a large group of normal individuals teaches us to appreciate the wide range of what is defined as normal(3). It also teaches us that the range of normal biologic data overlaps the range of abnormal biologic data. Accordingly, clinicians realize that one of their most difficult tasks is to differentiate *normal from abnormal.*

Figure 5.1 illustrates that although the height of different persons varies, most normal adults will be between x and y feet tall. There will be people, however, whose height is at either end of the bell-shaped curve, and for whom it will be impossible to state whether they are of normal height.

Figure 5.1 can also be used to illustrate that the size of the QRS complex recorded from a large number of normal adults will vary. It further illustrates that when the size of the QRS complex is located at either end of the bell-shaped curve, it will be impossible to state whether it is normal or abnormal.

Simply stated, the normal range of biologic data overlaps the abnormal range. This basic truth must always be remembered when electrocardiograms are interpreted.

PROBABILITIES

BAYES' THEOREM

Reverend Bayes pointed the way that eventually enabled the medical profession to formulate the following principle: *the predictive value of a test result for a particular disease is predetermined by the prevalence of the disease in the population being tested.* This basic principle is one of the few principles of medicine that must be understood and applied to all test results, including electrocardiographic abnormalities.

The following example shows the value of Bayes' theorem: suppose a clinician identifies an abnormal ST segment displacement in the exercise electrocardiogram of a 65-year-old man with vague chest discomfort. The probability (predictive value) that the ST segment displacement is due to myocardial ischemia is about 80 percent. On the other hand, suppose a clinician observes an ST segment displacement in the exercise electrocardiogram of a 40-year-old woman with similar chest discomfort. In this setting, the predictive value of the ST segment displacement for myocardial ischemia is about 50

---

*The emphasis here is on the words *complete* (2) and *cardiac.* These words are very different from electrocardiographic diagnoses, of which there are three types (see later discussion).

Note: As stated in several places in this book, the model presented here is a clinically useful approximation of the real situation within the heart. At times, the explanation moves beyond the known evidence. When this occurs, every effort has been made to extend the facts in a logical manner.

percent. The predictive value of the displacement differs in these two examples because 40-year-old women, as a population, have less coronary disease than 65-year-old men, and are therefore less likely to have myocardial ischemia.

PREDICTIVE VALUE

The predictive value for criteria used to determine the presence or absence of an abnormality can be calculated from the following formulae(3):

$$\text{Predictive value of a positive result} = \frac{\text{Number of true positives}}{\text{Number of true positives} + \text{number of false positives}}$$

$$\text{Predictive value of a negative result} = \frac{\text{Number of true negatives}}{\text{Number of true negatives} + \text{number of false negatives}}$$

SENSITIVITY

The sensitivity of a test result indicates the ability of the test to identify the individuals in a population who are truly positive for the test parameter(3). A sensitivity of 100 percent indicates that whenever the criteria for a positive test are fulfilled, the patient actually has the disease responsible for the abnormal measurement.

Suppose the clinician's criteria for left ventricular hypertrophy are defined as a QRS complex duration of 0.10 second or less, a mean QRS vector that is directed to the left and posteriorly, and a QRS voltage (amplitude) that occupies the entire vertical width of the electrocardiographic paper. Each time these criteria are met the clinician can state with certainty that left ventricular hypertrophy is present, because the sensitivity of the criteria is 100 percent. As the voltage demand is decreased, however, there comes a point at which the sensitivity of the criteria falls to 75 or 50 percent. In these ranges, the criteria for left ventricular hypertrophy begin to overlap the criteria for the size of a normal QRS complex.

The sensitivity of the criteria used to identify an abnormality can be calculated from the following formula (3):

$$\text{Sensitivity} = \frac{\text{Number of true positives}}{\text{Number of true positives} + \text{number of false negatives}}$$

There are two points to make here:

First, it is not wise to use criteria so rigid that left ventricular hypertrophy is not considered unless the QRS voltage (amplitude) meets a certain specified number of millivolts (see later discussion). Whenever the criteria for a QRS complex of normal size overlap the criteria for left ventricular hypertrophy in the electrocardiogram, the clinician should use other methods to examine the patient and determine whether there is any other clue to the presence of left ventricular hypertrophy. In other words, the clinician's strategy should be: (1) to consider the QRS complex as normal and, if no clue to left ventricular hypertrophy is found by other methods of examination, to accept the QRS as being normal or (2) to consider the QRS complex as abnormal due to left ventricular hypertrophy and, if a clue to left ventricular hypertrophy is found, to accept the QRS as being abnormal.

Second, the measurement of a phenomenon may have been on the low side of the normal range at one point in time and may be on the high side at a later point. The *change* of the two measurements, however, may be abnormal even though both are within the normal range. For example, the heart size may appear at the upper limit of normal on the chest x-ray film but may have been at the lower

limit of normal size in an earlier x-ray. The change in heart size, if artifacts can be excluded, may represent a significant and abnormal change. The same possibility exists for any of the deflections of the electrocardiogram.

SPECIFICITY

The problem with using a test that has 100 percent sensitivity is that it may fail to identify those individuals who have the abnormality for which the test is being done but in whom the test results do not meet the criteria for being abnormal. To determine this, we must know the specificity of the test. Specificity implies that the test can identify normal values and separate them from the abnormal values (3).

The formula for calculating the specificity of the criteria used to identify an abnormality is as follows:

$$\text{Specificity} = \frac{\text{Number of true negatives}}{\text{Number of true negatives} + \text{number of false negatives}}$$

In other words, the *sensitivity* of the criteria for a test result indicates the percentage of abnormals in a population that can be identified by the test while the *specificity* of the criteria of a test result indicates the percentage of normals in a population that can be identified by the test.

PROBLEMS WITH PROBABILITY DETERMINATIONS IN ELECTROCARDIOGRAPHY

While the criteria used to determine the probable presence of an electrocardiographic abnormality have improved over the years, much additional research is needed to enhance the accuracy of electrocardiographic interpretation. When possible, the predictive value of test results will be given whenever abnormalities are discussed later in this book. However, when scientific data are unavailable, an observational opinion may be given, based on the experience of the author.

Clinicians who correlate the data collected from the history, physical examination, electrocardiogram, and chest x-ray film are not bound to rigid electrocardiographic criteria because they can use minor clues as hints to diagnostic possibilities to be pursued using other methods of examination.

THE MEANING OF AN ABNORMALITY

It must be remembered that additional data are usually needed to determine the exact clinical importance of an abnormality. For example, many noses are anatomically unusual, but nevertheless serve their purpose of being able to smell with equal ability. So it is with certain electrocardiographic abnormalities; they may have no significance as far as the patient's future is concerned. Frank Wilson, the pioneer of electrocardiography in the United States, made the following statement about the faulty interpretation of an electrocardiogram. His admonition is reproduced here with the permission of the publisher (4).

In the last two decades there has been a tremendous growth of interest in electrocardiographic diagnosis and in the number and variety of electrocardiographs in use. In 1914, there was only one instrument of this kind in the state of Michigan, and this was not in operation; there were probably no more than a dozen electrocardiographs in the whole of the United States. Now there is one or more in almost every village of any size, and there are comparatively few people who are not in greater danger of having their peace and happiness destroyed by an erroneous diagnosis of cardiac abnormality based on a faulty interpretation of an electrocardiogram, than of being injured or killed by an atomic bomb.

THREE TYPES OF ELECTROCARDIOGRAPHIC DIFFERENTIAL DIAGNOSES

As discussed earlier, electrocardiographic abnormalities, or their absence, should be considered as the clinician reviews data collected from the history, physical examination, and chest x-ray film of a patient. The purpose of this discussion is to point out the three types of electrocardiographic differential diagnoses:

• The first type occurs as part of the analysis of an electrocardiogram, and involves identifying the *electrical abnormalities* that are present. Suppose, for example, that the QRS voltage (amplitude) is large. The differential diagnosis at this stage of analysis should be to consider whether the large QRS voltage is due to a thin chest wall, over-standardization of the recording, or disease of the heart.

• The second type occurs when an *electrophysiologic or anatomic designation* is assigned to the electrical abnormality detected in Step 1 above. For example, suppose it is determined that the large QRS voltage is due to heart disease; the question now is whether it is due to left ventricular hypertrophy or a left ventricular conduction defect. Let us assume that the clinician, using acceptable criteria, determines that it is due to left ventricular hypertrophy.

• The third type of differential diagnosis involves the assignment of *etiologic possibilities* to explain the abnormality found as a result of Steps 1 and 2. To continue with our example, it is wise to consider the following causes of left ventricular hypertrophy: systemic hypertension, aortic valve stenosis, aortic regurgitation, mitral regurgitation, or idiopathic hypertrophy. Having considered these, it is then wise to search for subtle clues in the ST and T waves that might reveal whether the condition is due to systolic or diastolic pressure overload of the left ventricle. Suppose that electrocardiographic abnormalities characteristic of diastolic overload of the left ventricle are discovered. This will enable the clinician to narrow the list of possible causes of the QRS voltage enlargement (increased amplitude) to aortic or mitral valve regurgitation, or congenital heart disease such as an interventricular septal defect or patent ductus arteriosus. Although only one example—that of a large QRS complex—has been used in this discussion, the same logic applies to all aspects of the electrocardiographic interpretation.

FIGURE 5.1

The distribution of the normal range of biologic phenomena. The range of normal human height or the size of the normal QRS complex in the electrocardiogram can be viewed in this manner. The majority of measurements will fall in the center of the figure, while low and high measurements will be at the extreme ends of the curve (x and y). It is easy to see that abnormal measurements would overlap the extreme ends of the normal range. (Reproduced with permission of the publisher and author; see Figure Credits.)

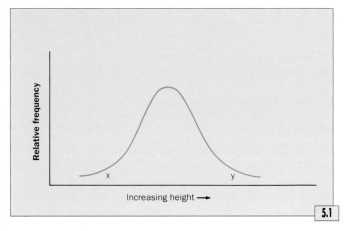

5.1

TABLE 5.1 DIFFERENTIAL DIAGNOSES AND THE CORRELATION OF DATA

	HISTORY	PHYSICAL EXAMINATION	ELECTROCARDIOGRAM	CHEST X-RAY FILM
ABNORMALITIES	• Syncope • Angina pectoris	• Harsh systolic murmur in 2nd right intercostal space • Decreased intensity of aortic valve closure sound • Sustained apical impulse	• Left ventricular hypertrophy with mean QRS vector directed at +65° and 45° posteriorly	• Calcification of aortic valve; slight left ventricular hypertrophy
DIFFERENTIAL DIAGNOSIS	• Aortic valve stenosis • Idiopathic hypertrophic subaortic stenosis • Coronary atherosclerosis plus arrhythmias	• Aortic valve stenosis	• Aortic valve stenosis • Systemic hypertension • Aortic regurgitation • Mitral regurgitation • Hypertrophic cardiomyopathy	• Aortic valve stenosis

Note: Aortic valve stenosis is mentioned in the differential diagnosis that follows the completion of each method of examination. This makes the diagnosis virtually certain. Although the diagnosis was made by radiography and physical examination, it was also listed in the differential diagnosis created after analyzing the history and electrocardiogram. The diagnostic possibilities considered to explain the abnormalities found in the history and electrocardiogram stimulate the thoughtful clinician to search for the proper clues on physical examination, and to look specifically for aortic valve calcification on the chest x-ray film. The cause of angina pectoris cannot be determined by the methods of examination listed here. Cardiac catheterization, including coronary arteriography, will be needed to determine the exact severity of an aortic valve stenosis and the presence of obstructive coronary atherosclerosis. Because syncope and left ventricular hypertrophy occurring in a patient with aortic valve stenosis signify severe aortic obstruction, cardiac catheterization is actually performed to determine the presence or absence of atherosclerotic coronary disease.

THE APPROACH TO THE ELECTROCARDIOGRAM

The electrocardiogram (see Fig. 5.2) should be approached in an orderly manner. The clinician should:

- Determine the heart rate and rhythm.
- Measure the duration of the P wave, PR interval, QRS complex, and QT interval.
- Measure the magnitude of the P waves; establish the direction of the mean P wave vector (Pm); identify the direction of the mean vectors representing the first half (P1) and last half (P2) of the P wave; identify the duration and depth of the second half of the P wave in lead V1; and determine the characteristics of the T wave of the P wave (Ta wave).
- Identify the duration of the QRS complex; measure its amplitude; establish the direction of the mean QRS vector; visualize the QRS loop; determine the directions of the mean initial and mean terminal 0.04–second QRS vectors and their relationship to the mean QRS vector; measure the intrinsicoid deflection of the QRS complex; and establish the relationship of the mean T vector to the mean QRS vector.
- Measure the duration of the T waves; identify their magnitude; establish the direction of the mean T vector and its relationship to the mean QRS vector (the QRS-T angle); calculate the ventricular gradient when possible.
- Measure the duration of the ST segment; determine the magnitude and direction of the vector representing it; establish the relationship of the mean ST vector to the mean T vector and mean QRS vector.
- Study the U wave.

THE NORMAL ELECTROCARDIOGRAM

THE HEART RATE AND RHYTHM

This book is concerned with the interpretation of the ventricular electrocardiogram rather than with the heart's rate and rhythm. However, the heart rate and rhythm can at times be used to assist in the interpretation of the ventricular electrocardiogram. For example, suppose the QRS complexes are abnormally small. The presence of sinus tachycardia in the electrocardiogram would support the interpretation of pericardial effusion or dilated cardiomyopathy of some type, whereas the presence of sinus bradycardia would support the presence of myxedema. As another example, suppose that an electrocardiogram shows a mean QRS vector that is directed vertically and slightly posteriorly, and that the P waves suggest a left atrial abnormality; the development of atrial fibrillation would support the diagnosis of mitral stenosis.

DETERMINATION OF THE HEART RATE AND RHYTHM: Normally, the heart of an adult is depolarized 60 to 90 times per minute. A depolarization rate lower than this is called *sinus bradycardia,* while one that is higher is called *sinus tachycardia.* The heart rate of the normal newborn is much higher than that of an adult.

The *heart rate* can be calculated by dividing the number of large squares, or fractions of large squares, separating two QRS complexes on the electrocardiograph paper into 300. When there is one large square (0.2 second) between two QRS complexes, the ventricular rate is 300 depolarizations per minute. When there are two large squares between two QRS complexes, the ventricular rate is 150 depolarizations per minute. Where there are three large squares, the ventricular rate is 100 depolarizations per minute. With experience, the clinician learns to estimate the rate of depolarization when portions of large squares are added to or subtracted from the large squares that are identified between the QRS complexes. For example, when two-and-one-half large squares are identified between the QRS complexes, the rate is about 120 depolarizations per minute. If more accuracy is needed, the R-R interval can be measured more precisely, and the rate of depolarization can then be determined by referring to tables constructed expressedly for this purpose (see Table 1 in the Appendix).

THE DURATION OF THE COMPLEXES AND INTERVALS

After determining the heart rate and rhythm, the clinician should measure the duration of the waves and intervals on the electrocardiogram. The waves and intervals, and the letters of the alphabet used to identify them, are illustrated in Figure 5.2.

THE P WAVE: The duration of the P wave is measured from the beginning of the P wave to the end. In normal adults, this period is usually less than 0.12 second; in neonates, it is less than 0.08 second. This is the time interval required for the wave of depolarization to spread through the atria and to reach the atrioventricular node.

THE PR INTERVAL: The PR interval represents the amount of time required for the depolarization process to spread from its origin in the sinus node, through the atria, to and through the atrioventricular node (where the impulses are delayed), down the bundle branches and their sub-branches (including the Purkinje fibers), and to the ventricular muscle. It is measured from the beginning of the P wave to the beginning of the QRS complex. In reality, this interval should be called the PQ interval, but convention holds that it is called the PR interval. When there is no Q wave, the measurement is made from the beginning of the P wave to the beginning of the R wave. The difference between the intervals as measured to the beginning of the Q wave, and as measured to the R wave, is usually about 0.02 second but may be as much as 0.04 second. The PR interval is less than 0.20 second in the normal adult and much less than this in normal children. The PR interval varies with the heart rate (see Table 2 in the Appendix).

THE DURATION OF THE QRS COMPLEX: The duration of the QRS complex represents the amount of time required for the depolarization of the ventricular musculature. It is measured from the beginning of the Q wave to the end of the S wave. In normal adults, the QRS duration is usually 0.10 second or less, and in children, it is usually less than 0.08 second.

THE DURATION OF THE ST SEGMENT: The duration of the ST segment represents the amount of time during which the ventricular musculature is depolarized. The depolarization process ends with the end of the QRS complex, and the repolarization begins with, or before, the beginning of the T wave. In some patients, the repolarization process begins during the ST segment (see later discussion). The ST segment duration is determined by measuring the interval of time from the end of the S wave to the beginning of the T wave. In practice, a prolonged ST segment is identified by detecting a prolonged QT interval while the duration of the T wave remains normal (see following discussion).

THE QT INTERVAL: The QT interval represents the amount of time required for depolarization of the ventricles, plus the amount of time during which the ventricles are excited (ST segment), plus the amount of time required for their repolarization (T wave). This interval represents the duration of electrical systole, which is different from the duration of mechanical systole (see later discussion). The QT interval is measured from the beginning of the Q wave of the QRS complex to the end of the T wave. The duration of the QT interval varies with age, gender, and heart rate. It should not exceed 0.40 second when the heart rate of an adult is 70 depolarizations per minute.

Refer to Table 1 in the Appendix in order to determine whether a QT interval is normal. When the interval is corrected for the heart rate, it is labeled as QTc for identification purposes.

A great deal of attention is currently being directed toward calculation of the corrected QT interval, since there is a known relationship between long intervals and ventricular arrhythmias. However, there are two problems with the measurement: (1) it is now recognized that interobserver variation in the measurement may be significant; and (2) Bazett's formula is often used by investigators to calculate the corrected QT interval (QTc), though it now appears that such a computation is not accurate when the heart rate is either slow or rapid. For example, ten formulae were recently tested by Puddu and colleagues(5), who concluded that Fridericia's equation was superior to Bazett's formula in middle-aged men. In practice, Bazett's formula is rarely used; the clinician simply refers to the tables shown in Table 1 in the Appendix.

THE DURATION OF THE T WAVE: The T wave is produced by the repolarization process. The duration of the T wave is measured from the beginning of the wave to the end. The repolarization process undoubtedly begins before the T wave and is sometimes quite visible as a displaced ST segment, which is referred to as "early repolarization." Although the duration of the normal T wave has been studied, and tables have been constructed using the data, the actual measurement is rarely performed in practice.

THE TQ INTERVAL: The TQ interval is measured from the end of the T wave to the beginning of the next Q wave. During this period the ventricles are polarized and waiting for the stimulation that initiates depolarization. This interval will be discussed in Chapter 6 in relation to epicardial injury.

THE U WAVE: The U wave can sometimes be seen following the T wave and preceding the P wave. Its origin and purpose are obscure, but it is probably due to the repolarization process.

THE P WAVE AND THE Ta WAVE

THE DEPLORIZATION OF THE ATRIA: The P wave is produced by the depolarization of the right and left atria. While there are "preferential electrical pathways" in the atria, none of the specialized cells are responsible only for conduction, as is the case in the ventricles. At this point, the reader should review this subject in Chapter 4.

The depolarization process does not appear to spread from the endocardium to the epicardium as it does in the ventricles; it spreads instead from the sinoatrial node in a laminar manner, through the atria, to the atrioventricular node and distant parts of the left atrium. An upright deflection is recorded when the depolarization process is directed toward the electrode attached to the positive pole of the electrocardiograph machine, and a negative deflection is recorded when this process spreads away from this electrode.

The characteristics of the depolarization process are controlled by the location, size, and thickness of the right and left atria, and the *preferential conduction*(6) system of the atria. The right atrium is located to the right and is anterior to the left atrium (see Fig. 4.6B). The left atrium is actually located posteriorly in the center of the chest, rather than on the left (see Fig. 4.6B). Exactly how much the thickness of the atria influences the magnitude of the P wave is unclear. P wave magnitude may, in fact, be determined more by overall atrial size than by wall thicknesses, but this has not been adequately studied. When the "preferential conduction pathways" in the atria are interrupted by various factors, the spread of electrical activity and the configuration of the P wave are both altered. It is highly likely that a prolonged P wave duration, notched and deformed P waves, and large P waves are due to an altered sequence of atrial depolarization. Recognizing this, I have, for the past 25 years, referred to abnormal P waves as indicators of right or left atrial abnormality rather than right or left hypertrophy or dilatation. To suggest that P wave abnormalities are due to one of the latter is to be more specific than our knowledge permits. An atrial abnormality may correlate with atrial hypertrophy or dilatation, but this is not the same as declaring that a P wave abnormality is caused by them.

The sinoatrial node (see Fig. 4.8) is located in the region of the right atrium where the latter joins the superior vena cava. This structure is located on the right, and is superior and slightly posterior to the remainder of the right atrium. Accordingly, the wave of depolarization spreads in a predominanty anterior direction through the right atrium, though it also moves posteriorly, inferiorly, and leftward on its way to the left atrium and atrioventricular node.

According to Dr. Lewis Katz, the wave of depolarization of the right atrium reaches the atrioventricular node at about the same time it reaches the left atrium(7). This is shown in a classic illustration created by Dr. Katz in 1941 (Fig. 5.3). The impulse is delayed by the atrioventricular node while left atrial depolarization continues. At this point, repolarization of the right atrium begins. The wave of depolarization then passes through the bundle of His, bundle branches, and Purkinje fibers, and into the ventricular septum and left and right ventricles, before the completion of left atrial repolarization. This is why it is reasonably accurate to consider the first half of the P wave (P1) as being due to right atrial depolarization and the second half of the P wave (P2) as being due to depolarization of the left atrium.

THE DURATION OF THE P WAVE: As stated earlier, the duration of the P wave in the normal adult is 0.12 second or less. It is less than 0.12 second in children and about 0.08 second or less in neonates.

THE AMPLITUDE OF THE P WAVES: The amplitude of the P waves of the normal adult is less than 2.5 mm in the extremity leads, and smaller than this in children. The amplitude of each half of the P wave is less than 1.5 mm in lead V1.

THE DIRECTION OF THE P VECTORS: The depolarization process of the atria of a normal adult, represented as a mean vector (Pm), is usually directed relatively parallel with lead axis II and either slightly anterior, parallel with, or slightly posterior to the frontal plane (Fig. 5.4A).

The analysis of P waves entails the creation of a mean vector that represents the first half of the P wave (P1, produced by depolarization of the right atrium) and one for the second half (P2, produced by depolarization of the left atrium)(8). In the normal adult, a mean vector representing the first half (P1) is directed more or less parallel with lead axis II, inferiorly, and parallel with or slightly anterior to the frontal plane (Fig. 5.4B). In the normal adult, the second half of the P wave (P2), represented as a mean vector, is directed inferiorly and more or less parallel with lead axis II. It is usually located to the left of P1 and is always slightly posterior to the frontal plane (Fig. 5.4B). The direction of the mean P vector (Pm) is the vector sum of P1 and P2.

SUMMARY OF CHARACTERISTICS OF Pm, P1, AND P2: *Normal right atrial depolarization produces a mean vector (P1) that is directed to the left, inferiorly, and parallel with or slightly anterior to the frontal plane. The duration of the P wave is less* than 0.12 second. The amplitude of the P wave is less than 2.5 mm in any lead. P1 is about the same size as P2 and is usually directed to the right of and slightly anterior to P2.

Normal left atrial depolarization produces a mean vector (P2) that is directed to the left, inferiorly, and parallel with or slightly posterior to the frontal plane. The duration of the P wave is less than 0.12 second, and its amplitude is less than 2.5 mm in any lead. P2 is about the same size as P1 and is usually directed to the left of and slightly posterior to P1. Morris and associates have emphasized the value of studying the P wave in lead V1 in order to identify the normality of P2(8). Jin and associates support their view (9). When the algebraic product achieved by multiplying the duration of P2, measured in seconds, by the amplitude of P2, measured in millimeters, is greater than -0.03 (mm-sec), it is considered abnormal, and signifies a left atrial abnormality (Fig. 5.5). A measurement of -0.03 mm-sec or less is considered normal. This technique enables one to make a refined judgment regarding the size and direction of P2. Morris and associates studied 100 normal subjects and 87 patients with aortic and mitral valve disease, and identified the normal and abnormal measurements shown in Table 5.2(8).

THE USE OF P WAVES IN THE INTERPRETATION OF THE QRS COMPLEX: Because this book deals primarily with the ventricular electrocardiogram, it is important to realize that the analysis of P waves may assist in the analysis of the QRS complexes and T waves. For example, the combination of a vertically-directed mean QRS vector and a left atrial P wave abnormality has a greater predictive value for mitral stenosis than does an isolated vertical mean QRS vector.

THE REPOLARIZATION OF THE ATRIA (THE Ta WAVE)

The repolarization of the atria begins in the area where depolarization was initiated. The electrocardiographic wave it produces is referred to as the Ta wave. Unlike the repolarization of the normal ventricles, this process in the atria seems to spread in the same direction as that of depolarization. The wave of repolarization produces a downward deflection when the process spreads toward an electrode that is attached to the positive pole of the electrocardiograph machine, and produces an upright deflection when it spreads away from such an electrode. This concept can be more easily understood when one studies the repolarization process in the hypothetical cell shown in Figures 3.3 and 3.4.

Theoretically, the repolarization wave of the atria (Ta) observed in the electrocardiogram is produced predominantly by repolarization of the left atrium. This is probably because the electrical forces created by depolarization of the left atrium dominate the electrical field during the repolarization of the right atrium. Accordingly, the wave produced by repolarization of the right atrium is obscured by that produced by depolarization of the left atrium. The Ta wave (Fig. 5.6) is not always detected, and when it is, it may not be seen in all leads. Accordingly, it is not possible to produce a mean vector that represents the electrical forces responsible for the Ta wave.

The Ta wave may be seen when the PR interval is long or when complete heart block is present, because these abnormalities increase the distance of the P wave from the QRS complex, making the Ta wave more easily visible. Ordinarily, however, the QRS complex masks the Ta wave. At times, especially when the PR interval is short, the Ta wave may be responsible for baseline depression following the J point of the QRS complex. This produces a displacement of the ST segment (Fig. 5.6).

It is interesting and valuable to study the illustration created by Katz (Fig. 5.3)(7). Note that repolarization of the left atrium is completed at about the same time as ventricular depolarization. Note, too, that repolarization of the right atrium is underway while depolarization of the left atrium continues.

More research is needed in order to understand the repolarization process of the atria. Practically, the study of the Ta wave is of limited value to the clinician, because it is usually not visible in all leads of the electrocardiogram.

FIGURE 5.2
The waves and intervals of the electrocardiogram. The PQRSTU complex on the left shows the waves and their identifying letters. The PQRSTU complex to the right shows the intervals and how to measure them.

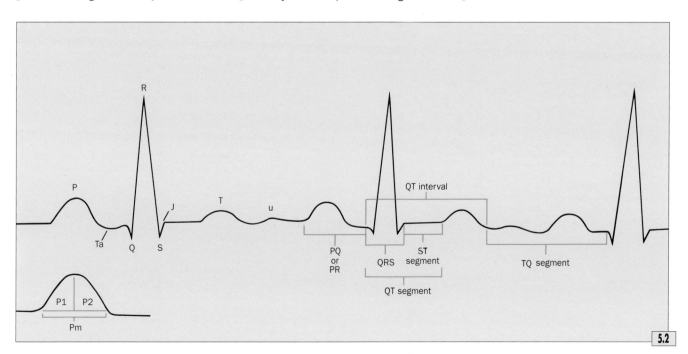

FIGURE 5.3
Depolarization and repolarization of the atria and ventricles, and their relationship to mechanical systole and diastole of the atria and ventricles. This figure was created by Dr. Louis Katz in 1941. Some of the details have undoubtedly changed since he conceived this illustration, but the concept still holds true today. In 1941, when Dr. Katz wrote this legend, the word *auricles* was used to identify atria.

Dr. Katz's legend is as follows:
A series of 32 diagrams to show the temporal correlation of electrical

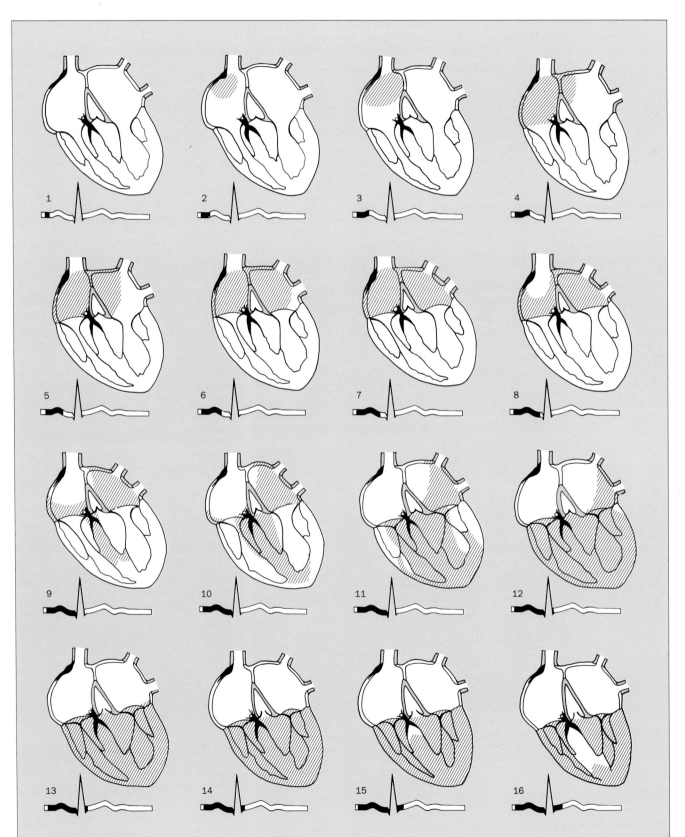

5.3

(Figure 5.3 continued.)
and mechanical events (above) with the electrocardiogram (below) in a human heart with a cycle of 0.76 second. The intervals between diagrams are 0.02 second apart except between 1 and 2, 6 and 7, 25 and 26, 26 and 27, 30 and 31, and 31 and 32, in which the interval is 0.04 second—this was necessary to permit the figure to be reproduced on a double page. The blacked out portion of the electrocardiogram shows how much of the record has been (Figure 5.3 continued on page 5.10.)

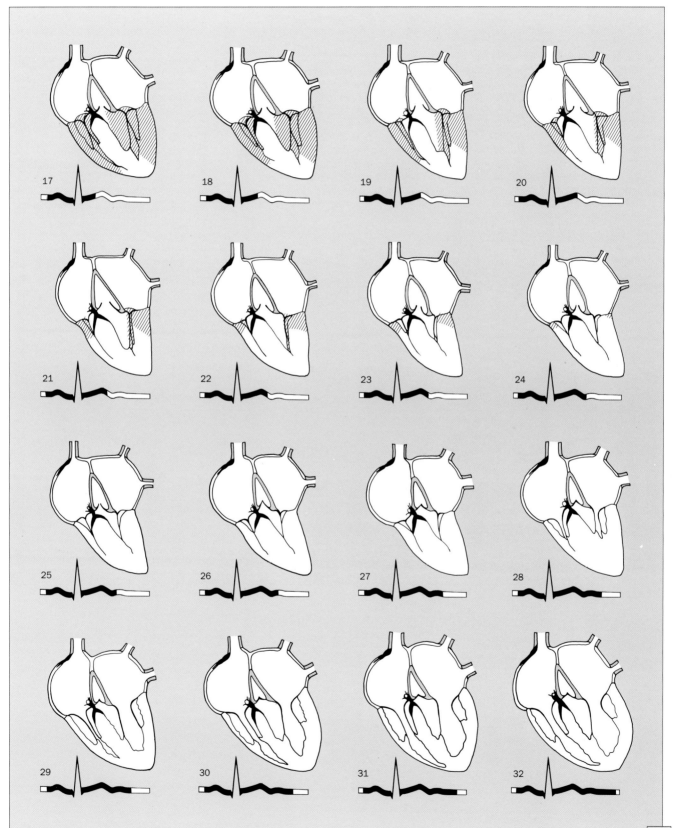

(Figure 5.3 continued.)
written up to the time represented by each diagram. For clarity, certain parts of the special conducting and nodal muscle systems have been omitted or altered in the diagrams. The location of the depolarized state in the heart is shown by cross-hatching and that of the polarized or repolarized stage by the absence of cross-hatching. The walls of the aorta and veins are stippled. The special muscular tissue, i.e., sinus and A-V nodes and the common bundle and its two branches are shown in black.

Attention should be paid to the changes in the size and shape of the cardiac chambers, aorta, superior vena cava, coronary sinus and the pulmonary veins, as well as to the changes in thickness of the walls of the auricles and ventricles and the opening and closing of the aortic and A-V valves in the successive diagrams. In constructing these charts they have been made as accurate as possible in the light of present knowledge. Note that the series starts at 1, with the heart in diastole, the A-V valves open, the semilunar valves closed and the impulse discharged in the sinus node still within the node. At 2, the impulse has begun to spread through the auricles. At 4, the auricles have begun to contract and cause A-V valves to close partially. At 7, stimulation of the auricles is completed. At 8, the repolarized state has begun to reappear in the auricles. At 9, the impulse has begun to spread in the ventricles. At 11 the A-V valves are closed as ventricular contraction begins. At 13, the ejection of the ventricles begins with the semilunar valves open, and stimulation of the ventricles is completed. At 14, repolarization in the auricles is completed. At 15, repolarization in the ventricles has begun. At 26, repolarization in the ventricles is completed, relaxation of the ventricles has begun, and the semilunar valves have closed. At 28, the A-V valves have again opened and filling of the ventricles has begun. At 32, the heart cycle is completed. (Reproduced with permission of the publisher; see Figure Credits).

FIGURE 5.4
The components of the P wave.
A. The mean P vector (Pm) is directed to the left, inferiorly and parallel with or slightly posterior to the frontal plane. The normal range for its frontal plane

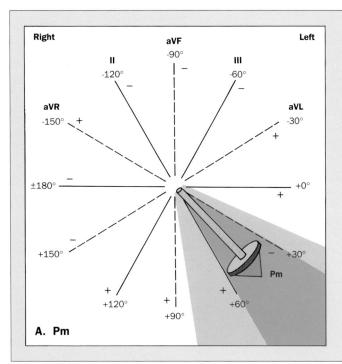

A. Pm

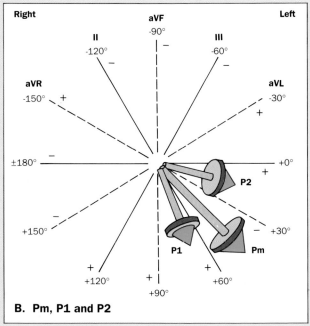

B. Pm, P1 and P2

5.4

(Figure 5.4 continued.) projection is shown in blue, with the darkest blue indicating its usual direction. **B.** The direction of the mean vectors produced by the first half of the P wave (P1), representing right atrial depolarization; the second half of the P wave (P2), representing left atrial depolarization; and their relationship to each other and to Pm.

FIGURE 5.5
The measurement of P2 in lead V1. Morris and associates reported the best method of analyzing the P wave for a left atrial abnormality (P2). When the amplitude of P2 is multiplied by its duration, the product is -0.03 mm-sec or less in normal adults(8).

FIGURE 5.6
Displacement of the PR interval and the ST segment by a prominent Ta wave. The displacement of the ST segment is more likely to occur when the PR interval is short.

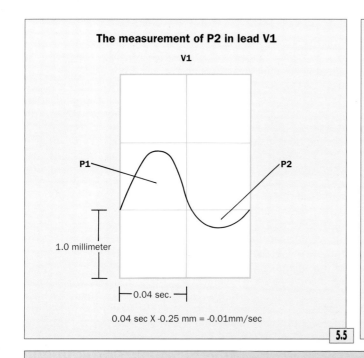

The measurement of P2 in lead V1

V1

P1   P2

1.0 millimeter

├─0.04 sec.─┤

0.04 sec X -0.25 mm = -0.01mm/sec

5.5

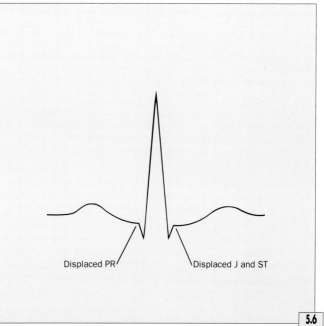

Displaced PR   Displaced J and ST

5.6

TABLE 5.2 P WAVE ANALYSIS IN LEAD V1

MEASURE	100 NORMAL SUBJECTS *	87 PATIENTS WITH AORTIC AND MITRAL DISEASE *
P initial duration (sec)	0.05±0.02	0.05±0.02
P initial amplitude (mm)	0.6±0.3	0.9±0.7
P initial vector (degrees)	55°±14°	50°±21°
P initial force (mm-sec)	0.03±0.02	0.05±0.04
P terminal duration (sec)	0.03±0.02	0.06±0.03
P terminal amplitude (mm)	-0.2±0.03	-1.2±0.8
P terminal vector (degrees)	+7°±12°	7°±15°
P terminal force (mm-sec)	0.01±0.01	0.08±0.06

*Mean ± 1 standard deviation.
Morris et al(8) concluded that the normal P terminal force in V1, caluclated by multiplying the last half of the P wave with the amplitude of the P wave, should be -0.03 mm-sec or less. (Reproduced with permission from the American Heart Association, Inc., and the author; see Figure Credits.)

THE QRS COMPLEX

THE DEPOLARIZATION OF THE VENTRICLES

The QRS complex is produced by depolarization of the ventricles of the heart. The various components of the QRS complex are shown in Figure 5.2. The magnitude, direction, and sense of the electrical forces of the ventricles, which can be represented by vectors, are determined by the location of the ventricles in the thorax, the thickness and integrity of the right and left ventricular walls, the ventricular conduction system, and the sensitivity of the electrocardiographic machine. It is important to recall that the action potential of the conduction tissue itself is not recorded in the surface electrocardiogram. The electrical impulse travels rapidly down the bundle of His, the right and left bundle branches, branches of the right bundle and the divisions of the left bundle, and the Purkinje system, to reach the working myocytes which actually produce the electrical forces responsible for the QRS complex seen in the electrocardiogram. The depolarization sequence of the ventricles has been studied for decades. I have accepted the work of Durrer and his colleagues(11), who, through a masterful experiment, accurately described this depolarization sequence. The diagram depicting ventricular depolarization shown in Figure 5.7 was created by Flowers and Horan(10), based on the works of Durrer and his colleagues.

Depolarization in the ventricles proceeds, for the most part, from the endocardium to the epicardium. This produces electrical forces that have the same direction as the wave of depolarization. The first portion of the heart to be depolarized is the left upper portion of the ventricular septum (Fig. 5.7). This is followed by the depolarization of the endocardial surfaces of the left and right ventricles. The electrical forces produced in the ventricles are almost perpendicular to the ventricular surface. The wall of the left ventricle is normally thicker than that of the right ventricle, and because of this, left ventricular electrical forces dominate the electrical field after right ventricular depolarization has been completed. The posterior-basilar portion of the left ventricle is the last part of the heart to depolarize. As stated earlier, it is the left ventricular conduction system that guides the depolarization sequence so that the process, when depicted as vectors, is directed to the left and posteriorly.

THE COMPONENTS OF THE QRS COMPLEX: The instantaneous electrical forces that produce the QRS complex influence each lead axis differently. These components are shown in Figure 5.2. The various waves are identified by letters of the alphabet. The letter Q is used to designate the downward deflection that is seen during the initial portion of the QRS complex. The letter R is used to designate the first upward deflection of the QRS complex. The letter S is used to designate the first downward deflection that projects below the baseline following the R wave. The second upright (positive) portion of the QRS complex is identified by the letter R'. The J point is located where the terminal portion of the QRS complex joins the ST segment.

THE DURATION OF THE QRS COMPLEX: The duration of the QRS complex in the normal adult is 0.06 to 0.10 second. In infants it may be as short as 0.045 second, and in older children it is as short as 0.09 second. When the QRS duration is greater than 0.10 second in adults, it is proper to consider the presence of some type of ventricular conduction defect.

AMPLITUDE OF THE MEAN QRS VECTOR: When the size of the QRS complex is evaluated, other variables must be considered in addition to ventricular hypertrophy. These include the thickness of the chest wall, the state of the pericardium and the pericardial space, the presence or absence of emphysema, and the standardization (calibration) of the electrocardiograph machine.

In the normal adult, the challenge is to determine when normal left ventricular preponderance ends and abnormal left ventricular hypertrophy begins. In the neonate and infant, one must determine when normal right ventricular preponderance ends and abnormal right ventricular hypertrophy begins.

THE UPPER LIMIT OF NORMAL QRS AMPLITUDE: Many electrocardiographic criteria have been created to indicate when normal left ventricular wall thickness ends and abnormal left hypertrophy begins (see Table 3 in the Appendix). However, none of the criteria are satisfactory(12,13). Romhilt and Estes created the criteria for left ventricular hypertrophy shown in Table 5.3, which are commonly used today(14). When the QRS amplitude is less than these values, it is believed to be normal. As emphasized earlier, however, the normal range is wide, and left ventricular hypertrophy may not be identified.

Recent emphasis has been on the use of the total 12-lead QRS amplitude to identify left ventricular hypertrophy. The method of measuring the QRS complex is shown in Figure 5.8. In recent autopsy studies of 30 subjects without cardiopulmonary disease, Odom and colleagues indicated that the normal range of the total QRS amplitude is 80 to 185 mm(15). As I have indicated earlier, I am opposed to the use of rigid criteria that claim to separate normal from abnormal, because such rigidity is against biologic principles, omits an understanding of the meaning of the normal range, and eliminates the variables that must be considered when a measurement is made. The sensitivity, specificity, and predictive value should be known for every biologic measurement. When the magnitude of the QRS complex appears to be large but could be normal, it is proper to search more carefully, using other methods of examination, to determine whether the left ventricle is actually enlarged or is of normal size.

While the mean QRS vector is directed to the right and anteriorly in the normal infant, such an orientation in an adult with a normal QRS complex duration is always abnormal. In such cases, the R wave is prominent in lead V1 and is usually larger than the Q wave or S wave; this is why the mean QRS vector is directed anteriorly. This abnormality may be caused by right ventricular hypertrophy or a right ventricular conduction abnormality, and since only the direction of the mean QRS vector is abnormal, a precise measurement of the size of the mean QRS complex is not needed. When the R wave is large in lead V1 but the S wave is larger, and the mean QRS vector is directed to the right, there may be right ventricular hypertrophy even if the mean QRS vector is not anteriorly directed. But what is an abnormally large R wave in V1? Table 3 in the appendix gives an estimate of the normal range of the R wave in various leads, including V1. When a large R wave is identified in lead V1 and the mean QRS vector is directed to the right, it is proper to consider the presence of right ventricular hypertrophy or a right ventricular conduction abnormality, regardless of the amplitude of the QRS complex.

Right ventricular hypertrophy may also be present when the mean QRS vector is directed vertically and posteriorly. This is especially likely when there is acquired right ventricular hypertrophy. This is discussed in Chapter 6.

THE LOWER LIMIT OF NORMAL FOR QRS AMPLITUDE: The normal QRS voltage may be as small as 5 to 7 mm, but it is usually greater than this (see Table 3 in the Appendix). It is generally accepted that the QRS voltage is definitely small when it measures 4 mm or less in all the extremity leads. When this occurs, it is wise to consider certain abnormalities (to be discussed in Chapter 6) as possible causes. According to Odom et al, the lower limit of normal for the total QRS amplitude is 80 mm(15).

I believe the clinician should consider the possible presence of certain cardiac conditions that are associated with a low QRS voltage when the QRS voltage is 5 mm or even 7 mm in the extremity leads and appears smaller than average in the precordial leads. Although the predictive value of the measurement is less than when the QRS voltage is 3 mm, the same diagnostic possibilities still exist. Under such circumstances, the clinician should use another method of examination to determine whether an abnormality is present (this is discussed further in Chapter 6).

THE DIRECTION OF THE MEAN QRS VECTOR: The thickness of the the right ventricle of the normal newborn is equal to or greater than that of the left ventricle. Accordingly, the mean QRS vector of the newborn will be directed to the right and anteriorly. The direction of the mean QRS vector of the normal infant is as shown in Figure 5.9A. Attention should be directed to the different shape of the thorax and the thickness of the chest wall of the newborn and infant, as compared with that of the adult. This produces a difference in the alignment of the chest electrodes in the infant. The heart of the infant is near the surface of the chest wall, making it impossible to apply rigid rules regarding the amplitude of the normal QRS complexes. The transitional pathway of electrical forces on the chest is wider in the infant than in the adult, and wide-swinging complexes are often recorded from a wider area of the chest than in the adult.

Figure 5.9A illustrates the difference in the direction of the normal mean QRS vector in a newborn, an infant, and an adolescent. Note in Figure 5.9B, that the mean QRS vector of the normal adult may be directed vertically, in the intermediate zone, or horizontally. The differences in direction of the mean QRS vector of the newborn, infant, adolescent, and adult arise as the myocardium of the normal left ventricle of the neonate gradually becomes thicker than that of the normal right ventricle, and as the chest contour changes from that of the infant to that of the adult.

The range of the frontal plane projection of the normal mean QRS vector in adults is from about +110° to -30°; it is usually directed somewhere between 0° to +60°. Factors other than the direction of the mean QRS vector itself must be considered in determining the normality of the measurement. For example, a mean QRS vector that is directed +90°, inferiorly, and slightly posteriorly in an adult should be correlated with the body build. A normal tall, thin person is more likely to have a mean QRS vector oriented in this direction than is a normal broad-chested, short person. Therefore, when a mean QRS vector is oriented vertically at +90° in a broad-chested short person, it is more likely to be abnormal than when it is oriented in this direction in a tall, thin person. On the other hand, a mean QRS vector that is directed -20° to the left is more likely to be abnormal in a tall, thin person than in a short, broad-chested individual.

TO SUMMARIZE: the mean QRS vector is directed to the right and anteriorly in the normal newborn (Fig. 5.9A). In the normal infant, it is directed vertically and parallel with the frontal plane (Fig. 5.9A). In the normal adolescent, it is directed vertically at about 45° and slightly posteriorly (Fig. 5.9A). The mean QRS vector in the normal adult is directed from -30° to +110° and moderately posteriorly (Fig. 5.9B). Horan and colleagues, using the precordial mapping technique, determined that the transitional pathway for the mean QRS vector of the normal adult passes near electrode position V3(17), indicating that the mean QRS vector of the normal adult is usually directed about 40° to 45° posteriorly.

A common error is to use the amplitude of the QRS complexes to compute the direction of the mean QRS vector. It is absolutely necessary to understand that the word *mean* implies that all of the electrical forces generated during the entire QRS cycle must be added together algebraically and assumed to be acting at one point in time. Accordingly, the area under the Q wave must be added to the area under the R wave, with this sum then added to the area under the S wave. For example, when the area of the Q wave and the area of the S wave are negative, their combined area is subtracted from the positive area under the R wave. In summary, it is necessary to use the resultant area contained within the QRS complex, rather than using the QRS amplitude alone to compute the direction of a vector. When there is no conduction abnormality, the amplitude of the QRS is used to determine the thickness of the left ventricle.

THE INSTANTANEOUS ELECTRICAL FORCES AND THE QRS LOOP: The QRS complex is produced by an infinite number of electrical forces. These forces, referred to as instantaneous forces (Fig. 5.10A) are generated in a sequence that is determined by the arrival time of the electrical stimulus at a particular portion of the myocardium. All of the instantaneous forces can be considered to originate at a central point in the chest, as in Figure 5.10B. (As stated in previous chapters, this concept is not precise, but is sufficiently accurate to be used for clinical purposes.) When a line is drawn to connect the termini of all of the instantaneous forces, the resulting figure is called the QRS loop (Fig. 5.10C). The frontal plane view of the QRS loop is shown in Figure 5.10C, and a transverse view is shown in Figure 5.10D. The QRS loop represents the sequence of depolarization of the ventricles, which in the normal adult heart takes about 0.08 to 0.10 second. It is the projection of the QRS loop onto the 12 lead axes that produces the various contours of the QRS complex.

The normal vertical QRS loop of an adult is inscribed in a clockwise manner. The normal intermediate QRS loop may be inscribed in a clockwise or counterclockwise manner. The normal horizontal QRS loop should be inscribed in a counterclockwise manner.

The normal range for the direction of the instantaneous QRS vectors is illustrated in Figure 5.11(18).

THE INITIAL AND TERMINAL MEAN INSTANTANEOUS QRS VECTORS: The frontal plane directions of the 0.01, 0.02, 0.04, 0.06, and 0.08–second instantaneous QRS vectors are shown in Figure 5.11(18).

The normal *initial* mean 0.04–second QRS vector should have a special relationship to the mean QRS vector. Recall that the area enclosed during the initial 0.04–second portion of the QRS complex is used to make the calculation. When the mean QRS vector is vertical, the initial mean 0.04–second vector should be to its left (Fig. 5.12A). This is because the normal vertical QRS loop is written in a clockwise direction. The normal initial mean 0.04–second QRS vector can be directed to the left or right of an intermediately directed mean QRS vector (Fig. 5.12B), because the normal intermediate QRS loop can be written in a clockwise or counterclockwise direction. When the mean QRS vector is directed leftward (horizontally), the initial mean 0.04–second QRS vector should be inferior to it (Fig. 5.12C). This is because the normal horizontal QRS loop of a normal adult is written in a counterclockwise direction. The *initial* mean 0.04–second QRS vector should *always* be anterior to the mean QRS vector in the normal subject. The direction of the normal initial mean 0.04–second QRS vector should be within 30 to 45° of the mean QRS vector.

The normal *terminal* mean 0.04–second QRS vector is usually located to the right of a vertical mean QRS vector (Fig. 5.13A). It may be on either side of an intermediate mean QRS vector (Fig. 5.13B), but it is usually superior to a leftward mean QRS vector (Fig. 5.13C). The mean terminal 0.04–second QRS vector is located posterior to, and within 30 to 45° of the mean QRS vector.

THE INTRINSICOID DEFLECTION: When an electrode is placed directly on the ventricular epicardium, it records the intrinsic QRS deflection, defined as the amount of time required for the depolarization process to spread from the endocardium to the epicardium. It is identified by measuring the time that elapses between the beginning of the QRS complex and the zenith of the R wave. The term intrinsicoid deflection is used when the same measurement is made with the electrode placed on the precordium; normally, it takes 0.04 second or less. Obviously, this time interval may be increased when the heart muscle is thicker than normal (see Chapter 6).

TABLE 5.3 POINT-SCORE SYSTEM OF ROMHILT AND ESTES FOR LEFT VENTRICULAR HYPERTROPHY [a]

FEATURE	POINTS	FEATURE	POINTS
Amplitude [b]	3	Left axis deviation [e]	2
ST-T segment abnormality [c]		QRS duration [f]	1
• Without digitalis	3	Intrinsicoid deflection [g]	1
• With digitalis	(1)	Maximum total (excluding	
Left atrial involvement [d]	3	ST-T segment abnormality with digitalis)	13

[a] A score of five points is read as left ventricular hypertrophy; a score of four points is read as probable left ventricular hypertrophy.
[b] Positive if any one of the following are present: (1) largest R or S wave in the limb leads ≥ 20mm, (2) S wave in V1 or V2 ≥ 30 mm, (3) R wave in V5 or V6 ≥ 30 mm.
[c] Positive if typical ST-T pattern of left ventricular strain is present (ST-T segment vector shifted in direction opposite mean QRS vector).
[d] Positive if the terminal negativity of the P wave in V1 is 1 mm or more in depth, with a duration of 0.04 sec or more.
[e] Positive if left axis deviation of -30° or more is present in frontal plane.
[f] Positive if QRS duration is ≥ 0.09 sec.
[g] Positive if intrinsicoid deflection in V5 or V6 is ≥ 0.05 sec.
(Reproduced with permission of the publisher and author; see Figure Credits.)

FIGURE 5.7

Sequence of ventricular depolarization as illustrated by Flowers and Horan (10). The illustration was modified from Durrer (11). The first portion of the ventricles to undergo depolarization is the left upper portion of the ventricular septum, followed by the left and right endocardial surfaces. The posterior basilar portion of the left ventricle is the last portion to depolarize. The light blue color indicates the portions of the heart that are depolarized last. Abnormalities of the myocardium in this area would not alter the initial portion of the QRS complex; any change would occur in the mid and late portions of the complex. Each number represents the milliseconds between the onset of the QRS complex, and the activation of the corresponding portion of the myocardium. (Reproduced with permission of the publisher; see Figure Credits.)

FIGURE 5.8

Measurement of the total QRS amplitude. This method of measurement was devised by Siegel and Roberts. (Reproduced with permission of the publisher and author; see Figure Credits.)

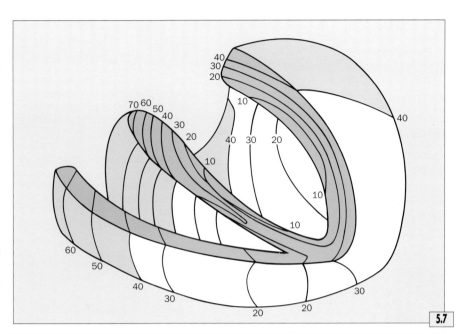

5.7

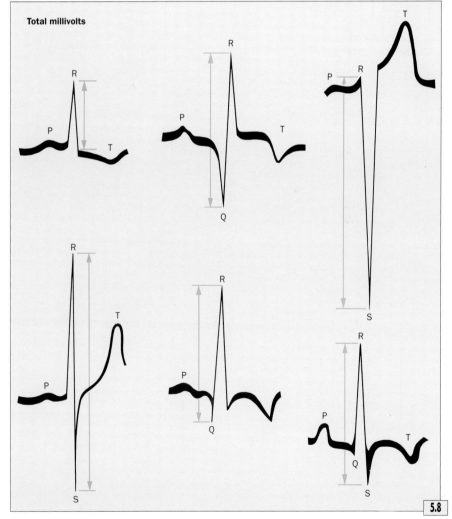

5.8

FIGURE 5.9
Direction of the mean QRS vector. **A**. The direction of the mean QRS vector in the normal newborn, normal infant, and normal adolescent. **B**. The mean QRS vector of the normal adult may be directed vertically, intermediately, or horizontally. This is partially determined by the body build of the patient. Note that the mean QRS vector gradually shifts from its rightward and anterior direction in the normal newborn, where it represents normal left ventricular preponderance. Note also that the mean T vector is to the left of the vertical mean QRS vector, to the left or right of the mean intermedi-

ate QRS vector, and inferior to a horizontal mean QRS vector. It is always anterior to the mean QRS vector in the normal adult. The QRS-T angle is about 45°. **C**. This diagram illustrates the direction of the mean QRS vector at different ages. (Part **C** reproduced with permission of the publisher and author; see Figure Credits.)

FIGURE 5.10
The QRS complex in the normal adult.
The QRS complex is created by an infinite number of instantaneous QRS forces; five of these forces are shown in **A**. Although it is not strictly accurate,

one can assume that the instantaneous forces originate in the center of the heart and chest, as shown in **B**. A line drawn around the termini of the instantaneous QRS forces creates the QRS loop. The direction of the sequence of depolarization is indicated by the small arrow. The frontal plane projection of the QRS loop is shown in **C**. The transverse view is shown in **D**.

FIGURE 5.11
The direction of the normal mean QRS vector and the instantaneous QRS vectors in the normal adult. **A**. The direction of
(Figure 5.11 continued on page 5.18.)

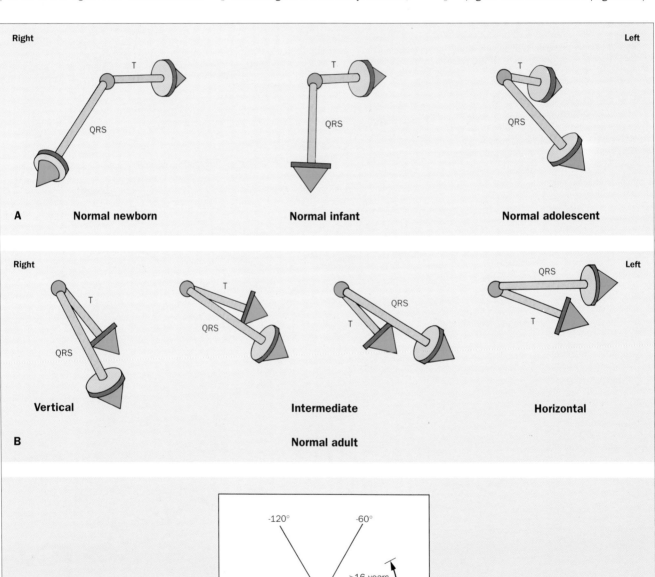

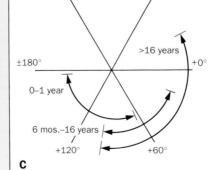

Direction of mean QRS vector at different ages

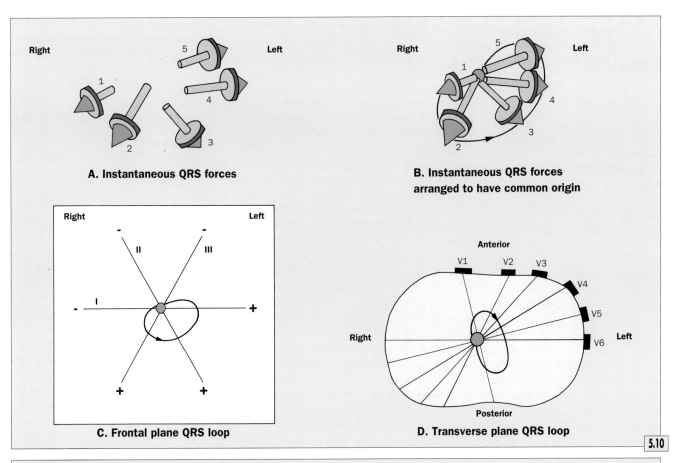

A. Instantaneous QRS forces

B. Instantaneous QRS forces arranged to have common origin

C. Frontal plane QRS loop

D. Transverse plane QRS loop

5.10

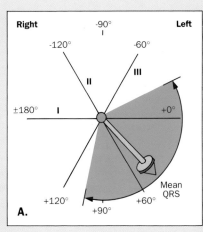

A.

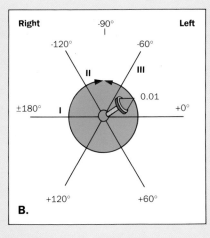

B.

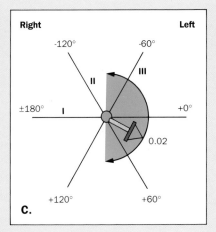

C.

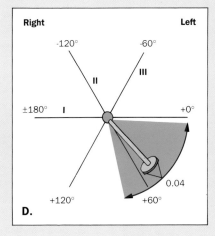

D.

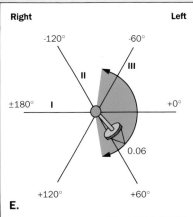

E.

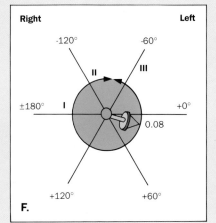

F.

5.11

(Figure 5.11 continued.)
the mean QRS vector in the normal adult. **B.** The direction of the instantaneous vector at 0.01 second. **C.** The direction of the instantaneous vector at 0.02 second. **D.** The direction of the instantaneous vector at 0.04 second. **E.** The direction of the instantaneous vector at 0.06 second. **F.** The direction of the instantaneous vector at 0.08 second.

The blue area indicates the normal range for the instantaneous vector. The vector itself depicts the average or usual direction. (Modified and reproduced with permission from the publisher; see Figure Credits.)

FIGURE 5.12

The relationship of the initial mean 0.04–second QRS vector to the mean QRS vector. **A.** The initial mean 0.04–second QRS vector should normally be directed to the left of, and anterior to a vertical mean QRS vector. **B.** The initial mean 0.04–second QRS vector is normally directed to either side of, and anterior to an intermediate mean QRS vector. **C.** The initial mean 0.04–second QRS vector should normally be directed inferior and anterior to a horizontal mean QRS vector. Note that the angle between the mean QRS vector and initial mean 0.04–second QRS in the adult is normally about 30° to 45°.

FIGURE 5.13

The relationship of the terminal mean 0.04–second QRS vector to the mean QRS vector. **A.** The normal terminal mean 0.04–second QRS vector is usually directed to the right of, and posterior to a vertical mean QRS vector. **B.** The normal terminal mean 0.04–second QRS vector can be directed on either side of, and posterior to an intermediate mean QRS vector. **C.** The normal terminal mean 0.04–second QRS vector is usually directed superior and posterior to a horizontal mean QRS. Note that the angle between the mean QRS vector and terminal 0.04–second QRS vector is normally about 30° to 45°.

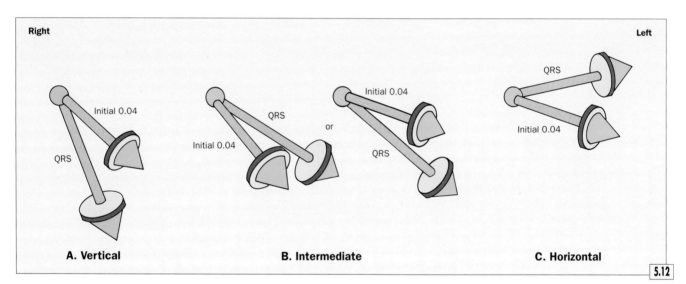

A. Vertical   **B. Intermediate**   **C. Horizontal**

5.12

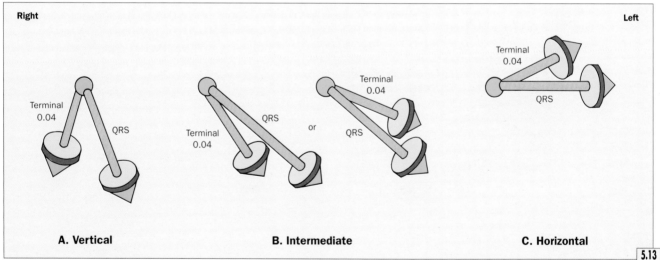

A. Vertical   **B. Intermediate**   **C. Horizontal**

5.13

THE T WAVE

THE REPOLARIZATION PROCESS

In the hypothetical cell discussed in Chapter 3, the repolarization process began, after a quiescent period, at the same point at which the depolarization process began. The wave of repolarization occurred in one direction, but unlike the wave of depolarization, it produced electrical forces that were oriented in the opposite direction. The wave of depolarization in the hypothetical cell recorded an upright (positive) deflection because the electrical forces were directed toward the electrode attached to the positive pole of the measuring device. Although the wave of repolarization occurred in the same direction, it produced electrical forces directed away from the electrode attached to positive pole. Accordingly, the wave of repolarizaiton produced a downward (negative) deflection.

If the conditions existing in the hypothetical cell were present in the human heart, the T wave would tend to be inverted whenever the QRS complex was upright. Although this does tend to be the case with newborns (Fig. 5.14) and young children, it is not true in older subjects. The reason for this has always been the subject of speculation.

As noted earlier, the depolarization process of the normal adult heart begins largely in the endocardium and spreads to the epicardium. The repolarization process should also begin in the endocardium, but it does not. It actually begins in the epicardium. Why does this occur(19)? The best of several explanations is that the repolarization process actually begins during late mechanical systole (Figs. 5.3 and 5.15). The duration of electrical systole is smaller than that of mechanical systole; the T wave is written when the left and right ventricles are still contracted, during the stage of isometric relaxation(20). During this period of ventricular systole, the pressure within the ventricular wall is greatest in the endocardial area and least in the epicardial area. It is theorized that the pressure gradient across the ventricular wall reverses the endocardial-to-epicardial direction of the repolarization process (Fig. 5.16). This is reminiscent of the hypothetical cell when cooled on the left side, as shown in Figure 3.5. Recall that the cell was cooled on the right side, where depolarization began. The cooling did not alter the sequence of depolarization but reversed the sequence of repolarization. Similarly, in the adult human heart the repolarization process begins at the epicardium and spreads toward the endocardium, producing electrical forces that are oriented in an opposite direction. This creates a T wave that is usually upright (positive) in the leads where the QRS complex is also upright (positive).

THE DURATION OF THE T WAVE: The exact measurement of the duration of the T wave is rarely made in clinical practice. It is important, however, to separate the T wave from the U wave when they are adjacent to each other.

THE MAGNITUDE OF THE T WAVE: The area encompassed by the T wave may be a little smaller or a little larger than that encompassed by the QRS complex; it is usually about two-thirds that of the latter. Characteristically, the upstroke of the normal T wave is less steep than the downstroke.

THE DIRECTION OF THE MEAN T VECTOR: The mean T vector of the normal newborn, infant, adolescent, and adult has a special relationship to the mean QRS vector (see Fig. 5.9). In the normal adult, the frontal plane direction of the mean T vector usually lies between 0° and +60°. It can be more accurately defined in terms of its relationship to the mean QRS vector (Fig. 5.9). The normal mean T vector should be to the left of a vertical mean QRS vector (Fig. 5.9). It can be located on either side of an intermediate mean QRS vector (Fig. 5.9), but it should be inferior to a horizontal mean QRS vector (Fig. 5.9). It should always be anterior to the mean QRS vector, and the QRS-T angle should be about 45° or less in normal adults. The QRS-T angle may be almost 180° in the normal newborn, and may be 90° in the normal child.

THE VENTRICULAR GRADIENT: Frank Wilson conceived, named, and defined the ventricular gradient as the measurement of the extent to which the repolarization process does not follow the same time sequence as the depolarization process(22). In the hypothetical cell the ventricular gradient is zero, implying that the repolarization process follows the same time sequence as the depolarization process. The T wave is downward (negative) when the QRS complex is upright (positive).

In the normal adult, the ventricular gradient can be estimated by visualizing the direction and magnitude of the mean QRS and mean T vectors. The areas of the QRS complexes and T waves must be carefully estimated, and the length of the arrows representing them must be determined as accurately as possible. A parallelogram should be constructed by visualizing the mean T vector as displaced in such a way that it is directed from the tip of the arrowhead representing the mean QRS vector. The QRS vector is visualized as being displaced so that it is directed from the tip of the arrowhead representing the mean T vectors. A diagonal line should then be drawn from the origin of the vectors to the most distant angle of the parallelogram (Fig. 5.17A). The diagonal line represents the ventricular gradient.

The terminus of the normal ventricular gradient of the adult lies in the left lower quadrant of the hexaxial reference system, between 0° and +90° (Fig. 5.17B)(23). It is either parallel with the frontal plane or directed slightly posteriorly. As one can surmise, much of the information inherent in the concept of the ventricular gradient is incorporated in the earlier discussion of the mean T vector and its relationship to the mean QRS vector and the QRS-T angle. The practical value of calculating the ventricular gradient is that it is sometimes useful in distinguishing between secondary and primary T wave abnormalities (see Chapter 6). The ventricular gradient is directed away from the area of the heart where repolarization is delayed.

In general, normal T waves are subject to more hour-to-hour or day-to-day variations than are the QRS complexes. Some patients who exhibit normal T wave variability have shorter than average QT intervals and are more sensitive to changes in the autonomic nervous system, body position, and heart rate. The range of normal for T waves in the black population is greater than in the white population.

FIGURE 5.14

Depolarization and repolarization in the newborn. **A**. In a hypothetical cell, depolarization proceeds in one direction, producing electrical forces in the same direction. Repolarization begins in the same area where depolarization was initiated, and spreads across the cell in the same direction as the wave of depolarization. However, unlike the latter, it produces electrical forces that are in the opposite direction (see Figs. 3.3 and 3.4). Note the upward (positive) QRS complex, and the downward (negative) T wave. **B**. The depolarization and repolarization process in the myocardium (mainly the right ventricle) of the neonate. Theoretically, the sequence of depolarization and repolarization is the same as in the hypothetical cell because the transmyocardial pressure gradient is small. This is represented by the grey color of the myocardium. Note that this shade is the same in both the endo- and epicardium.

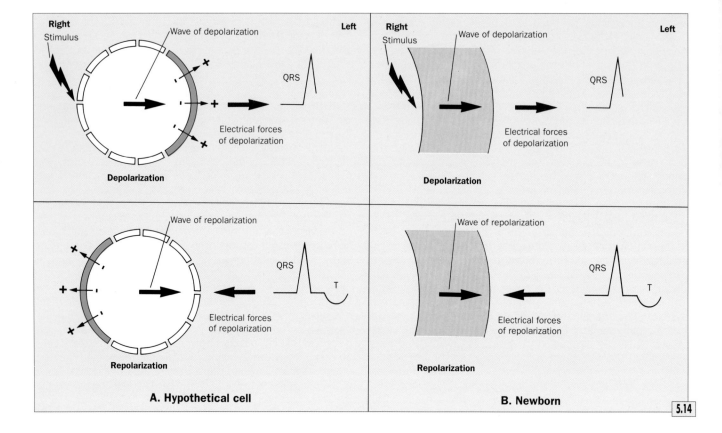

A. Hypothetical cell   B. Newborn

5.14

FIGURE 5.15

Relationship of electrical systole in the electrocardiogram to mechanical systole. This diagram and legend were prepared by Dr. Robert Schlant. The diagram shows the pressure curves of the great vessels and cardiac chambers, valvular events and heart sounds, left ventricular volume curve, jugular pulse wave, apex cardiogram (Sanborn piezo crystal), and the electrocardiogram during the cardiac cycle. For illustrative purposes, the time intervals between the valvular events have been modified, and the Z point has been prolonged.

Valve motion: MC and MO denote mitral closure and opening; TC and TO, tricuspid closure and opening; AC and AO, aortic closure and opening; PC and PO, pulmonic closure and opening.

Apex cardiogram: IC denotes isovolumetric contraction wave; IR, isovolumetric relaxation wave; O, opening of mitral valve; RFW, rapid-filling wave; SFW, slow-filling wave. (Reproduced with permission of the publisher and author; see Figure Credits.)

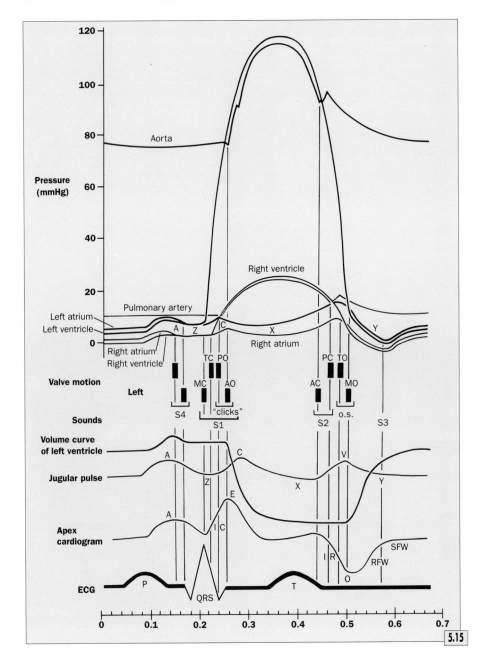

FIGURE 5.16
Depolarization and repolarziation in the normal adult. **A**. In a hypothetical cell that has been cooled on one side, the sequence of depolarization remains the same as in Figure 5.14, producing an upright QRS complex. Repolarization, however, does not follow the sequence of depolarization. Instead, it is initiated in an area of the cell that is the least cooled. As usual, the wave of repolarization progresses in one direction, producing electrical forces in an opposite direction. This produces an upright T wave in the hypothetical cell.
B. In ventricular muscle (the left ventricle of an adult), the depolarization process stimulates myocardial contractility. The repolarization process occurs during the late stage of mechanical systole (see Fig. 5.15). During this period there is a transmyocardial pressure gradient that is greatest in the endocardial area (dark grey) and least in the epicardial area (light grey). This pressure gradient is responsible for the initiation of repolarization in the epicardium. Accordingly, the repolarization process spreads from epicardium to endocardium, producing electrical forces in an opposite direction. This produces an upright T wave and QRS complex, similar to what occurs after cooling one side of the hypothetical cell shown in **A**.

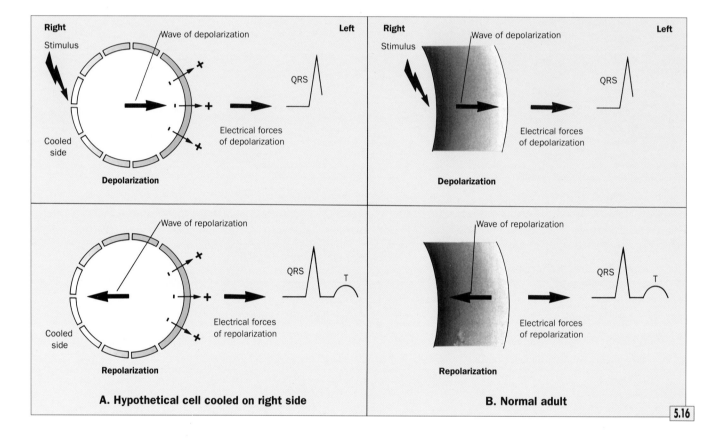

A. Hypothetical cell cooled on right side

B. Normal adult

5.16

FIGURE 5.17
The ventricular gradient. **A**. This diagram shows the relationship between the normal depolarization and repolarization processes. The ventricular gradient is a measure of the extent to which the sequence of repolarization is predetermined by the sequence of depolarization. It is constructed by creating a parallelogram of which the mean T vector and mean QRS vector are two sides, and drawing a line from the origin of electrical activity to the most distant angle of the figure. The gradient is directed away from the area of the heart where the repolarization is most delayed. **B**. The blue area indicates the normal range for the direction of the ventricular gradient in the adult. It is normally parallel with the frontal plane or directed slightly posteriorly. (Adapted and reproduced with permission of the publisher and author; see Figure Credits.)

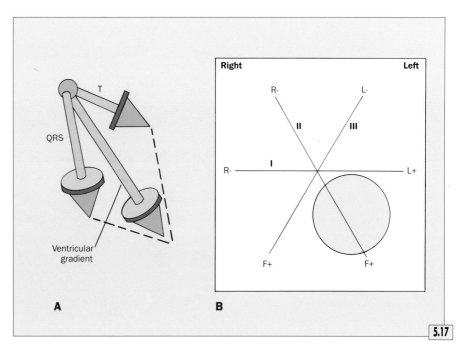

THE ST SEGMENT

The normal ST segment is usually isoelectric (occurring directly along the baseline). There may be a normal ST vector that is parallel to the mean T vector (Fig. 5.18). This is usually associated with a rather large T wave, and is thought to represent the electrical forces of early repolarization. In such a patient, early repolarization may actually begin during the QRS complex, and may be seen as ST segment displacement just after the QRS complex is completed.

THE U WAVE

The origin of the U wave is not known, but it is related to the repolarization process(24). The U wave may be observed in the electrocardiograms of patients with no other evidence of heart disease. It is usually less than one-quarter the size of the preceding T wave and about 0.5 mm in height in the extremity leads; it may be as large as 2 mm in height in leads V1 and V2. The U wave is normally upright. Its mean direction cannot be determined because it cannot be seen in all leads.

AFTER-POTENTIAL

Special equipment is needed to identify the electrical potential that follows the QRS complex. A signal-averaging technique is used for this purpose (Fig. 5.19)(25). Normally, very little potential can be identified following the QRS complex.

EXAMPLES OF NORMAL ELECTROCARDIOGRAMS

The electrocardiograms shown in Figures 5.20 through 5.22 are normal. The mean QRS vector is vertical in Figure 5.20, intermediate in Figure 5.21, and horizontal in Figure 5.22.

COMMENTS ABOUT THE APPARENTLY NORMAL ELECTRO-CARDIOGRAM

Considerable heart disease can be present without being revealed by the electrocardiogram. The best example is the patient with severe atherosclerotic heart disease who has been successfully resuscitated from an episode of ventricular fibrillation and has a normal resting electrocardiogram. I also wish to emphasize once again that not all electrocardiographic abnormalities are serious; data from other sources are usually needed to determine the seriousness of an abnormality.

FIGURE 5.18

ST segment displacement. **A.** The normal adult electrocardiogram may not exhibit any displacement of the ST segment. **B.** At times the ST segment may be displaced from the baseline of a normal electrocardiogram. This type of displacement accompanies a large but normal T wave, and the mean ST vector is parallel with the mean T vector.

FIGURE 5.19

This figure illustrates a normal signal-averaged electrocardiogram. The QRS duration is normal (87 msec) and the voltage content in the last 40 msec of the QRS complex is normal at 93.2 V. Note that there are normally no deflections (after-potential) following the completion of the QRS complex. (I thank Dr. Paul Walter of Emory University for providing this illustration.)

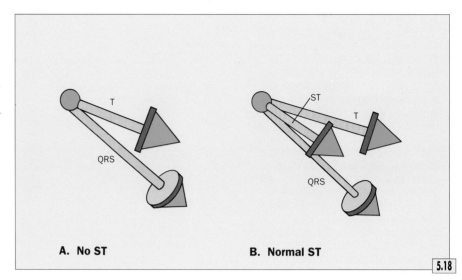

A. No ST   **B. Normal ST**

5.18

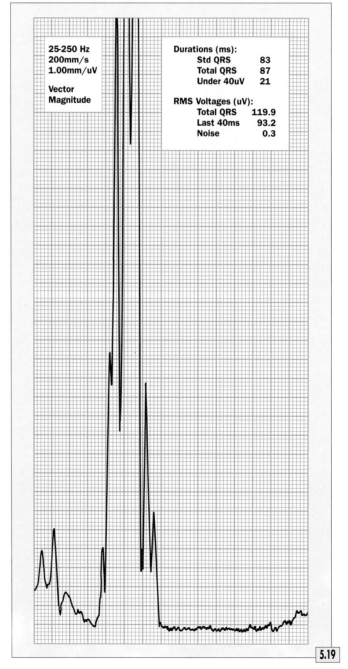

| 25-250 Hz |
| 200mm/s |
| 1.00mm/uV |
| Vector Magnitude |

Durations (ms):	
Std QRS	83
Total QRS	87
Under 40uV	21

RMS Voltages (uV):	
Total QRS	119.9
Last 40ms	93.2
Noise	0.3

5.19

FIGURE 5.20
The electrocardiogram of a normal, tall, 37-year-old male with a vertical mean QRS vector. Note that the electrodes at positions V4, V5, and V6 are located near the transitional pathway for the mean QRS vector. Accordingly, the QRS complex is nearly diphasic in all of these leads. Note the relationship of the mean initial 0.04-second QRS vector and the mean T vector to the mean QRS vector. (I thank Dr. Philip Gainey for providing this electrocardiogram.)

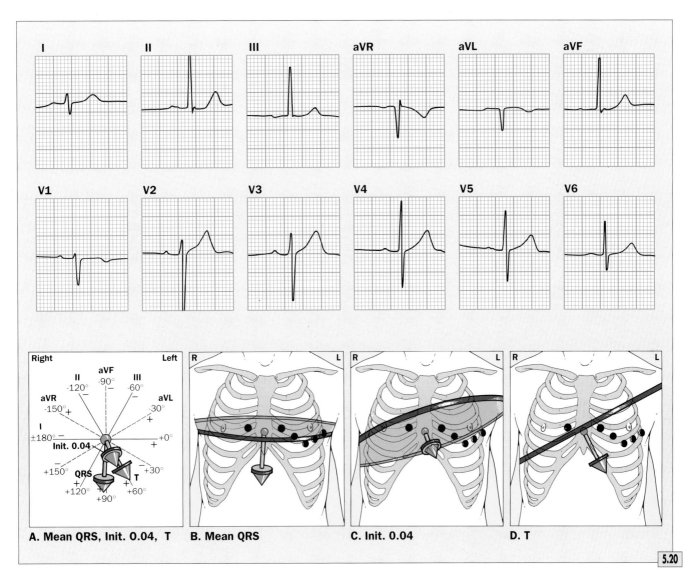

FIGURE 5.21

The electrocardiogram of a normal, medium-sized 27-year-old male with an intermediate mean QRS vector.

The magnetic resonance images shown in Figures 4.5 through 4.7 are of the same subject. Note the relationship of the mean initial 0.04-second QRS vector and the mean T vector to the mean QRS vector. (I thank Dr. Mark Lowell for providing this electrocardiogram.)

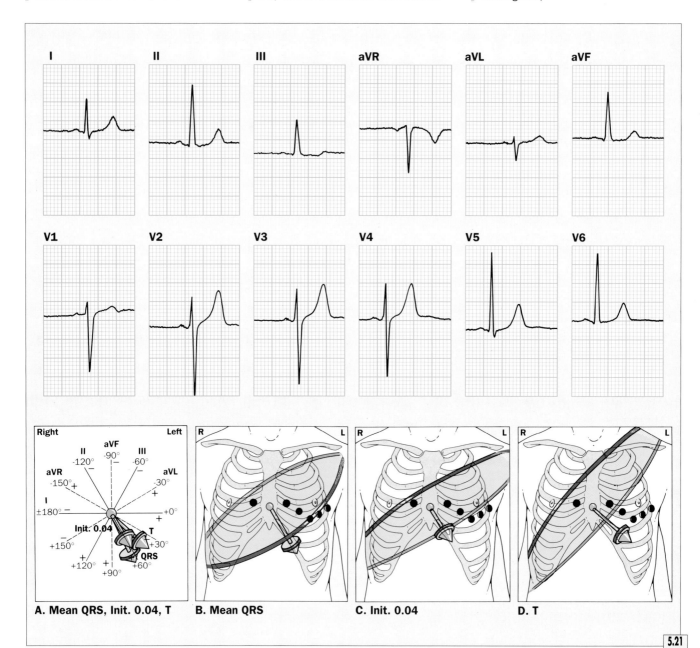

A. Mean QRS, Init. 0.04, T   B. Mean QRS   C. Init. 0.04   D. T

5.21

FIGURE 5.22
The electrocardiogram of a normal, heavy-set, broad-chested 31-year-old male with a horizontal mean QRS vector. Note the relationship of the mean initial 0.04-second QRS vector and the mean T vector to the mean QRS vector (I thank Dr. Curtis Weaver for providing this electrocardiogram.)

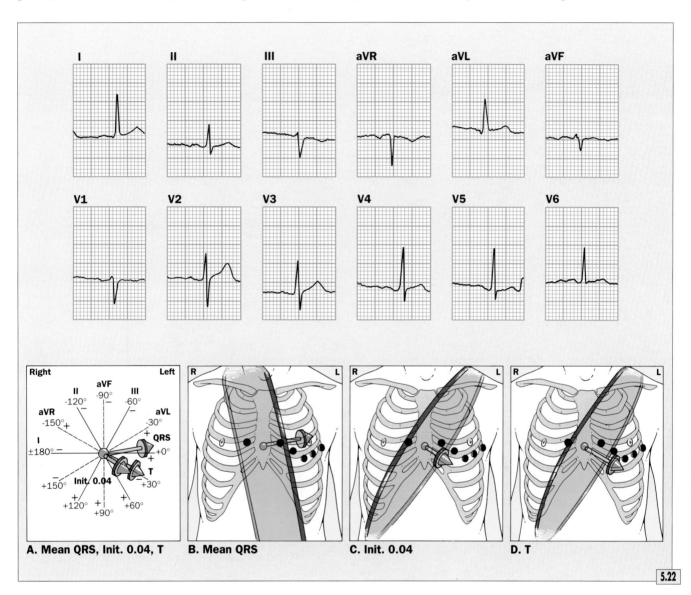

A. Mean QRS, Init. 0.04, T   B. Mean QRS   C. Init. 0.04   D. T

REFERENCES

1. Hurst JW: The physician's approach to the patient: goals and cardiac appraisal, in Hurst JW (ed.): *The Heart*, Ed. 7. New York: McGraw-Hill, 1990, p. 115.
2. The Criteria Committee of the New York Heart Association: *Nomenclature and Criteria for Diagnosis of Diseases of the Heart and Great Vessels*, Ed. 8. Boston: Little, Brown and Co, 1979.
3. Leaverton PE: *A Review of Biostatistics: A Program for Self-Instruction*, Ed. 2. Boston: Little, Brown and Co, 1978.
4. Wilson F: Foreword, in Lepeschkin E (ed.): *Modern Electrocardiography*. Baltimore: Williams and Wilkins, 1951, vol. 1, p. 5.
5. Puddu PE, Jouve R, Mariotti S, et al: Evaluation of 10 QT prediction formulas in 881 middle-aged men from seven countries study: emphasis on the cubic root Fridericia's equation. *J Electrocardiol* 1988; 21(3):219.
6. Becker AE: Personal letter to JWH, May 20, 1988.
7. Katz LN: *Electrocardiography: Including an Atlas of Electrocardiograms*. Philadelphia: Lea & Febiger, 1941.
8. Morris JJ, Estes EH Jr, Whalen RE, et al: P wave analysis in valvular heart disease. *Circulation* 1964; 29:242.
9. Jin L, Weisse AB, Hernandez F, et al: Significance of electrocardiographic isolated abnormal terminal P wave force (left atrial abnormality): an echocardiographic and clinical correlation. *Arch Intern Med* 1988. 148(7):1545.
10. Flowers NC, Horan LG: Mid and late changes in the QRS complex, in Schlant RC, Hurst JW (eds.): *Advances in Electrocardiography*. New York: Grune & Stratton, 1972, vol. 1, p. 331.
11. Durrer E: Electrical aspects of human cardiac activity: a clinical physiological approach to excitation and stimulation. *Cardiovasc Res* 1968; 2:1.
12. Griep AH: Pitfalls in the electrocardiographic diagnosis of left ventricular hypertrophy: a correlative study of 200 autopsied patients. *Circulation* 1959; 20:30.
13. Romhilt DW, Bove KE, Norris RJ, et al: A critical appraisal of the electrocardiographic criteria for the diagnosis of left ventricular hypertrophy. *Circulation* 1969; 40:185.
14. Romhilt DW, Estes EH Jr: A point-score system for the ECG diagnosis of left ventricular hypertrophy. *Am Heart J* 1968; 75(6):752.
15. Odom H II, Davis JL, Dinh HA, et al: QRS voltage measurements in autopsied men free of cardiopulmonary disease: a basis for evaluating total QRS voltage as an index of left ventricular hypertrophy. *Am J Cardiol* 1986; 58:801.
16. Hurst JW, Woodson GC Jr: *Atlas of Spatial Vector Electrocardiography*. New York: Blakiston, 1952.
17. Horan LG, Sridharan MR, Hand RC, et al: Variation in the precordial QRS transition zone in normal subjects. *J Electrocardiol* 1988: 21(1):25.
18. Grant RP: *Clinical Electrocardiography*. New York: McGraw-Hill, 1957, p. 49.
19. Burgess MJ: V. Miscellaneous effects upon the electrocardiogram: physiologic basis of the T wave, in Schlant RC, Hurst JW (eds.): *Advances in Electrocardiography*. New York: Grune & Stratton, 1972, vol. 1, p. 367.
20. Schlant RC: Normal anatomy and function of the cardiovascular system, in Hurst JW, Logue RB (eds.): *The Heart*, Ed. 1. New York: McGraw-Hill, 1966.
21. Burger HC: A theoretical elucidation of the notion "ventricular gradient." *Am Heart J* 1957; 53:240.
22. Wilson FN, MacLeod AG, Barker PS, Johnston FD: The determination and the significance of the areas of the ventricular deflections of the electrocardiogram. *Am Heart J* 1934; 10:46.
23. Burch G, Winsor T: *A Primer of Electrocardiography*. Philadelphia: Lea & Febiger, 1945.
24. Lepeschkin E: Physiologic basis of the U wave, in Schlant RC, Hurst JW (eds): *Advances in Electrocardiography*. New York: Grune & Stratton, 1972, vol. 2, p. 353.
25. Breithhardt G, Borggrefe M: Pathophysiological mechanism and clinical significance of ventricular late potentials. *Eur Heart J* 1986; 7:364.

FIGURE CREDITS

Figure 5.1 From Leaverton PE: *A Review of Biostatistics: A Program for Self-Instruction*, Ed. 2. Boston: Little, Brown and Co, 1978, p 95.

Table 5.2 From Morris JJ, Estes EH, Whalen RE: P wave analysis in valvular heart disease. *Circulation* 1964; 29:245.

Table 5.3 From Romhilt DW, Estes EH Jr: A point-score system for the ECG diagnosis of left ventricular hypertrophy. *Am Heart J* 1968; 75(6):754.

Figure 5.3 From Katz LN: *Electrocardiography: Including an Atlas of Electrocardiograms*. Philadelphia: Lea & Febiger, 1941, p. 62-63.

Figure 5.7 From Durrer E: Electrical aspects of human cardiac activity: a clinical physiological approach to excitation and stimulation. *Cardiovasc Res* 1968;2:5.

Figure 5.8 From Siegel RJ, Roberts WC: Electrocardiographic observations in severe aortic valve stenosis: correlative necropsy study to clinical, hemodynamic, and ECG variables demonstrating relation of 12-lead QRS amplitude to peak systolic transaortic pressure gradient. *Am Heart J* 1982; 103:210.

Figure 5.9C. From Ferrer MI: *Electrocardiographic Notebook*, 4th ed. Mt. Kisco, NY: Futura, 1973.

Figure 5.11 From Grant RP: *Clinical Electrocardiography*. New York: McGraw-Hill, 1957, p. 49.

Figure 5.15 From Schlant RC: Normal anatomy and function in the cardiovascular system, in Hurst JW, Logue RB (eds.): *The Heart*, Ed. 1. New York: McGraw-Hill, 1966.

Figure 5.17B From Burch G, Winsor T: *A Primer of Electrocardiography*. Philadelphia: Lea and Febiger, 1945, p. 186. (Burch and Winsor created the diagram after studying the reports of Robert Bayley.)

CHAPTER SIX

The Abnormal Ventricular Electrocardiogram

This book is concerned with the electrical forces produced by the ventricular myocardium(1). It is not primarily concerned with cardiac arrhythmias. However, cardiac arrhythmias may be mentioned from time to time if they contribute to the analysis of the ventricular electrocardiogram. The same is true for the P wave itself. The P wave is discussed here because, at times, its characteristics contribute to the analysis of the ventricular electrocardiogram.

HEART RATE AND RHYTHM

The average heart rate for the normal adult atria and ventricles ranges from 60 to 90 depolarizations per minute. *Sinus bradycardia* is said to be present when the rate is less than 60 depolarizations per minute, and *sinus tachycardia* is said to be present when there are more than 90 depolarizations per minute. The heart rate of the trained athlete may be as low as 40 depolarizations per minute. The heart rate in a newborn or child is much faster than it is in an adult.

SINUS BRADYCARDIA

Sinus bradycardia, which is commonly present in the elderly, is often due to an early stage of the "sick sinus syndrome." Such patients may also have a "sick atrioventricular node." The precise cause of the condition is not known, but it is commonly related to aging.

When low voltage of the QRS complexes accompanies sinus bradycardia it is appropriate to consider myxedema as a possible cause of the two abnormalities. Sinus bradycardia may also be caused by beta-blocking drugs.

SINUS TACHYCARDIA

Sinus tachycardia may be caused by endogenous or exogenous catecholamines, or by blood loss, shock of any cause, or hyperthyroidism. Cardiac tamponade may produce sinus tachycardia and low voltage in all components of the electrocardiogram. Sinus tachycardia may alter the T waves, ST segments, and conduction in the bundle branches.

ATRIAL FIBRILLATION

Atrial fibrillation may occur when no heart disease can be discovered and, in such cases, the rhythm is referred to as *lone atrial fibrillation*. However, it may also accompany mitral valve disease. A vertical mean QRS vector of +90° is more likely to be abnormal when it occurs with atrial fibrillation, the combination suggesting mitral stenosis. Right ventricular conduction delay of the QRS complex plus atrial fibrillation in a young person is likely to be due to an ostium secundum type of atrial septal defect. Right bundle branch block with left anterior-superior division block and atrial fibrillation in a child is likely to be due to an ostium primum septal defect. Atrial fibrillation may be associated with coronary disease, constrictive pericarditis, cardiomyopathy, and any advanced form of heart disease. Atrial tachycardia or atrial fibrillation may be associated with pre-excitation of the ventricles, in the condition referred to as Wolff-Parkinson-White syndrome(2).

The ventricular rate in an untreated, resting patient with atrial fibrillation is usually 140 to 160 depolarizations per minute.

When it reaches 180 to 200 ventricular depolarizations per minute, it is wise to consider thyrotoxicosis, although other causes, such as acute heart failure, shock, and blood loss, are more common.

When the ventricular rate is 220 to 300 in a patient with atrial fibrillation, a bypass tract outside the atrioventricular node is usually present; this commonly occurs in patients with the Wolff-Parkinson-White syndrome(2). Such a tract prevents the atrial impulses from passing through the atrioventricular node, where many of them are normally blocked so that they do not reach the ventricles. The rapid ventricular rate may make it difficult to identify the QRS abnormality associated with bypass tracts.

Finally, whenever atrial fibrillation occurs in an untreated patient and the ventricular rate is 60 to 80 depolarizations per minute, it is likely that disease of the atrioventricular node is present. When digitalis is used to control the ventricular rate of a patient with atrial fibrillation, the QT interval may become shorter, the U wave may become prominent, and an abnormal ST segment vector may develop (see Chapter 12).

THE DURATION OF THE COMPLEXES AND INTERVALS

THE P WAVE

The first clue to an atrial abnormality may be the duration of the P wave. When this is longer than 0.12 second in an adult or 0.08 second in a newborn, it is proper to consider a left atrial abnormality. Morris and his colleagues(3) were among the first to suggest that an abnormality of the second half of the P wave represented a left atrial abnormality (see later discussion). A right atrial abnormality is more likely to be recognized by an increased amplitude of the first half of the P wave rather than an increased duration of the P waves (see later discussion).

THE PR INTERVAL

The normal range for the PR interval is shown in Table 2 in the appendix. When PR interval prolongation occurs, it is referred to as first-degree atrioventricular block. The PR interval may be prolonged by digitalis medication; acute myocarditis, especially due to acute rheumatic fever; coronary disease; severe heart disease of any cause; degenerative disease of the atrioventricular node; beta-blocking drugs; and verapamil.

Pericarditis may produce PR segment displacement. The mean vector representing the PR interval usually has a direction opposite that of the mean P vector(4).

THE QRS DURATION

The duration of the normal QRS complex in adults is 0.10 second or less, and in children it is 0.08 second or less. In neonates, it is about 0.06 second. In adults, it may be slightly prolonged by right and left ventricular hypertrophy, but usually does not exceed 0.10 second. It is almost always prolonged to 0.12 second by right or left bundle branch block, but it rarely exceeds 0.10 second when there is anterior-supe-

---

Note: As stated in several places in this book, the model presented here is a clinically useful approximation of the real situation within the heart. At times, the explanation moves beyond the known evidence. When this occurs, every effort has been made to extend the facts in a logical manner.

rior or posterior-inferior division block of the left bundle branch system. It may be prolonged by pre-excitation of the ventricles, as observed in the Wolff-Parkinson-White syndrome. Finally, the QRS duration may be prolonged when there is accidental hypothermia.

THE ST SEGMENT DURATION

Measurement of the ST segment duration is seldom made in clinical practice because the same information is usually provided by measurement of the QT interval. Hypocalcemia is one condition, however, that can be suspected when the duration of the ST segment is prolonged because of a delay in the appearance of the T wave. This condition is often caused by hypoparathyroidism. A long QU interval, which is often due to hypokalemia, should not be misinterpreted as a long QT interval.

THE QT INTERVAL

The QT interval is a measure of the duration of electrical systole. Accordingly, it is greatly influenced by the heart rate. The duration of the normal QT interval associated with different heart rates is shown in Table 1 in the appendix.

The ability to determine whether a corrected QT interval is normal or abnormal when the heart rate is rapid or slow is now under question (see Chapter 5).

PROLONGATION OF THE QT INTERVAL: Prolongation of the QT interval may be caused by the following conditions:

THE "LONG QT SYNDROME," which must not be overlooked because it may be accompanied by serious ventricular arrhythmias. Drugs that prolong the QT interval may cause serious consequences in these patients. The Romano-Ward syndrome is the term assigned to this congenital anomaly(5,-5A). The Jervell, Lange-Nielsen syndrome is said to be present when congenital deafness accompanies the long QT interval(6).

HYPOCALCEMIA due to hypoparathyroidism causes a long QT interval(7,8). The T waves usually appear to be normal but are delayed in appearance (the ST segment is prolonged).

HYPERKALEMIA,, which prolongs the QT interval(9). Hypokalemia also prolongs the QT interval. The U wave becomes prominent and fuses with the T wave; this contributes to the appearance of a long QT interval. The condition is often recognized by identifying what is believed to be long, low T waves.

VARIOUS TYPES OF HEART DISEASE, including atherosclerotic coronary heart disease, myocarditis and cardiomyopathy, and any advanced heart condition, may also prolong the QT interval.

SUBARACHNOID HEMORRHAGE may do so as well, because of the long duration of the large, abnormal T waves that occur in this condition(11).

The following drugs can prolong the QT interval: quinidine, procainamide (Pronestyl), disopyramide (Norpace), amio-darone (Cordarone), tricyclic drugs used to treat depression, and phenothiazides.

Systemic conditions including hypothyroidism or hypothermia may also prolong the QT interval.

SHORTENING OF THE QT INTERVAL: Little is written about a short QT interval. Three points can be made here: first, I have noted that normal subjects with normal hearts who have QT intervals on the short side of the normal range may have labile T waves. The T waves in such patients may be altered to a remarkable degree with tachycardia or a change in posture. I have termed this condition "an inherent ability to repolarize quickly." It seems that any factor capable of shortening the QT interval by creating earlier repolarization will, in these patients who already show shortened QT intervals, cause a change in the sequence of the repolarization process. This, in turn, may alter the direction of the mean T vector.

Second, digitalis medication may shorten the QT interval by encouraging the repolarization process to begin earlier than usual (12). It is generally known that digitalis may prolong the PR interval, but it is far more likely that the QT interval will become shorter after the administration of the drug than that the PR interval will become longer. The effect of digitalis on the ventricular electrocardiogram is discussed in Chapter 12.

Third, hypercalcemia related to hyperparathyroidism or renal disease may produce a QT interval duration that is on the low side of the normal range. In these cases, the ST segment may resemble that seen in patients taking digitalis.

THE DURATION OF THE T WAVE

The duration of the T wave may be prolonged by hyperkalemia, subarachnoid hemorrhage, other acute cerebral vascular events, and drugs that prolong the QT interval. Hypokalemia makes a prominent U wave, which, when it joins with a low-amplitude T wave, may be misinterpreted as a prolonged T wave.

THE U WAVE

The U wave may become more prominent in certain conditions, but its duration is not necessarily prolonged (see later discussion)(13).

THE P WAVE AND TA WAVE

THE P WAVE

The size, shape, and location of the atria in the thorax, the preferential conduction system within the atria, and the depolarization and repolarization sequence of the right and left atria are discussed in Chapter 4. The characteristics of the normal P wave (including Pm, P1, and P2) are discussed here and in Chapter 5(3,14).

Analysis of the P waves may at times assist in the analysis of the QRS complex. Unfortunately, it is not as easy to identify the P and Ta waves as it is to identify the components of the QRS complex and T wave. The electrical forces responsible for the former are smaller, and the stylus of the direct-writing electrocardiograph machine seems to blur the small deflections, possibly eliminating valuable information. This makes one consider the value, though untested, of increasing the sensitivity of the machine and running the paper at double speed in an effort to record the P and Ta waves so that they can be analyzed more readily. There is undoubtedly more information contained in both the P wave and Ta wave than we are currently extracting from our studies of them.

As will be discussed, there are a few abnormalities of the P waves that indicate specific cardiac conditions; the predictive value of these is high. Many apparent P wave abnormalities, however, overlap the normal range for P wave characteristics, have no known cause, and are not accompanied by any other evidence of heart disease. Accordingly, when minor P wave abnormalities are identified, it is wise to consider the etiologic possibilities they suggest, but to recognize that their predictive value is low.

It is useful to divide P wave abnormalities into three groups. Group one is composed of electrocardiograms from adults in which the P waves have a duration of less than 0.12 second but an amplitude, especially of P1, that is greater than 2.5 mm. In group two, the P waves are broad and notched and have a duration greater than 0.12 second due to a prominent, prolonged P2 component. A third group is created when both of the preceding abnormalities occur in the same electrocardiogram.

I have used the term *atrial abnormality* for 25 years. I prefer this to "atrial hypertrophy," "dilatation," or "enlargement" because it is less specific than the latter terms. Although such anatomic correlations may occasionally be present, I believe that they are indirect and cannot be made in many cases. I suggest that many P wave abnormalities are caused by conduction abnormalities within the walls of the atria.

RIGHT ATRIAL ABNORMALITIES: A right atrial abnormality is characterized by P waves that are taller than 2.5 mm and that show, in adults, durations of 0.12 second or less. Such an abnormality was formerly called P pulmonale; this terminology, which is no longer used, became popular before the era when the clinical features of congenital heart disease began to be recognized. The electrocardiographic abnormality was called P pulmonale because lung disease was well-recognized at that time.

The P wave is not usually notched. The mean P vector (Pm) is commonly directed from +60° to +90° and is directed anteriorly (Fig. 6.1). The first half of the P wave (P1), when represented as a mean vector, is large, and often directed to the right of, and anterior to the mean P vector. The second half of the P wave (P2), when represented as a mean vector, is smaller, directed to the left, and posterior to the mean P vector.

Right atrial abnormalities occur in patients with cor pulmonale, pulmonary hypertension (due to any cause), pulmonary valve stenosis, Ebstein's anomaly, and tricuspid atresia. Examples of electrocardiograms having right atrial abnormalities are shown in Figure 7.2.

LEFT ATRIAL ABNORMALITIES: A left atrial abnormality is characterized by P waves that are greater than 0.12 second in duration. They are often notched at about the halfway mark, and the mean P vector (Pm) is directed about +30° to +60° in the frontal plane. It is parallel with the frontal plane or directed slightly posteriorly (Fig. 6.2). The first half of the P wave (P1), when represented by a mean vector, is directed to the right of, and anterior to the mean P vector. The second half of the P wave (P2), when represented as a mean vector, is directed to the left of, and posterior to the mean P vector. When the amplitude (depth) of P2 in lead V1 is multiplied by its duration in that lead in an adult, it should not normally be greater than -0.03 mm-sec. The predictive value of the measurement indicating a left atrial abnormality increases as the number increases; -0.06 mm-sec has a greater predictive value than -0.03 mm–sec (Fig. 5.5).

When the signals from all 12 electrocardiograph leads are recorded simultaneously, it is possible to measure backward from the Q wave to the beginning of the P wave, and to identify the right and left atrial contributions to the P wave by comparing the deflections observed in one lead with those of another.

Left atrial abnormalities may occur in patients with mitral stenosis, mitral regurgitation, aortic stenosis, aortic regurgitation, and all types of cardiomyopathy. An example of an electrocardiogram showing a left atrial abnormality is shown in Figure 7.3.

In teaching, I have used the diagrammatic metaphor shown in Figure 6.3 for many years, in an effort to emphasize the notion that there are cases in which P wave abnormalities should force the clinician to auscultate the heart carefully for mitral stenosis.

COMBINED RIGHT AND LEFT ATRIAL ABNORMALITIES: Right and left atrial abnormalities may appear in the same electrocardiogram. They produce abnormalities of the mean P vector (Pm), the vector representing the first half of the P wave (P1), and the vector representing the second half of the P wave (P2). Examples of electrocardiograms showing bi-atrial abnormalities are shown in Figures 7.4 and 7.5.

THE TA WAVE

The repolarization of the atria produces electrical forces that are opposite in direction to those generated during depolarization. Accordingly, these forces create a negative deflection (the Ta wave) when they are directed away from the electrode attached to the positive pole of the electrocardiograph machine.

The Ta wave is not seen in all leads. Therefore, it is not possible to identify the spatial direction of a mean vector that represents it. The Ta wave is more likely to be identified when the PR interval is long or when there is complete heart block. The normal Ta wave may influence the PR interval and even the J point of the QRS complex (Fig. 5.6). When this occurs, the clinician may be misled into believing an abnormality is present.

FIGURE 6.1
Right atrial abnormality.

The duration of the P wave in lead II of an adult is about 0.12 second or less, and its amplitude is 2.5 mm or greater. Its amplitude in lead V1 may also be 2.5 mm. The mean P vector (Pm) is directed inferiorly and anteriorly. The first half of the P wave, produced by right atrial electrical forces, is represented by a mean vector (P1) directed inferiorly (+60° to +90°) and anteriorly. P1 is directed to the right of and always anterior to Pm. P1 may be larger than P2, which represents the second half of the P wave.

FIGURE 6.2
Left atrial abnormality.

The duration of the P wave in lead II of an adult is greater than 0.12 second, and its amplitude may be 2.5 mm. It is often notched at the halfway point. The mean P vector (Pm), directed at +60° or less, is parallel with the frontal plane or directed slightly posteriorly. The second half of the P wave is produced by left atrial electrical forces and is represented by a mean vector (P2) directed to the left and posteriorly. It is directed to the left of and posterior to Pm and P1. When the amplitude (depth) of the second half of the P wave in V1 is multiplied by its duration, the product is greater than -0.03 mm-sec; the greater the measurement, the more likely there is to be a left atrial abnormality.

FIGURE 6.3
Diagrammatic metaphor for the left atrial abnormality secondary to mitral stenosis.

A. Note the large, broad, notched P wave, the configuration of the QRS complex, and the first part of the T wave. **B.** The notched P wave is assumed to be a letter **M**. A dot is placed above the first small upright deflection of the QRS complex, which is then assumed to be an **i**. The second large upright deflection of the QRS complex is crossed and assumed to be a **T**. The T wave is assumed to be an **R**. When joined together, the letters produce **MITR**, the first four letters of **mitral**.

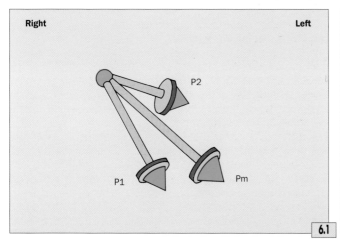

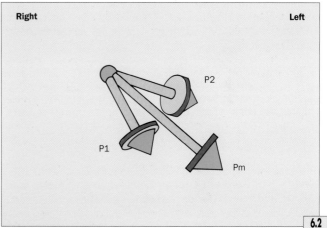

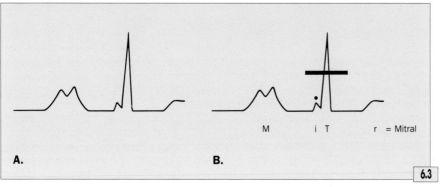

THE QRS COMPLEX

ABNORMAL QRS COMPLEX WITH NORMAL QRS DURATION

NORMAL DIRECTION OF THE MEAN QRS VECTOR: Normally, the mean QRS vector in an adult is directed somewhere between -30° and +110°. It is usually directed between -10° and +80° (Fig. 5.9), and *always* slightly posteriorly. The reasons for this are discussed in Chapter 5. The direction of the mean QRS vector in the adult is also governed by the body build of the subject. A tall person is more likely to have a vertically-directed mean QRS vector, while a broad-chested or obese person is more likely to have this vector directed horizontally. Examples of electrocardiograms of normal adults, showing vertical, intermediate, and horizontal mean QRS vectors are illustrated in Figures 5.20, 5.21, and 5.22.

The mean QRS vector in the normal newborn is directed to the right and anteriorly. It is directed +90° to +100° in the child, in whom it may be parallel with the frontal plane. Simply stated, as the newborn grows older, the normal mean QRS vector gradually shifts from right to left ventricular dominance (Fig. 5.9).

The term *axis deviation* is often used to identify the direction of the mean QRS vector. Actually, this term can be used to refer to the direction of the mean P vector, QRS vector, ST vector, T vector, or any portion of any of them. It matters not which term is used. What does matter is that the deviation of the axis (or vector) from the zero position be stated in degrees.

THE DIRECTION OF THE MEAN QRS VECTOR IN RIGHT VENTRICULAR HYPERTROPHY: When the mean QRS vector is directed from +90° to +110° and *slightly posteriorly,* it is appropriate to consider the possibility that *acquired* right ventricular hypertrophy may be present (Fig. 6.4A). Acquired diseases, such as mitral stenosis, gradually developing Eisenmenger syndrome, gradually developing primary pulmonary hypertension, and left ventricular failure with pulmonary hypertension may produce right ventricular hypertrophy that, in the early stages of the disease, causes only a rightward shift of the mean QRS vector; the mean QRS vector may retain its posterior direction. This is because the gradually increasing right ventricular hypertrophy must overcome the normal left ventricular dominance in such patients. Because the most powerful electrical forces produced by the normal left ventricle are located posteriorly, it is easier for the mean QRS vector that results from acquired right ventricular hypertrophy to shift to the vertical position before it rotates anteriorly. When the mean QRS vector is directed to the right and anteriorly as well, it signals the presence of advanced acquired disease.

When right ventricular hypertrophy is due to *congenital heart disease,* such as pulmonary valve stenosis, the tetralogy of Fallot, or many other defects, the right ventricular dominance of the newborn is never lost, and left ventricular forces never dominate the electrical field. Accordingly, the mean QRS vector in such a patient is directed to the *right and anteriorly,* toward the anatomic location of the right ventricle (Fig. 6.4B)(15).

The exact size of the mean QRS vector is less useful in determining the presence of right ventricular hypertrophy than in determining the presence of left ventricular hypertrophy.

The amplitude of the R wave in lead V1 does, however, assist the clinician in determining the number of degrees to which the mean QRS vector is directed anteriorly.

The upper limit of normal for the amplitude of the R wave in lead V1 is shown in Table 3 in the appendix.

Right ventricular hypertrophy is not the only condition producing a mean QRS vector directed to the right, inferiorly, and anteriorly. This vector may be directed more than +90° to the right by lateral myocardial infarction, right ventricular conduction delay, and left posterior-inferior division block, and it may be directed anteriorly when there is an inferior-posterior or true posterior infarction.

Examples of electrocardiograms showing right ventricular hypertrophy are shown in Chapter 9.

THE DIRECTION OF THE MEAN QRS VECTOR IN LEFT VENTRICULAR HYPERTROPHY: The mean QRS vector may be directed from -30° to about +75° in patients with left ventricular hypertrophy; it is always directed posteriorly. However, the direction of this vector alone does not enable the clinician to identify left ventricular hypertrophy.

When the mean QRS vector is directed 0° to -30° to the left and posteriorly, it is proper to consider the possibility of left ventricular hypertrophy. However, this finding alone is not an adequate indicator of this condition, which may be caused by systemic hypertension, aortic stenosis or regurgitation, mitral regurgitation, or cardiomyopathy.

A mean QRS vector that is directed more than -30° to the left is usually due to a left ventricular conduction defect. The QRS duration may be a little longer than average but is not longer than 0.10 second. This conduction defect is called left anterior-superior division block and will be discussed later. While it may be associated with left ventricular hypertrophy, there are also other causes for left anterior-superior division block.

Examples of electrocardiograms showing left ventricular hypertrophy are shown in Chapter 9.

AN ABNORMAL INCREASE IN QRS AMPLITUDE: The mean QRS vector is directed to the right and anteriorly in the normal neonate. It may be directed inferiorly and parallel with the frontal plane in normal children. It is directed to the left and posteriorly in normal adults.

Right ventricular hypertrophy caused by acquired heart disease may, during its early stage, produce a mean QRS vector that is directed inferiorly and posteriorly. Right ventricular hypertrophy, caused by *congenital or advanced acquired heart disease* (Chapter 9), can be identified in adults when the mean QRS vector is directed to the right and anteriorly (Fig. 6.4). The contour of the QRS complex in V1 is useful in identifying an anterior direction of the mean QRS vector; when the mean QRS vector is directed to the right and the R wave is larger than the S wave in lead V1, the mean QRS vector is directed anteriorly. The mean QRS vector is never directed anteriorly in the normal adult. Note that it is the *amplitude* of the R wave in lead V1 that assists in determining the direction of the mean QRS vector.

Right ventricular hypertrophy can be suspected when the mean QRS vector is located between 90° and 110° and is directed slightly posteriorly (Fig. 6.4). As emphasized earlier, this direction of the mean QRS vector may be the only sign of right ventricular hypertrophy in the *early stages of acquired disease*. An added clue may be an R wave in lead V1 whose *amplitude* is greater than 5 to 10 mm, even though it is smaller than the S wave. The list of diseases capable of producing such abnormalities includes mitral stenosis, cor pulmonale, pulmonary arteriolar disease, primary pulmonary hypertension, pulmonary hypertension in patients with an interventricular septal defect or patent ductus arteriosus (Eisenmenger's physiology), and pulmonary hypertension due to disease and failure of the left ventricle. Examples of electrocardiograms showing right ventricular hypertrophy are given in Chapter 9.

Left ventricular hypertrophy is usually associated with a mean QRS vector that is directed between +75° and -30° in the frontal plane. This vector is always posteriorly directed. An increase in the *amplitude* of the mean QRS vector is crucial to the identification of left ventricular hypertrophy, and over the years many criteria have been developed for recognizing this. However, none of these has been satisfactory(16). The Romhilt and Estes criteria are often used (Table 5.3)(17), but I have pleaded for less rigidity because each set of criteria has its own sensitivity, specificity, and predictive value. In addition to this, the body build, especially the thickness of the chest wall, influences the amplitude of the QRS vector. At times, however, the amplitude of the mean QRS vector will be so large that its predictive value is 100 percent in indicating left ventricular hypertrophy. More frequently, though, the amplitude of the mean QRS vector is borderline; it could be normal because the normal range is wide. In such cases, it is necessary to seek other electrocardiographic clues to left ventricular hypertrophy, such as ST and T wave changes (to be discussed later), or to determine its presence by physical examination or from a chest x-ray film.

As will be discussed in Chapter 9, the mean QRS vector may be directed vertically or horizontally, but it must be directed posteriorly. There must be an increase in amplitude of the QRS complexes or evidence of the ST and T wave changes of left ventricular hypertrophy to make the diagnosis.

Recent studies have tested the value of the 12-lead total QRS amplitude in determining the presence of left ventricular hypertrophy. The method of measuring the total QRS voltage is shown in Figure 5.8. The upper limit of normal for the 12-lead total QRS amplitude as determined by Odom and associates was 185 mm(18). The total 12-lead QRS voltage was found to be 245±56 mm in patients with aortic stenosis(19) and 274±87 mm in patients with aortic regurgitation(20).

Left ventricular hypertrophy occurs in patients with systemic hypertension, aortic valve stenosis, subvalvular aortic stenosis, congenital tricuspid atresia, aortic regurgitation, mitral regurgitation, and cardiomyopathy (especially the hypertrophic type), and rarely in patients with the compensatory hypertrophy of myocardial infarction. The rare cardiac condition known as *glycogen storage disease* may produce an extremely large QRS voltage because the abnormal tissue seems to transmit electrical forces with great ease.

Examples of electrocardiograms showing left ventricular hypertrophy are shown in Chapter 9.

Combined right and left ventricular hypertrophy can occur: certain congenital defects produce right, left, or balanced ventricular hypertrophy. For example, a patient with patent duc-

tus arteriosus or an interventricular septal defect may have a normal initial electrocardiogram, or one showing left ventricular hypertrophy alone. Later tracings may show combined hypertrophy or only right ventricular hypertrophy alone as the patient develops Eisenmenger's physiology. Patients with truncus arteriosus have large, wide-swinging QRS complexes because both the right and left ventricles are equally affected by the peripheral resistance when the pulmonary arteries arise from the common trunk.

An Abnormal Decrease in QRS Amplitude: The QRS amplitude is said to be decreased when, in the extremity leads, it is decreased to 3 mm. This figure has always seemed too low to me. As stated earlier, the range of normal voltage for the QRS complex is wide, and if one chooses the figure of 3 mm to represent an abnormal QRS complex, one risks overlooking a large number of patients with low QRS voltages measuring 4 to 5 mm. It is wise to consider the conditions that produce low voltages even when the magnitude of the QRS is 5 to 7 mm.

The lower limit of normal for the amplitude of the QRS complexes is shown in Table 3 in the appendix. Odom and associates found the lower limit of normal for the 12-lead QRS voltage to be 80 mm(18). Examples of electrocardiograms showing low QRS and T voltage are shown in Chapters 9 and 13.

Patients with *pericardial effusion* of any cause may exhibit low voltage in the electrocardiogram (see Chapter 10). Occasionally, one may see *electrical alternans* in such patients(21). This condition, which is unrelated to mechanical alternans, is said to be present when the QRS complexes alternate in magnitude. It is euphemistically called "cardiac nystagmus," a term originally used by Dr. David Lippman of Boston to imply that the heart swings more when surrounded by pericardial fluid and consequently presents a different electrical field to the thorax on every other beat. The T waves also alternate in magnitude, but this is more difficult to identify. Normal rhythm or sinus tachycardia is usually present.

Constrictive pericarditis may produce low voltage in the electrocardiogram (see Chapter 9). This occurs because the thick pericardium acts as a barrier to the transmission of electrical forces to the chest wall.

Patients with *dilated cardiomyopathy* may show low voltage because the myocardium is replaced with fibrous tissue or a material such as amyloid, which conducts poorly and does not generate electrical forces. Low voltage would undoubtedly be observed more often in patients with dilated cardiomyopathy, but they tend to develop ventricular conduction defects which are often associated with an increased QRS voltage.

The QRS voltage may be low in patients with *obstructive lung disease* and *considerable emphysema* (Chapter 13) because the chest itself becomes "barrel-shaped" and the hyperinflated lung tissue blankets the electrical field. Whenever this occurs, there are usually other electrocardiographic signs of the lung disease, including a right atrial abnormality and rightward deviation of the mean QRS vector (see Fig. 13.1).

Myxedema may be responsible for a low QRS-T voltage (Chapter 13). As a rule, sinus bradycardia will be present in such patients. The low voltage is due to an excess of pericardial fluid, increased skin resistance, and myocardial changes.

ALTERNATING CHANGE IN SIZE OF THE QRS COMPLEX: As discussed above, patients with pericardial effusion may exhibit electrical alternans; the QRS voltage decreases in amplitude with every other ventricular depolarization because the heart "swings" more than it does normally. Electrical alternans may also be observed in patients with *paroxysmal atrial tachycardia*(21); the exact cause of this has not been determined.

DECREASE IN VOLTAGE OF THE LEFT PRECORDIAL LEADS: A large amount of fluid in the left pleural space may result in a diminished QRS-T voltage in leads V4, V5, and V6. This occurs because the pleural fluid blankets the transmission of the electrical field.

ABNORMAL COMPONENTS OF THE QRS COMPLEX
Abnormalities of the initial or terminal portions of the QRS complex may be small and may not alter the direction of the mean QRS vector. On the other hand, they may be sufficiently large to produce significant changes in the mean vector direction.

ABNORMALITIES OF THE INITIAL PORTION OF THE QRS COMPLEX: When the initial component of the QRS complex is negative, it is referred to as a Q wave. All normal subjects have an area on the body from which Q waves can be recorded.

Accordingly, a Q wave abnormality is defined not only in terms of its presence, but also in terms of the location and size of the Q wave area on the chest(15). A Q wave is analyzed by determining the direction and magnitude of the mean vector responsible for it, and through the relationship of this vector to the direction and amplitude of the mean QRS vector.

An abnormal initial QRS vector, which produces abnormal Q waves in the electrocardiogram, should not lead to an automatic, reflexive assumption that it is caused by myocardial infarction due to coronary atherosclerosis: there are many causes of abnormal initial QRS forces. They may be due to left or right ventricular hypertrophy; myocardial infarction due to coronary atherosclerosis; myocardial infarction due to other forms of coronary disease such as coronary spasm, dissection of the coronary arteries, coronary embolism, coronary thrombosis, or Kawasaki disease; acute myocarditis; dilated cardiomyopathy; hypertrophic cardiomyopathy; restrictive cardiomyopathy; primary or secondary neoplastic disease of the heart; amyloid disease; sarcoid of the heart; acute pulmonary embolism; Wolff-Parkinson-White syndrome; cardiac trauma; and certain types of congenital heart disease. Examples of these abnormalities are shown in Chapters 11 and 13.

The frontal plane projections of the normal 0.01, 0.02, 0.04, 0.06, and 0.08-second QRS vectors are shown in Figure 5.11. Normally, the initial 0.01 to 0.02-second QRS vectors are anterior to the subsequent QRS vectors. The vertical QRS loop should have a clockwise direction. The normal intermediate QRS loop can be directed in a clockwise or counterclockwise manner, and a normal horizontal QRS loop should be directed counterclockwise. The initial mean 0.01 or 0.02-second vector is abnormal whenever it is posterior to the subsequent QRS forces (Fig. 6.5). When directed to the right of a vertical mean QRS vector, identifying a counterclockwise rotation of the QRS loop, or located superior to a horizontal QRS loop, identifying a clockwise rotation of that loop, it is likely to be abnormal.

Whenever the mean initial 0.04-second QRS vector is directed to the right of a vertical mean QRS vector, or superior to a horizontal mean QRS vector, it is abnormal (Fig. 6.6). It is also abnormal when it is posterior to the mean QRS vector. This vector may normally be directed to either side of an intermediate mean QRS vector, but the angle between the two should be about 45°. Whenever the initial mean 0.04-second QRS vector is directed 60° or more away from the mean QRS vector it is likely to be abnormal.

MYOCARDIAL INFARCTION: Abnormal Q waves may be caused by myocardial infarction(15). This statement must not be interpreted as implying that all abnormal Q waves are due to myocardial infarction, or that abnormal Q waves, when due to infarction secondary to coronary disease, are always the result of coronary atherosclerosis: several types of coronary disease may cause myocardial infarction. Neither should the statement imply that myocardial infarction, regardless of the type of coronary disease causing it, always produces abnormal Q waves. In fact, the electrocardiogram may remain normal or show only T wave or ST-T wave abnormalities following myocardial infarction.

The mechanism responsible for the abnormal Q waves of myocardial infarction is best understood in terms of the anatomic characteristics of the left ventricle, the conduction system, and the depolarization sequence. The normal left ventricle is located to the left and slightly anteriorly; it rests on the left leaf of the diaphragm. The septum is anatomically continuous with the left ventricle, and the ventricular muscle at the apex is thinner than at the superior portions of the heart. There is little ventricular muscle opposite the apex of the left ventricle; the mitral and aortic valve orifices are located there. The superior portion of the left side of the septum is the first area of the myocardium to undergo depolarization; this is responsible for the initial 0.01-second vector. By 0.04 second, the depolarization process has spread through the endocardial area of both ventricles, and by 0.06 to 0.08 second, there are fewer right ventricular forces and more left ventricular forces dominating the electrical field. The terminal QRS forces are produced by the superior basilar portion of the left ventricle.

The abnormal Q waves of myocardial infarction are produced when early QRS forces are removed from one portion of the myocardium, permitting the early QRS forces generated by the myocardium on the opposite side of the ventricle to dominate the electrical field. Most infarctions involve the left ventricle of the heart, although the right ventricle can be involved by inferoseptal left ventricular infarction. Infarction of the right ventricle may occasionally occur without involvement of the left ventricle, and atrial infarction may also occur, but this is seldom recognized.

Abnormal Q waves develop in the electrocardiogram when an infarction occurs in the endocardial region, because the initial forces of the QRS complex are normally produced by this region of the left and right ventricles. The area of infarction must be sufficiently large and located in a proper site within the left ventricular endocardium for the QRS forces produced by the opposite ventricular wall to dominate the electrical field.

Unfortunately, for some obscure reason, it became common practice to refer to infarctions as *subendocardial* when the electrocardiogram showed T wave abnormalities but no Q waves. Today, this is more properly referred to as a non-Q wave infarction. It has also been customary to refer to an electrocardiogram exhibiting abnormal Q waves as revealing a transmural infarction. It is more accurate to say that it shows a Q wave infarction. Figure 6.7 illustrates how the location of an infarction of the left ventricle influences the direction of the mean initial 0.04-second vector, and how, in turn, this vector would determine the location of Q waves in the various leads of the electrocardiogram. Note in the illustration, that the Q wave actually results from electrical forces generated by the myocardium located opposite the area of infarction.

Somehow the notion has been perpetuated that a Q wave must be 0.04 second wide and be one fourth the size of the QRS complex to be considered abnormal. Although there is some merit to these requirements, it must be stressed that Q waves of 0.02 or 0.03 second duration may be abnormal when the mean vector representing them is: (A) directed to the right of a vertical mean QRS vector, (B) 60° away from a mean intermediate QRS vector, (C) superior to a mean horizontal QRS vector or (D) posterior to the vector representing the subsequent electrical forces (see Fig. 6.6).

It is important to remember that intramural infarcts can occur without producing Q wave abnormalities. Q waves may decrease in size as time passes, and an apical infarct may not be associated with an abnormal Q wave because there is no myocardium opposite it. Left bundle branch block may make it impossible to recognize initial force abnormalities. The more infarcts a patient has had, the fewer new electrocardiographic abnormalities appear after a new infarction.

The electrocardiographic abnormalities produced by myocardial infarctions are shown in detail in Chapter 11.

LEFT VENTRICULAR HYPERTROPHY VERSUS SEPTAL INFARCTION: Abnormal Q waves with a QRS complex of normal duration may be seen in patients with left ventricular hypertrophy. The initial 0.04-second QRS vector may be large in patients with large QRS vectors, and this is due to septal hypertrophy. The initial 0.04-second QRS vectors may be directed posteriorly in patients with horizontal mean QRS vectors. In such cases, the initial 0.04-second QRS vector is anterior to the mean QRS vector, as it should be, but it is posteriorly directed, so that no R waves are recorded in leads V1, V2, or even V3 (Fig. 6.8). When this phenomenon is seen, the observer should recognize that left ventricular hypertrophy alone can cause it. Certainly septal infarction can cause such an abnormality as well, but other data will be needed to prove it. Frequently, no explanation for the abnormality can be found by other methods of examination, including coronary arteriography.

The cause of absent R waves in leads V1, V2, and V3 in the absence of left ventricular hypertrophy or septal infarction is unknown, but it may be due to an initial QRS conduction defect. It should be emphasized that the absence of R waves in leads V1, V2, and V3 does not signify septal infarction nearly as definitely as the absence of R waves in leads V1 and V2 with a Q followed by an R and an S wave in lead V3 (see Fig. 6.5B). The Q wave in the latter circumstance indicates that the initial QRS forces are posterior to the subsequent QRS forces.

RIGHT VENTRICULAR HYPERTROPHY: Abnormal Q waves with a QRS complex of normal duration may also be seen in patients with right ventricular hypertrophy. An abnormal initial 0.04-second QRS vector may develop in patients with right ventricular hypertrophy, presumably because the direction of the septal electrical forces and the subsequent electrical forces becomes altered as a result of remodeling of the right ventricular architecture, including the septum itself. Normally, the septum is continuous with the left ventricle, but when right ventricular hypertrophy develops, the septum begins to conform to the circular shape of the right ventricle. When this occurs, the electrical forces generated by the septum and the endocardial layers of the two ventricles produce abnormal Q waves, presumably because the position of the septum changes (see Chapter 9).

MYOCARDITIS: Abnormal Q waves with a QRS complex of normal duration may, on rare occasions, be seen in patients with myocarditis. This occurs because the severe, extensive, inflammatory process of myocarditis destroys myocytes. When the destroyed myocytes are situated in the proper location, the result is no different from that occurring in a myocardial infarction; the electrical forces produced by the opposite myocardium dominate the electrical field.

CARDIOMYOPATHY: The electrocardiograms of patients with dilated, hypertrophic, or restrictive cardiomyopathy may exhibit abnormal Q waves with normal QRS durations (see Chapter 9). The abnormal Q waves of both dilated and restrictive cardiomyopathy are produced when a sufficient number of myocytes are replaced by fibrous tissue or some other substance such as amyloid, iron, or eosinophilic material. As with myocardial infarction, the myocardium opposite the abnormal tissue produces the abnormal electrical forces. The abnormal Q waves associated with hypertrophic cardiomyopathy are produced by a different mechanism. The hypertropic myocytes are often arranged in an abnormal fashion, referred to as myocardial cellular disarray. It is postulated that the Purkinje-myocyte unit is disordered, producing an early QRS conduction defect that gives rise to abnormal Q waves.

PULMONARY EMBOLISM: Abnormal Q waves and a QRS complex of normal duration may be produced by acute pulmonary embolism (see Fig. 13.2)(22). The initial QRS forces may be directed to the left and parallel with the frontal plane, and the terminal QRS forces may be directed to the right and anteriorly. This is due to an abrupt increase in pulmonary artery pressure, which results in the development of acute right ventricular wall stress and a delay in the right ventricular conduction system. The unbalanced electrical forces are directed far to the left during the early period of depolarization and to the right during the last period.

PENETRATING OR BLUNT TRAUMA: Penetrating or blunt trauma to the heart may produce abnormal Q waves through damage to a coronary artery or to the myocardium itself. The mechanism by which abnormal Q waves are produced is the same as for myocardial infarction due to coronary disease.

NEOPLASTIC DISEASE, AMYLOID DISEASE, SARCOID, AND OTHER SUBSTANCES: Primary and metastatic neoplastic heart disease may be associated with abnormal Q waves. The neoplastic tissue displaces normal myocytes, and the electrical forces produced by the opposite myocardial wall generate abnormal Q waves. Sarcoid, amyloid, and other substances may, when located in the proper site in the myocardium, produce abnormal Q waves. These substances displace normal myocytes, and the electrical forces produced by the opposite myocardial wall generate abnormal Q waves.

CONGENITAL DISEASE: Congenital disease of the coronary arteries may produce abnormal Q waves due to myocardial infarction. Other types of congenital heart disease may produce abnormal Q waves with normal QRS conduction. The cause is either right or left ventricular hypertrophy or a conduction defect. The electrical forces produced by the septum may be redirected so as to produce an abnormal Q wave, because the septum itself is often remodeled in such patients.

PRE-EXCITATION OF THE VENTRICLES: The initial QRS forces are abnormal when pre-excitation of the ventricles occurs. The abnormal Q waves may be misinterpreted as being caused by an anterior or posterior myocardial infarction. The QRS duration may be as short as 0.10 second or longer than 0.16 second. The PR interval is 0.12 second or less, and the initial portion of the QRS complex is slurred; this characteristic feature is called a *delta wave*. There are many types of this condition; the reader is referred to Chapter 8 for further discussion. Patients with this conduction disorder experience episodes of atrial tachycardia or uncontrolled atrial fibrillation with a ventricular rate of 200 to 300 ventricular depolarizations per minute. When the electrocardiographic abnormalities are associated with episodes of atrial tachycardia or fibrillation, the condition is called the Wolff-Parkinson-White syndrome(2). No associated disease may be detected, but the clinician should look for an atrial septal defect, Ebstein's anomaly, and hypertrophic cardiomyopathy, because the anomaly occurs more often in these conditions.

LEFT VENTRICULAR CONDUCTION DELAY:: The electrocardiographic abnormalities of *left ventricular conduction delay* resemble those of left bundle branch block except that the QRS duration is 0.10 or occasionally 0.11 second rather than 0.12 second as it is in left bundle branch block. The initial QRS vectors are directed to the left and posteriorly; no Q wave is seen in lead I or in lead V6, and the R wave is often absent in lead V1. The mean terminal 0.04-second vector is directed to the left and posteriorly; however, it is not so far to the left that the mean QRS vector is shifted beyond -30°. The condition is discussed further in Chapter 8. Left ventricular hypertrophy is commonly present, but the initial QRS abnormality is similar to that of left bundle branch block.

ABNORMALITIES OF THE TERMINAL PORTION OF THE QRS COMPLEX

RIGHT VENTRICULAR CONDUCTION DELAY: Right ventricular conduction delay(15) is characterized by a QRS complex duration of less than 0.10 second, with the mean QRS vector directed vertically or located in the intermediate zone. The terminal mean 0.04-second QRS vector is directed to the right and anteriorly, producing a prominent secondary R wave in lead V1. In brief, the electrocardiographic abnormalities in right ventricular conduction delay resemble those in right bundle branch block, as discussed later in this chapter, but the QRS duration is normal rather than prolonged. The reader is referred to Chapter 8, and to the discussion of diastolic overload of the right ventricle in Chapter 9.

Right ventricular conduction delay is a common abnormality and is not usually associated with other disease, in which case it is unimportant. It may, however, be associated with an atrial septal defect.

S1, S2, S3 PATTERN: The S1, S2, S3 pattern is a type of right ventricular conduction delay with a QRS complex of normal duration(23). The abnormality may be due to an unimportant conduction defect in the right ventricle, or it may be caused by cor pulmonale and emphysema. It may also be seen with mild pulmonary valve stenosis, although it is unexplained in this condition. The reader is referred to Chapter 8(15,23).

LEFT ANTERIOR-SUPERIOR AND LEFT POSTERIOR-INFERIOR DIVISION BLOCK: In order to understand the development of an abnormal mean terminal 0.04-second vector, it is necessary to review the direction of the normal third vector shown in Figure 6.9. This third vector is, for the most part, produced by the vector sum of the electrical forces generated by the left ventricular myocytes after their stimulation by the left anterior-superior and posterior-inferior divisions of the left bundle branch conduction system. The electrical forces produced by the myocytes controlled by these two divisions are generated simultaneously. The forces produced by the myocytes under the normal control of the anterior-superior division are directed inferiorly and anteriorly. Those produced by the myocytes under the control of the posterior-inferior division are directed superiorly and posteriorly. Vector three is the diagonal produced when the sides of a parallelogram are made of the vectors produced when the myocytes are stimulated by the two divisions of the left ventricular conduction system (Fig. 6.9).

Left anterior-superior division block(24) occurs when conduction is blocked in the anterior-superior division of the left bundle branch conduction system. The initial portion of the QRS complex is normal, and the QRS duration does not exceed 0.10 second. The direction of the mean QRS vector is greater than -30° in the frontal plane, because the posterior-inferior system conducts normally and the area of myocardium normally controlled by the anterior-superior division of the left conduction system, including the Purkinje branches, depolarizes in a direction almost opposite to normal. Although the depolarization process continues to be from endocardium to epicardium, the stimulus arrives at the endocardial area slightly later than it does normally, because it must spread from the region of endocardium serviced by the posterior-inferior division to the area normally serviced by the anterior-superior division. This produces a terminal mean 0.04-second QRS vector that is directed superiorly, to the left, and posteriorly (Fig. 6.9C).

Such a conduction block can be associated with, but is not due to, left ventricular hypertrophy. The defect may be caused by degeneration of the anterior-superior division, such as occurs in elderly persons when no other evidence of disease is found. It may occur in patients with dilated, hypertrophic, or restrictive cardiomyopathy; hypertension; calcific aortic stenosis; myocarditis; and acute or chronic coronary heart disease. It may also be produced by surgical replacement of the aortic valve. While the defect is usually located in the more distal portion of the left anterior-superior division, it may also be due to a precisely located defect within the common left bundle branch itself.

Left anterior-superior conduction block produces a mean QRS vector that is directed -30° or more to the left and a QRS duration at the upper limit of normal, about 0.10 second. This degree of left axis deviation must be differentiated from that due to inferior myocardial infarction, Wolff-Parkinson-White syndrome in which the QRS duration is normal, and tricuspid atresia (see Chapter 8).

Left posterior-inferior division block(24) occurs when conduction is blocked in the posterior-inferior division of the left ventricular conduction system. The initial portion of the QRS complex is normal, and the QRS duration does not exceed 0.10 second. The direction of the mean QRS vector is usually beyond +110°. I have arbitrarily required it to be at +120°, in order to distinguish these patients from the occasional normal subject whose mean QRS vector is directed +110° to the right.

When the posterior-inferior division of the left bundle branch system fails to conduct, the myocardium serviced by this portion of the conduction system is depolarized downward from above rather than upward from below, as occurs when the posterior-inferior division conducts normally. The electrical forces follow this direction because the wave of depolarization controlled by the anterior-superior division is intact (Fig. 6.9B). The wave of depolarization ordinarily controlled by the posterior-inferior division is directed opposite its normal orientation.

Left posterior-inferior division block may be caused by degeneration of the posterior-inferior division, such as occurs in elderly patients; myocarditis; cardiomyopathy; or coronary disease. Theoretically, the defect could occur if a precise segment of the common portion of the left bundle branch were damaged.

It is not possible to identify left posterior division block unless a previously recorded electrocardiogram is available for comparison. It is impossible to separate the development of this block from the vertical QRS loop of a tall, thin, normal subject. It is also necessary to exclude right ventricular hypertrophy, right ventricular conduction delay, pulmonary emphysema, and infarction of the lateral wall of the left ventricle as sources of a mean QRS vector that is directed +90° to +120° to the right.

HYPOTHERMIA: Hypothermia may produce a peculiar type of terminal QRS abnormality. The unusual defect is called an Osborn wave and is seen in patients who develop hypothermia as a result of exposure to extremely cold weather(25). The terminal depolarization abnormality is probably produced by the left ventricle, since one would think that its outer superior portion would be cooler than the other regions of the heart (see Fig. 8.22).

ABNORMAL QRS COMPLEX WITH PROLONGED QRS DURATION

The duration of the QRS complex of the normal adult is 0.10 second or less. As stated above, left anterior-superior division block or left posterior-inferior division block of the left conduction system causes a slight increase in the duration of the QRS complex, from its normal average of 0.08 to 0.09 second to 0.10 second, but not to 0.11 or 0.12 second(24).

LEFT BUNDLE BRANCH BLOCK: Left bundle branch block occurs when conduction is blocked in the proximal portion of the left bundle system(24). The QRS duration is usually 0.12 second in adults but may be prolonged to 0.14 or 0.16 second (see later discussions). The initial depolarization of the septum is from the right rather than the left ventricular surface. The mean QRS vector is directed to the left and posteriorly, and the mean initial 0.01 to 0.04-second QRS vectors are directed to the left and posteriorly. The terminal mean 0.04-second vector is directed to the left and posteriorly because the last portion of the heart to undergo depolarization is the basal region of the left ventricle (Fig. 6.10B).

I use the term *uncomplicated* to refer to the electrocardiogram when: the duration of the QRS complex is no more than 0.12 second; the mean QRS vector is not directed more than -30° to the left; the mean ST vector is relatively parallel with the mean T vector; and the T wave vector is due to a secondary repolarization abnormality (Fig. 6.10B). The conduction defect is usually located in the common bundle in such cases. Left bundle branch block is said to be *complicated* when: the QRS duration is greater than 0.12 second (it may be 0.14 or even 0.16 second);the mean QRS vector is directed more than -30° to the left (in such cases the mean terminal 0.04-second QRS vector may be directed as far as -100° to the left because there is associated left anterior-superior division block) (Fig. 6.10C); the mean ST vector is not parallel with the mean T vector; or there is an associated primary repolarization abnormality (primary T wave abnormality). The conduction defects in these patients are located in the more distal portions of the conduction system, and it is more likely that there will be damaged myocytes as well.

Normally, the first portion of the left bundle branch supplies small sub-branches to the left-superior side of the interventricular septum, and the first portion of the ventricles to depolarize is the left-superior portion of the septum. This is not possible when there is uncomplicated left bundle branch block; rather, the depolarization spreads from right to left and begins a little lower on the septum than normal. During the period from 0.01 to 0.02 second, the mean vector representing the electrical forces is directed to the left and posteriorly; no Q wave is written in lead I or V6, and no R wave is written in lead V1. The depolarization of the right ventricle proceeds normally, but the depolarization of the left ventricle is delayed by 0.03 to 0.04 second. This occurs because the depolarization process, spreading from right to left, must find its way into the intact left anterior-superior and posterior-inferior divisions of the left bundle branch conduction system. The terminal QRS forces are unopposed by other QRS forces. These leftward and posterior terminal QRS forces do not, however, cause the mean QRS vector to be shifted to the left as far as -30°. In fact, the mean QRS vector of uncomplicated left bundle branch block is usually in the intermediate or horizontal range (0 to + 60°). The number of degrees to which the mean QRS vector is directed to the left is determined, in part at least, by its direction prior to development of the left bundle branch block. In general, however, one should not expect the mean QRS vector to shift to the left more than 30° in uncomplicated left bundle branch block.

Uncomplicated left bundle branch block may be caused by myocardial infarction; congestive cardiomyopathy; aortic stenosis with impingement of calcium on the conduction system; aortic regurgitation; mitral annular calcification; surgical replacement of the aortic or mitral valve; sclerosis of the cardiac skeleton (Lev's disease)(26); Lenegre's disease (primary disease of the conduction system)(27); or drug toxicity. Since there are many causes of left bundle branch block, the common practice of using this electrocardiographic abnormality as a specific sign of coronary atherosclerosis is not wise. Even when coronary atherosclerotic heart disease is identified by coronary arteriography, the left bundle branch block may at times be due to some other disorder. Uncomplicated left bundle branch block may occur in the absence of any other identifiable heart disease.

Complicated left bundle branch block, as defined above, is often due to associated myocardial disease with its related distal conduction defects. It may be caused by all of the conditions responsible for uncomplicated left bundle branch block, but, as just stated, the myocardium itself is often diseased. I have observed that patients with complicated bundle branch block generally have more serious disease and a poorer prognosis than those with the uncomplicated condition.

Left bundle branch block, because of the altered sequence of depolarization, obscures the initial 0.04-second QRS vector abnormality produced by myocardial infarction.

Examples of electrocardiograms exhibiting left bundle branch block are shown in Chapter 8.

LEFT BUNDLE BRANCH BLOCK PLUS LEFT ANTERIOR-SUPERIOR DIVISION BLOCK.: This type of complicated left bundle branch block has the following features: the QRS duration is 0.12 second or greater, the mean QRS vector is directed -30° or more to the left and posteriorly, and the mean terminal 0.04-second QRS vector may be directed as much as 100° to the left and posteriorly. This combination of defects occurs because the spread of depolarization is from the right side of the septum into the portion of the left ventricle where the myocytes are normally stimulated by the left posterior-inferior division of the left bundle branch system.

The causes of this conduction defect include all of those listed in the discussion of complicated left bundle branch block. An example of this combination of conduction defects is shown in Chapter 8.

RIGHT BUNDLE BRANCH BLOCK: Right bundle branch block occurs when conduction is blocked in the proximal portion of the right bundle system(24). The QRS duration is usually 0.12 second but may be 0.10 second in young patients and 0.11second in some adults. The requirement for a QRS duration of 0.12 second is not as rigid as it is for left bundle branch block, and a QRS duration of 0.14 to 0.16 second is less likely to occur in this condition.

When there is right bundle branch block, the initial depolarization of the septum occurs normally and the initial QRS forces are directed normally. The mean QRS vector is directed to the right and anteriorly (Fig. 6.11B). The terminal mean 0.04-second QRS vector is directed to the right and anteriorly because the last portion of the heart to undergo depolarization is the anterior portion of the right ventricle. This delay in depolarization of the right ventricle occurs because depolarization must spread through the septum and gain access to the more distal portion of the right bundle branch system, a process that requires about 0.03 second.

I use the term *uncomplicated* right bundle branch block when: the mean QRS vector is directed less than +120° to the right; the initial mean 0.04-second QRS vector is almost normally directed; the QRS duration is 0.11 or 0.12 second; the terminal 0.04-second QRS vector is directed to the right and anteriorly; the mean ST vector is relatively parallel with the mean T vector; and the mean T vector is due to a secondary repolarization abnormality (Fig. 6.11B). Right bundle branch block is said to be *complicated* when: the mean QRS vector is directed more than +120° to the right; the mean initial 0.04-second QRS vector is abnormally directed (right

bundle branch block does not mask the mean initial 0.04-second abnormality of myocardial infarction); the mean terminal 0.04-second vector is directed far to the right and anteriorly; the QRS duration is greater than 0.12 second; the mean ST vector is not parallel with the mean T vector; or the mean T vector is due to a primary repolarization abnormality (Fig. 6.11C).

Uncomplicated right bundle branch block may be caused by or associated with cardiomyopathy, coronary disease, aortic stenosis, long-standing mitral regurgitation, severe right ventricular hypertrophy, pulmonary embolism, Lev's disease(26), Lenegre's disease(27), atrial septal defect, surgical repair of a congenital heart disease, such as ventricular septal defect, or drug toxicity. It may occur when there is no other evidence of heart disease. *Complicated* right bundle branch block may be due to any of the causes just mentioned, but whenever it is present, additional myocardial disease should be considered.

RIGHT BUNDLE BRANCH BLOCK PLUS LEFT ANTERIOR-SUPERIOR DIVISION BLOCK: In right bundle branch block plus left anterior-superior division block (Fig. 6.12), the QRS duration is 0.12 second or longer, and the mean QRS vector is directed more than -30° to the left and anteriorly or is parallel with the frontal plane(24). It is the anterior direction of the mean QRS vector that separates this abnormality from left bundle branch block. The mean initial 0.04-second QRS vector may be normal, as it is in isolated right bundle branch block. It is the direction of the terminal QRS vector that distinguishes the abnormality from uncomplicated right bundle branch block. In the latter, this vector is directed to the right and anteriorly. In isolated left anterior-superior division block, it is directed far to the left and posteriorly, because this portion of the left ventricle must be depolarized upward from below, as dictated by the intact posterior-inferior division of the left bundle branch system. In right bundle branch block *plus* left anterior-superior division block, the summation of these two terminal QRS vectors creates a terminal 0.04-second QRS vector that is often directed superiorly, parallel with the frontal plane, or anteriorly. This also redirects the mean QRS vector to the left and anteriorly

This unique variety of conduction system abnormality is commonly seen in patients with *sclerosis of the cardiac skeleton* as described by Lev(26). The sclerosis and calcification may impinge upon the conduction system, producing left bundle branch block, right bundle branch block, or complete atrioventricular block. Such patients may have calcification of the mitral or aortic valve annulus. Right bundle branch block and left anterior-superior division block may also be caused by: primary disease of the conduction system (Lenegre's disease)(27), which commonly progresses to complete heart block; multiple myocardial infarctions from coronary disease; dilated hypertrophic or restrictive cardiomyopathy; and a congenital endocardial cushion defect such as an ostium primum.

RIGHT BUNDLE BRANCH BLOCK PLUS LEFT POSTERIOR-INFERIOR DIVISION BLOCK: It is difficult to identify the combination of right bundle branch block plus left posterior division block (Fig. 6.13)(24), because it is never possible to be certain that the portion of the QRS complex attributed to left posterior division block is actually due to this condition or to some other disorder. The duration of the QRS complex is 0.12 second or greater. The mean QRS vector is directed to the right and is either parallel with, or anterior to, the frontal plane; it is also directed farther to the right than in uncomplicated right bundle branch block, but there is no sharp separation between the two conditions. The mean initial 0.04-second QRS vector is directed normally, as it is in right bundle branch block alone. The mean terminal 0.04-second QRS vector is directed far to the right and parallel with, or anterior to, the frontal plane.

When there is uncomplicated right bundle branch block, the terminal mean 0.04-second QRS vector is created by a normal vector 3 (Fig. 6.9D) plus the electrical forces generated by the right ventricle. When there is right bundle branch block and left posterior-inferior division block, the mean terminal 0.04-second QRS vector is directed farther to the right than in right bundle branch block alone; this redirects the mean QRS vector to more than +120° to the right. Accordingly, the mean QRS vector is directed further to the right than it is in isolated right bundle branch block (Fig. 6.11). This poses a difficult situation: it is not possible to state the exact number of degrees that define a condition as being due to right bundle branch block plus posterior division block, or to exclude other causes of the rightward deviation of the terminal QRS forces. For example, right ventricular hypertrophy plus right bundle branch block may be associated with a rightward mean terminal 0.04-second QRS vector that overlaps the extent of rightward deviation seen in right bundle branch with left posterior-inferior division block.

The diseases responsible for this combination of conduction defects are similar to those that produce right bundle branch and left anterior-superior division block, with the exception of endocardial cushion defects. Right bundle branch plus left posterior-inferior division block is rare, but when it occurs it is more likely to progress to complete heart block than is right bundle branch block alone (see Chapter 8).

RIGHT BUNDLE BRANCH BLOCK WITH PARTIAL OR COMPLETE ATRIOVENTRICULAR BLOCK AND BLOCKAGE OF EITHER DIVISION OF THE LEFT SYSTEM: This condition is recognized when *atrioventricular block* is added to the signs of right bundle branch block plus left anterior-superior or left posterior-inferior division block(24).

This combination of conduction defects is extremely serious, and complete heart block is likely to develop. It may be caused by the conditions listed in the section that deals with right bundle branch block plus left anterior-superior division block.

PRE-EXCITATION OF THE VENTRICLES: Pre-excitation of the ventricles occurs when an anomalous conduction pathway between the atria and ventricles produces early depolarization of the ventricles. The PR interval is short, and the QRS duration may be 0.10 to 0.16 second. The early portion of the QRS complex is slurred; this is called a *delta wave*. The direction of the terminal QRS electrical forces may also be altered simply because the depolarization sequence is profoundly altered. The condition is referred to as the Wolff-Parkinson-White syndrome when episodes of atrial tachycardia or atrial fibrillation occur(2). In the latter case there may be 200 to 300 ventricular depolarizations each minute.

DIFFUSE DISTAL CONDUCTION DEFECT: A poorly defined type of conduction defect occurs when many areas of the distal portions of the conduction system are damaged. This produces a QRS duration of 0.12 second or more. However, the configuration of the QRS complex does not conform to any of the usual conduction defects described above.

A diffuse distal conduction defect is caused by a condition that affects the ventricular muscle, such as cardiomyopathy, myocarditis, coronary disease, severe heart disease of any kind, hyperkalemia, or drug intoxication.

THE ELIMINATION OF CONFUSING TERMINOLOGY

In the past, the conduction system was often spoken of as having three fascicles: the right bundle branch, the left anterior-superior division branch, and the left posterior-inferior division branch. Strangely, the left bundle itself was omitted by some writers. Unifascicular block was said to be present when there was evidence of right bundle branch block, left anterior division block, or left posterior-inferior division block. Bifascicular block was said to be present when there was evidence of either left bundle branch or right bundle branch block plus left anterior-superior or left posterior-inferior division block. Trifascicular block included atrioventricular block plus left bundle branch block, atrioventricular block plus right bundle branch and left anterior-superior division block, or atrioventricular block plus right bundle branch and left posterior-inferior division block. This confusing terminology can be eliminated by identifying the location of the conduction defect(s) and omitting the words *unifascicular*, *bifascicular*, or *trifascicular*.

The terms *left anterior hemiblock* and *left posterior hemiblock* are often used to describe left anterior-superior or left posterior-inferior division conduction defects. This is inaccurate because the term "hemiblock" implies that 50 percent of the left conduction system is blocked. Tarawa described the conduction system on the left side as a tripartite rather than bipartite system (Fig. 4.10). It is true that the middle part of the system is initially related to the anterior-superior division, but it is more accurate to remember the tripartite nature of the left system, which is more like a fan than separate branches. Another reason to eliminate the term "hemiblock" is that beginners sometimes believe it means that conduction in the division is half blocked. Here again, the confusion is eliminated when the location of the conduction defect is specified.

The term *parietal block* is confusing and is replaced by the term left anterior-superior division block(12). The term *peri-infarction* block has been eliminated from terminology, but it may retain a place because there appear to be conduction defects associated with myocardial infarction that do not conform to the description of the conduction defects detailed above(28). In such cases, the mean initial 0.04-second QRS vector is directed away from the infarction, and the mean terminal 0.04-second QRS vector tends to be directed toward the infarction, because depolarization of the area of epicardium beyond the infarction is delayed.

FIGURE 6.4

The direction of the mean QRS vector due to right ventricular hypertrophy.

A. Acquired right ventricular hypertrophy may produce a mean QRS vector that is directed inferiorly or slightly to the right. The mean QRS vector may remain directed posteriorly. The QRS duration is 0.10 second or less.
B. Congenital heart disease, such as pulmonary valve stenosis or advanced acquired disease, produces a mean QRS vector that is directed more than +110° to the right and anteriorly. The QRS duration is 0.10 second or less.

FIGURE 6.5

The problem of "absent R waves" in leads V1, V2, and sometimes V3.

A. Transverse plane showing a normal QRS loop and normal QRS deflections in the chest leads. **B**. Transverse plane showing an abnormal QRS loop in which the initial QRS forces are posterior to the subsequent QRS forces; this produces an absent R wave in leads V1 and V2 and a Q wave followed by an R wave in lead V3. This abnormality is usually caused by anteroseptal infarction, and must be distinguished from the absent R wave due to left ventricular hypertrophy, as illustrated in Figure 6.8.

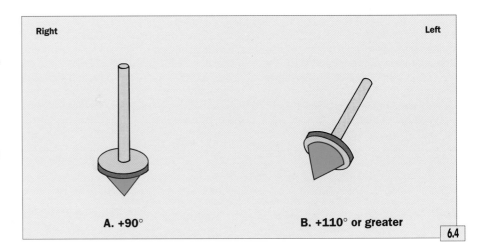

A. +90°   **B. +110° or greater**

6.4

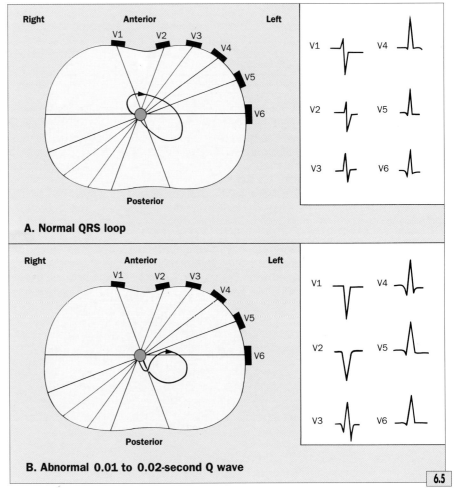

A. Normal QRS loop

B. Abnormal 0.01 to 0.02-second Q wave

6.5

FIGURE 6.6

Abnormal relationships between the mean initial 0.04-second QRS vector and the mean QRS vector.

A. The mean initial 0.04-second QRS vector is directed too far to the right of the vertical mean QRS vector to be considered normal; it should normally be directed to the left of the vertical mean QRS vector. It is also directed too far posteriorly; it should normally be anterior to the mean QRS vector. The angle between the mean initial 0.04-second QRS vector and the mean QRS vector is less than 60°, but its location is abnor-

mal. **B.** When the mean QRS vector is in the intermediate position, the mean initial 0.04-second QRS vector may be to the left or right of it. The angle between the two is abnormal when it is greater than 60°. The mean initial 0.04-second vector is abnormal when it is posterior to the vectors representing the subsequent QRS forces. **C.** When the mean initial 0.04-second QRS vector is directed far to the left (superior) of the horizontal mean QRS vector, it is abnormal. It should normally be directed to the right (inferior) of a horizontally directed mean QRS vector. In this illus-

tration, the mean initial 0.04-second QRS vector is directed posteriorly, which is usually abnormal. **D.** The mean initial 0.04-second QRS vector, directed to the left and posteriorly, is definitely abnormal because it is more posterior than the mean QRS vector. When its posterior orientation is smaller than is shown here, it is necessary to study the relationship of the mean initial 0.04-second vector or even the mean initial 0.02-second or 0.03-second vectors to the mean QRS vector to determine whether the initial QRS forces are posterior to the subsequent ones.

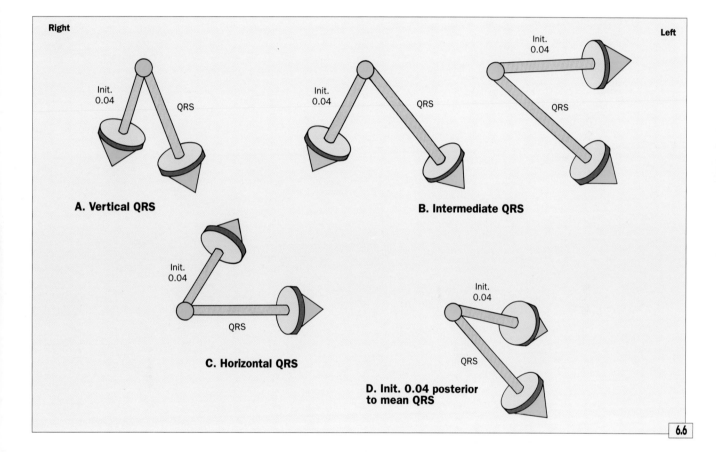

A. Vertical QRS

B. Intermediate QRS

C. Horizontal QRS

D. Init. 0.04 posterior to mean QRS

6.6

FIGURE 6.7

The effect of the location of a dead zone due to myocardial infarction on the direction of the mean initial 0.04-second QRS vector. The dead zone, shown in dark blue, is largest in the endocardium and decreases in size as it nears the epicardium. The area of injury is shown in medium blue; it is larger in the epicardium than in the endocardium. The area of ischemia is shown in light blue; it is larger in the epicardium than in the endocardium.

A. The infarction is located inferiorly. The mean initial 0.04-second QRS vector is directed away from the dead zone. The mean ST vector points toward the area of predominant epicardial injury, and the mean T vector is directed away from the area of predominant epicardial ischemia. This produces abnormal Q waves in leads II, III, and aVF, as well as elevated ST segments and inverted T waves in leads II, III, and aVF; the R wave in lead V1

might be prominent. **B.** The effect of an apical infarction on the mean initial 0.04-second QRS vector. Because there is no myocardium opposite the apex, the normal mean initial 0.04-second QRS vector is simply diminished in size; the ST segment vector points toward the epicardial injury surrounding the infarction, making the ST segment vector of apical infarction somewhat similar to that of pericarditis. The mean T vector may become smaller or, if the

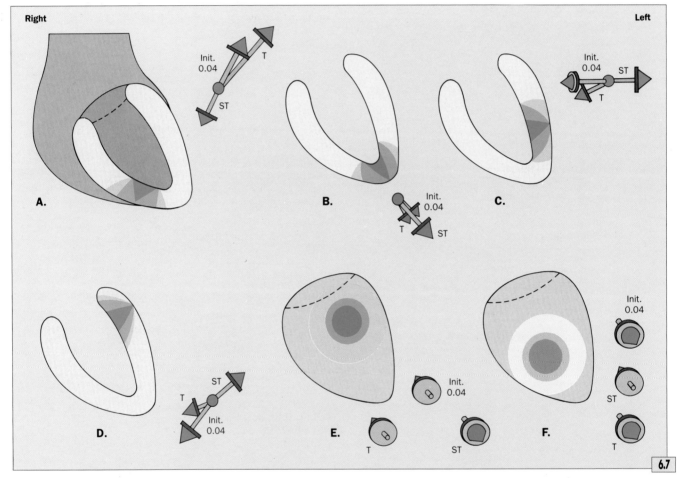

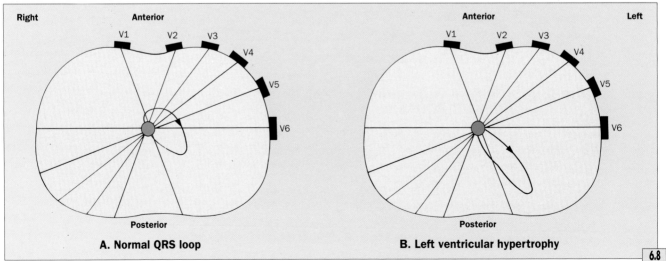

A. Normal QRS loop

B. Left ventricular hypertrophy

(Figure 6.7 continued.)
epicardial ischemia does not perfectly surround the apex, abnormally directed. **C.** The effect of a lateral infarction on the mean initial 0.04-second QRS vector, the mean ST vector, and the mean T vector. The electrocardiogram would show abnormal Q waves in leads I, II, aVL, V4, V5, and V6. **D.** The effect of a superior (basilar) lateral infarction on the mean initial 0.04-second QRS vector, the mean ST vector, and the mean T vector. The electrocardiogram of this unusual infarction would show abnormal Q waves in leads I and aVL. The direction of the mean initial 0.04-second QRS vector in the precordial leads would vary according to whether the 0.04-second vector was directed anteriorly or posteriorly. **E.** The infarction is located anteriorly. The mean initial 0.04-second QRS vector is directed posteriorly, the mean ST vector is directed anteriorly, and the mean T vector is directed posteriorly. The electrocardiogram would show abnormal Q waves in leads V1,V2, V3, V4, and sometimes V5; ST segment elevation and T wave inversion would appear in leads V1, V2, V3, V4, and sometimes V5. **F.** The infarction is located in the posterior portion of the left ventricle—a true posterior infarc-

tion. The mean initial 0.04-second QRS vector is directed anteriorly, the mean ST vector is directed posteriorly, and the mean T vector is directed anteriorly. The electrocardiogram would show abnormally tall R waves in leads V1 and V2; depressed ST segments in leads V1, V2, perhaps V3, and rarely V4; and prominent T waves in leads V1 through V3 or V4.

FIGURE 6.8
The influence of the shape and location of the QRS loop of left ventricular hypertrophy on the precordial electrodes, so that no initial R waves are recorded in leads V1, V2, or V3.
A. The QRS loop of a normal person as viewed in the transverse plane. There would a small R wave in lead V1, which would gradually increase in size as recordings were made with leads V2, V3, V4, V5, and V6. **B.** The QRS loop of a patient with left ventricular hypertrophy as viewed in the transverse plane. The QRS loop is larger than normal and may be directed posteriorly, so that no R waves are recorded in leads V1, V2 or V3. Though such an abnormality may be due to septal infarction, it is usually due to left ventricular hypertrophy. This is quite differ-

ent from the absence of R waves in leads V1, V2, and V3 described in Figure 6.5B.

FIGURE 6.9
The creation of vector 3.
A. Vector 1 is produced by depolarization of the superior portion of the ventricular septum. Vector 2 is produced by endocardial-subendocardial depolarization of the right and left ventricles. Vector 3 is composed of the electrical forces generated by the myocytes serviced by the anterior-superior division (A-S) and the posterior-inferior (P-I) division of the left conduction system. **B.** The electrical forces generated by the myocytes serviced by the superior-inferior division. **C.** The electrical forces generated by myocytes serviced by the posterior-inferior division. **D.** The formation of vector 3 when the depolarization process occurs simultaneously in the anterior-superior and posterior-inferior divisions of the left ventricular conduction system. Note that vector 3 is the diagonal for the parallelogram whose sides are made up of forces produced by myocytes serviced by the A-S and P-I divisions of the left ventricular conduction system.

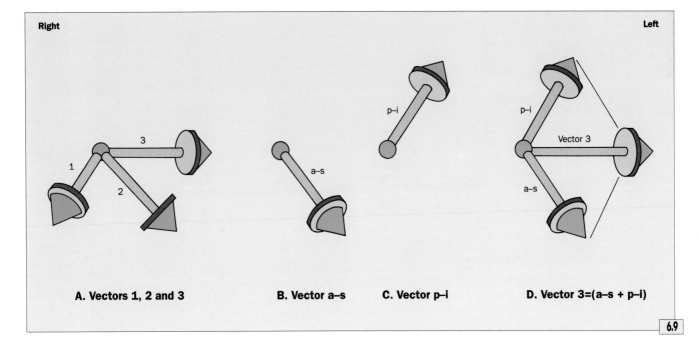

Right   Left

A. Vectors 1, 2 and 3   B. Vector a–s   C. Vector p–i   D. Vector 3=(a–s + p–i)

F I G U R E   6 . 1 0
Left bundle branch block.

A. Normally, the duration of the QRS complex is 0.10 second or less. The mean QRS vector may be directed from -30° to the left to +110°. The normal mean initial 0.04-second QRS vector is directed to the left of a vertical mean QRS vector, inferior to a horizontal mean QRS vector, and on either side of an intermediate QRS vector. The normal mean initial 0.04-second QRS vector is always anterior to the mean QRS vector. The terminal mean 0.04-second QRS vector is usually directed to the right of a vertical mean QRS vector, superior to a horizontal mean QRS vector, and on

either side of an intermediate mean QRS vector (the angle between the two should be less than 60°). It should be posterior to the mean QRS vector. **B.** In uncomplicated left bundle branch block, the duration of the QRS complex is 0.12 second, and the initial mean 0.04-second QRS vector is shifted to the left and posteriorly; no Q wave is seen in leads 1 and V6 because the depolarization of the septum is from right to left rather than left to right. This prevents the identification of the dead-zone effect of myocardial infarction. The mean QRS vector should be directed less than -30° to the left and posteriorly. The terminal 0.04-second QRS vector is directed to

the left and posteriorly but is not so far to the left that the mean QRS vector is shifted more than -30°. **C.** In complicated left bundle branch block the duration of the QRS complex is greater than 0.12 second, and the initial mean 0.04-second QRS vector is directed to the left and posteriorly; no Q wave is seen in leads I and V6. The terminal mean 0.04-second QRS vector may be shifted so far to the left and posteriorly that it influences the mean QRS vector to be directed more than -30° to the left.

This type of electrocardiogram is usually produced by left bundle branch block plus left anterior-superior division block at distal sites in the myocardium.

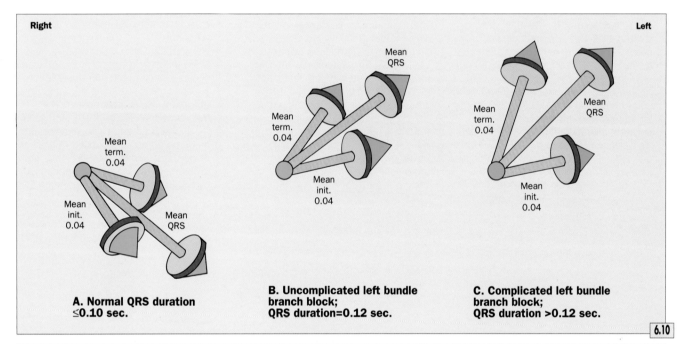

A. Normal QRS duration ≤0.10 sec.

B. Uncomplicated left bundle branch block; QRS duration=0.12 sec.

C. Complicated left bundle branch block; QRS duration >0.12 sec.

6.10

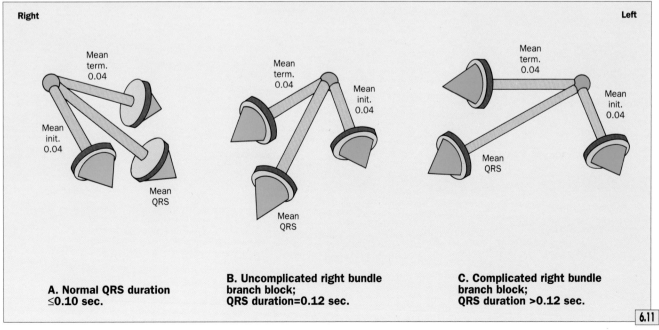

A. Normal QRS duration ≤0.10 sec.

B. Uncomplicated right bundle branch block; QRS duration=0.12 sec.

C. Complicated right bundle branch block; QRS duration >0.12 sec.

6.11

FIGURE 6.11

Right bundle branch block.

A. The normal duration of the QRS complex is 0.10 second or less. The mean initial 0.04-second QRS vector is directed inferiorly and slightly anteriorly. The mean QRS vector is directed inferiorly and posteriorly, and the mean terminal 0.04-second QRS vector is directed to the left of and posterior to it.

B. Uncomplicated right bundle branch block. The duration of the QRS complex is 0.12 second. The mean initial 0.02-second QRS forces are directed normally because the first part of the septum is depolarized normally; early branches of the left bundle branch supply the conduction pathway for the stimulus that depolarizes the first part of the septum. The direction of the mean initial 0.04-second QRS vector may appear normal in that the vector may be directed inferiorly and probably a little to the right of its usual direction. It is directed anteriorly. Because the early forces are nearly normal, it is possible to identify the dead-zone effect of myocardial infarction. Left ventricular hypertrophy may be identified when the mean 0.06-second QRS vector is large. The direction of the mean QRS vector is usually less than +120° to the right. The terminal mean 0.04-second QRS vector is directed to the right and anteriorly, but not so far that it influences the mean QRS vector to shift beyond +120° to the right.

C. Complicated right bundle branch block.

The duration of the QRS complex is greater than 0.12 second, and the mean initial 0.02-second QRS vector is normal. The mean initial 0.04-second vector is shifted a little more to the right than usual, but remains directed inferiorly and anteriorly. The mean QRS vector may be directed more than +120° to the right and anteriorly. The terminal mean 0.04-second QRS vector is shifted far to the right and anteriorly, redirecting the mean QRS vector more than +120° to the right. This type of electrocardiogram may be caused by right bundle branch block and left posterior-inferior division block.

FIGURE 6.12

Right bundle branch block plus left anterior-superior division block.

The QRS duration is 0.12 second or greater, and the initial 0.04-second QRS vector may be directed normally. The mean QRS vector is directed more than -30° to the left and anteriorly, and the terminal 0.04-second QRS vector is directed superiorly (more than -90°) and anteriorly. This occurs because the anterior-superior division of the left bundle branch system is blocked. Therefore, the depolarization of the left ventricle is guided by the posterior-inferior division, producing a mean vector that is directed far to the left. In addition to this, the myocardium ordinarily served by the left

anterior-superior system is depolarized in a reversed fashion. Both of these together, when added to the terminal QRS vectors associated with right bundle branch block which are directed to the right and anteriorly, cause the mean QRS vector and the terminal 0.04 second vector to be directed to the left, superiorly and anteriorly.

FIGURE 6.13

Right bundle branch block plus left posterior-inferior division block.

The QRS duration is 0.12 second or greater, and the mean initial 0.04-second QRS vector is directed vertically and anteriorly. The terminal 0.04-second vector is directed far to the right and anteriorly, to the degree that it influences the mean QRS vector to be shifted more than +120° to the right. This occurs because the posterior-inferior division is blocked, leaving the depolarization of the left ventricle under the control of the left anterior-superior division of the left bundle branch system. Further, the area of myocardium serviced by the left posterior-inferior division depolarizes in a reverse fashion. When the electrical forces produced in this manner are added to the terminal forces produced by the right bundle branch block, the mean terminal 0.04-second QRS vector will be directed far to the right, and the mean QRS vector will be +120° or more to the right.

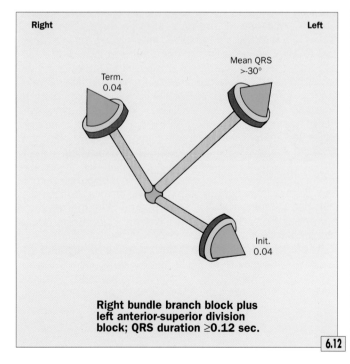

Right bundle branch block plus
left anterior-superior division
block; QRS duration ≥0.12 sec.

6.12

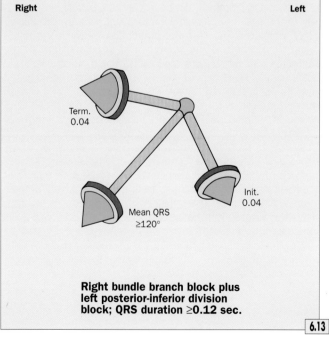

Right bundle branch block plus
left posterior-inferior division
block; QRS duration ≥0.12 sec.

6.13

THE ST SEGMENT

Normally the ST segment does not deviate from the baseline of the electrocardiogram. However, it may occasionally deviate slightly, because in certain circumstances the Ta wave may influence the early part of the ST segment. It may also deviate from the baseline when early, but normal, repolarization occurs. In these cases, the T waves are large and the mean ST vector is parallel with the large mean T vector. There is little day-to-day change, unlike the ST segment displacement of pericarditis or myocardial ischemia. This normal "early repolarization" is common in athletes (see Chapter 13).

THE ST SEGMENT VECTOR ASSOCIATED WITH VENTRICULAR HYPERTROPHY OR BUNDLE BRANCH BLOCK

The direction of the mean ST segment vector associated with right or left ventricular hypertrophy tends to be parallel with that of the mean T vector (see Chapter 9). This is true for ventricular hypertrophy due to systolic or diastolic pressure overload of the left ventricle.

The mean ST vector associated with bundle branch block tends to be relatively parallel with the mean T vector.

THE ST SEGMENT VECTOR OF PERICARDITIS

Pericarditis is rarely localized to a small patch of pericardium; it is usually diffuse, involving the entire pericardium(4). In this condition, it is the damaged epicardial surface of the ventricles that produces the electrocardiographic abnormalities; the pericardium generates no electrical energy. When pericardial fluid is present, the amplitude of the QRS and T waves may be diminished and electrical alternans may be present (see Chapter 10). Initially, a mean ST vector is apparent; it is directed toward the centroid of the damaged epicardium and points toward the anatomic apex of the left ventricle (Fig. 6.14). This produces an ST segment vector that is usually directed parallel with the frontal plane projection of the normal mean QRS vector. It is, however, usually directed anteriorly to the mean QRS vector. This occurs because the generalized epicardial injury is not influenced by the conduction system that controls the sequence of depolarization of the ventricles and directs the mean QRS vector to the left and posteriorly. The mean ST vector, representing generalized pericarditis, is directed toward the anatomical apex of the left ventricle, which is located slightly anterior to the mean QRS vector. The abnormality of the ST segment vector gradually subsides, and as it does, the abnormality of the mean T vector becomes more pronounced. The mean T vector becomes directed away from the centroid of epicardial damage and away from the anatomic apex of the left ventricle. It eventually decreases in size and returns to normal, but it may be permanently decreased in amplitude. The evolution of the four electrocardiographic phases associated with pericarditis is illustrated in (Fig. 6.15).

In the past, it was taught that the ST-T abnormalities of pericarditis produced no "reciprocal changes," while those of myocardial infarction were accompanied by "reciprocal changes." For example, a reciprocal change was said to be present when an ST segment elevation in lead III was accompanied by a depressed ST segment in lead I or vice versa. When ST segment elevation occurred in all of the bipolar extremity leads and aVF, the electrocardiogram was said to exhibit no reciprocal change. The clinician memorized the deviation (up or down) of the ST segment displacement in all other extremity and precordial leads. Such memorization is not necessary if one recalls that the mean ST segment vector points toward an area of epicardial injury, and the mean T vector points away from the area of epicardial ischemia. When the damage is due to hypoxia, as occurs with coronary disease, it tends to be localized to a specific area of the left ventricle, either inferiorly, posteriorly, laterally, or anteriorly. The mean ST and mean T vectors are *not* parallel with the mean QRS vector; they are often directed 90° or more away from the mean QRS vector. It is this arrangement that produces reciprocal changes.

Pericarditis does not cause reciprocal changes because the mean ST segment vector tends to point toward the centroid of diffuse epicardial injury produced by generalized epicardial damage (Fig. 6.14). Consequently, the mean ST vector points toward the anatomic apex of the left ventricle and is relatively parallel with the mean QRS vector, and the mean T vector becomes directed away from the mean QRS vector. Accordingly, the ST segment tends to be elevated in the extremity leads, with the exception of lead aVR, and in the precordial leads, except leads V1 and possibly V2.

The mechanism responsible for the ST segment elevation associated with pericarditis is probably similar to that causing the ST segment displacement of epicardial injury due to intense myocardial ischemia. As will be discussed in the next section, the electrical forces responsible for the latter occur during the TQ as well as the ST segment interval.

THE ST SEGMENT VECTOR OF MYOCARDIAL ISCHEMIA

Tradition holds that myocardial infarction due to obstructive coronary disease of any type *may* produce abnormal Q waves, ST segment abnormalities, and T wave abnormalities. The Q wave abnormality has been ascribed to a *dead zone effect* that removes certain depolarization forces from the endocardial-subendocardial area of the left ventricle, permitting the forces of the diametrically opposite myocardium to dominate the electrical field (Fig. 6.7). The ST segment abnormality has been attributed to an *injury current* that is thought to be secondary to more intense hypoxia surrounding the dead zone. The T wave abnormality is due to *ischemia* and is produced by hypoxia that is less intense than that responsible for the injury current. Thus, myocardial hypoxia due to coronary disease is thought to result in *dead myocardial cells* that give rise to *abnormal Q waves*, injured cells that produce *abnormal ST segments*, and ischemic cells that produce *abnormal T waves*.

The purpose of this section is to discuss the ST segment displacement, referred to as injury, that is caused by myocardial hypoxia. This displacement, caused by intense myocardial ischemia (injury), has captured the interest of many investigators. There is no question that the mean ST segment vector points toward the area of predominant epicardial injury. But why? Three theories have been advanced to explain this phenomenon, but in order to understand them, it is necessary to recall that electrical systole of the ventricles occurs during the QT interval of the electrocardiogram, and that electrical diastole occurs during the TQ segment. The QT interval is defined as the interval that begins with the onset of the Q wave and ends with the end of the T wave; the TQ segment is the interval that begins with the end of the T wave and ends with the beginning of the Q wave.

The depolarization and repolarization of the ventricles occur during the QT interval. The ST segment of the electrocardiogram represents the time at which the ventricular myocytes are depolarized. The T wave itself is due to the repolarization. Undoubtedly, the repolarization of a few cells begins just after the QRS complex ends, but as a rule this number is insufficient to alter the ST segment. At times, with normal early repolarization or when the T wave is altered by ventricular hypertrophy or bundle branch block, the forces of repolarization appear earlier than usual (during the ST segment) and follow the course of the T wave abnormality.

The TQ segment represents a period when almost all of the ventricular myocytes have been repolarized and are waiting for the stimulus that initiates depolarization. During this period, the myocytes are electrically "at rest." While the U wave, to be discussed subsequently, represents a poorly understood salvo of repolarization forces that occur during the TQ segment, the majority of myocytes have repolarized prior to the U wave.

The theories that have been postulated to explain why the mean ST segment vector points toward the area of predominant epicardial injury have been beautifully discussed by Holland and Brooks(29). They are as follows:

• *Current Produced During Electrical Diastole.*
Several investigators have suggested that epicardial injury produces displacement of the baseline during the TQ segment. When an area of myocardium is injured by severe ischemia, it cannot repolarize normally. Therefore, during ventricular repolarization, the damaged myocytes fail to repolarize normally or, if you will, continue to be depolarized as compared with the surrounding muscle. When this occurs, the flow of current is from the injured cells to the normal cells. The electrical forces responsible for the current, represented as vectors, are directed away from the injured tissue, creating a downward displacement of the TQ segment. An artifact is then produced because the electrocardiograph machine uses an alternating current coupled with amplifiers that sense the displacement of the QT segment and interject an equal and opposite electrical force sufficient to bring the stylus of the machine back to the baseline. This eliminates the TQ segment shift. Following this, the depolarization process produces the QRS complex, and the electrical charges on the myocytes are lost. At this time the machine-induced force becomes apparent during the ST segment. However, the displacement of the baseline during the

ST segment is opposite in direction to the displacement during the TQ segment, because it is produced by the machine-induced artifact used earlier to "neutralize" the ST segment displacement of the TQ interval.
• *Current Produced During Electrical Systole*(29).
Some investigators believe that the muscle injured by myocardial ischemia cannot become completely depolarized. The electrical forces can be represented as vectors directed toward the injured muscle.
• *Combination of the Previously Listed Mechanisms.*
Many investigators believe that the combination of a diastolic current, with its machine-induced artifact, plus a systolic current produces the ST segment displacement associated with injured myocytes(29).

Holland and Brooks created the excellent diagram reproduced with permission in Figure 6.16(29). It shows the possible causes of the ST segment displacement of localized epicardial injury.

Figure 6.7 illustrates the usual areas involved with epicardial injury due to obstructive coronary disease. Note that the mean ST vector is directed toward the area of epicardial injury. The reader is also referred to Figure 6.17.

The ST segment displacement of pericarditis is probably due to the same mechanisms as described in myocardial ischemia, but the injury tends to be more generalized. The ST segment vector of epicardial injury related to myocardial infarction is directed toward the area of epicardium that is involved, which is usually 90° or more away from the direction of the mean QRS vector. On the other hand, the mean ST vector of pericarditis points toward the centroid of generalized epicardial injury; the ST vector is directed almost parallel with the mean normal QRS vector (Fig. 6.14).

The electrocardiographic representation of subendocardial injury due to coronary disease differs significantly from that of epicardial injury. The mean ST segment vector is directed away from the area of subendocardial injury(12) and tends to be directed away from the mean QRS vector (Fig. 6.18). Subendocardial injury is likely to be generalized. It often occurs with spontaneous angina pectoris, during a positive exercise test or global myocardial ischemia. It can be secondary to hypotension in a patient with coronary disease, and it is more likely to occur in patients who also have left ventricular hypertrophy or increased left ventricular diastolic pressure. When subendocardial injury persists for hours, the electrocardiographic abnormality is likely to give way to the QRS, ST, and T wave changes typical of infarction, which reveal evidence of epicardial injury and ischemia with or without Q waves.

Some years ago, a myocardial infarct that showed ST and T wave abnormalities, or a T wave abnormality alone, was referred to as a subendocardial infarct. This type of infarct is currently and more properly referred to as a non-Q wave infarct; the anatomic correlate, which is not known, should not be specified. This is proper because some non-Q wave infarcts are transmural and some Q wave infarcts are nontransmural.

F I G U R E   6 . 1 4

The epicardial injury of pericarditis compared with the myocardial injury of myocardial infarction.

A. Pericarditis.

The epicardial damage caused by pericarditis is generalized. Accordingly, a mean ST segment vector produced by injured epicardium will be directed toward the centroid of epicardial damage; it is directed toward the anatomic cardiac apex. The mean ST vector will be directed to the left, inferiorly and parallel with the frontal plane, producing an elevated ST segment in leads I, II, III, aVF, V2, V3, V4, V5, and V6. The mean ST vector is directed relatively parallel with, but usually anterior to, the frontal plane direction of the normal mean QRS vector. **B**. The epicardial injury surrounding a myocardial infarction is located predominantly in the epicardium. The injury does not involve the entire epicardium of the left ventricle; rather, it is localized to various segments. This illustration shows an infarction of the lateral left ventricular wall. The mean ST vector is directed to the left and superiorly; this produces an elevated ST segment in lead I, an isoelectric ST segment in lead II, and a downward displacement of the ST segment in lead III. The ST segment would be elevated in lead aVL, displaced downward in lead aVF, and slightly depressed in lead aVR. The influence of the epicardial injury on the precordial leads would depend upon how anteriorly or posteriorly the injury was located.

F I G U R E   6 . 1 5

The four electrocardiographic phases of pericarditis.

A. Normal. The mean QRS and mean T vectors are directed normally. **B**. Phase 1 of pericarditis. The ST segment vector is directed toward the centroid of generalized epicardial injury. The mean QRS vector is not altered unless pericardial fluid is present; the voltage may be diminished when this occurs. The mean T vector may or may not be altered; if it is, it will be diminished in size.

C. Phase 2 of pericarditis. The mean ST segment vector and mean T vector may decrease in size but retain the same direction as shown in part B.
D. Phase 3 of pericarditis. The mean ST segment vector becomes smaller, but its direction does not change. The mean T vector is opposite the centroid of generalized epicardial damage; the

epicardial injury is giving way to generalized epicardial ischemia. **E**. Phase 4 of pericarditis. The electrocardiogram returns to normal, or the T waves may be smaller than they were prior to the pericarditis. Should the epicardial damage become localized, the mean T vector may change direction, and at times the T waves may remain inverted.

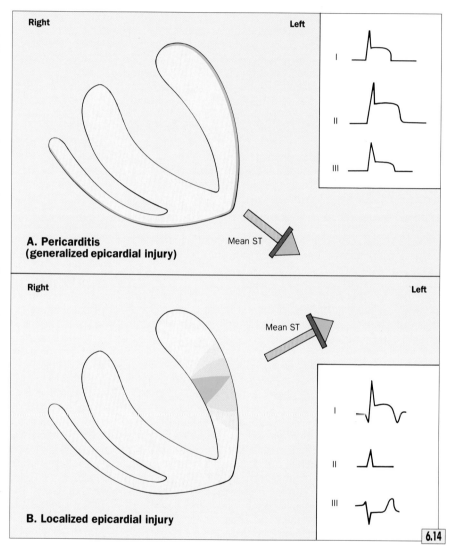

A. Pericarditis (generalized epicardial injury)

B. Localized epicardial injury

6.14

FIGURE 6.16

Top left: Transmembrane potentials of ischemic (broken curve) and normal (solid curve) tissue. Numbers indicate phases 0 to 4. Phase 0 = initial rapid upstroke; phase 1 = phase of early rapid repolarization; phase 2 = plateau phase of slow repolarization; phase 3 = terminal phase of rapid repolarization; phase 4 = diastolic period. **Bottom left**: Electrocardiogram recorded by an electrode overlying the ischemic tissue. The TQ segment is located below the isoelectric line (broken), and the ST segment above. **Top right**: Potential gradients existing at the boundary between normal (-90 mv) and ischemic (-70 mv) tissue during electrical dias-tole. **Bottom right**: Potential gradients existing at the boundary between normal (+5 mv) and ischemic (-15 mv) tissue at mid systole. Arrows indicate the direction of current flow (positive to negative) at the boundary. (Figure and legend reproduced with permission from the publisher and author; see Figure Credits.)

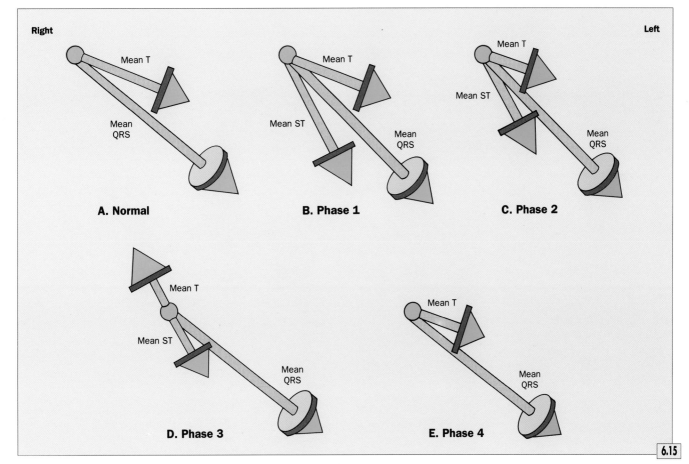

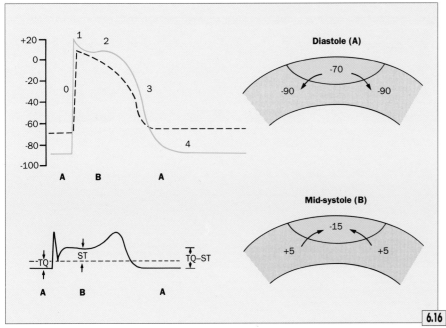

FIGURE 6.17

The influence of myocardial infarction on the mean QRS vector, the initial mean 0.04-second QRS vector, the mean ST vector, and the mean T vector.

A. Infarction of the lateral-superior segment of the left ventricle. Only the frontal plane view is shown, but the area of damage could also be located anteriorly or posteriorly. Note that the dead zone

(dark blue) is largest in the endocardial area; the area of injury (medium blue) and the area of ischemia (light blue) are largest in the epicardium. **B.** This figure shows the mean QRS vector, the mean initial 0.04-second QRS vector, the mean ST vector, and the mean T vector produced by the myocardial infarction located as shown in part A. **C.** Lead I of an electrocardiogram recorded from a

patient with a myocardial infarction as shown in part A.

FIGURE 6.18

Subendocardial injury.

The mean ST vector produced by subendocardial injury is directed away from the centroid of such injury; subendocardial injury due to hypoxia is likely to be generalized.

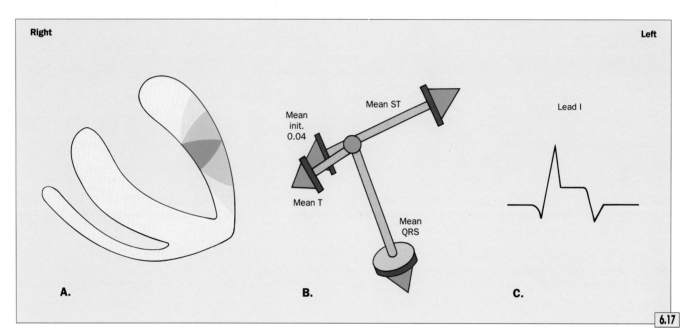

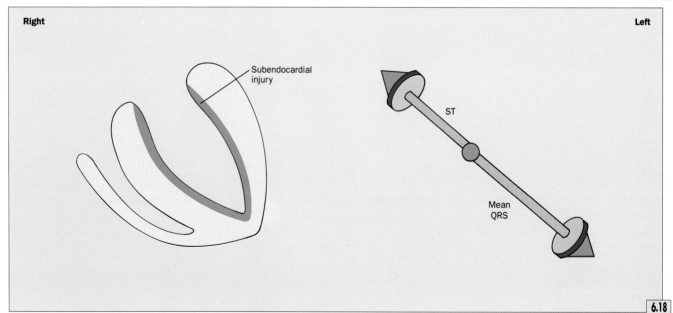

T WAVE ABNORMALITIES

THE DURATION AND SIZE OF THE T WAVE

HYPERKALEMIA: As a result of hyperkalemia, the amplitude of the T wave becomes greater than normal, and the ascending and descending limbs of the T wave tend to be equally slanted (9). This produces a "tent-like" T wave.

HYPOKALEMIA: The T wave becomes longer and smaller and joins a prominent U wave in hypokalemia(10). Sometimes the U and T waves unite in a perfect blend so that they cannot be separated. When this occurs, the QT interval is longer than normal, and the T wave also appears longer than average. Examples of electrocardiograms reflecting hyperkalemia and hypokalemia are shown in Chapter 13.

UNEXPLAINED LOW T WAVES: Occasionally an electrocardiogram is seen in which the T waves may be smaller than average but the direction of the mean T vector may be normal. T waves may even be imperceptible in rare cases. More often than not, the cause of this finding is not discovered, and it is often benign.

ALTERATION OF THE DIRECTION OF THE MEAN T VECTOR: THE QRS-T ANGLE

THE MEAN T VECTOR IN LEFT VENTRICULAR HYPERTROPHY:

DIASTOLIC PRESSURE OVERLOAD OF THE LEFT VENTRICLE(30,31): such as occurs with aortic regurgitation, mitral regurgitation, patent ductus arteriosus, or ventricular septal defect, may produce a large T wave vector that is directed about 45° to 60° or more away from the mean QRS vector. In such cases, the mean vector representing the ST segment tends to be parallel with the large mean T vector (Fig. 6.19). It must be emphasized that these abnormalities occur during the early stages of the disease process. During the later stages, the ST and T vectors assume the characteristics of left ventricular systolic pressure overload.

The cause of the ST-T wave abnormality associated with diastolic overload is poorly understood. The ST segment and T wave are both due to repolarization and are produced during the late stage of left ventricular mechanical systole. However, the after load against which the ventricle contracts is less than in systolic pressure overload. The direction of the repolarization process continues to be from epicardium to endocardium. As the diastolic pressure in the left ventricle increases secondary to diastolic pressure overload, the transmyocardial systolic pressure gradient of late-stage mechanical ventricular systole increases, producing the electrocardiographic characteristics of systolic pressure overload (see Chapter 9).

SYSTOLIC PRESSURE OVERLOAD OF THE LEFT VENTRICLE(30,31): occurs with aortic valve stenosis, systemic hypertension, hypertrophic cardiomyopathy, or advanced diastolic overload of the left ventricle. The mean T vector tends to rotate away from the mean QRS vector, so when the latter is directed to the left and posteriorly, the former begins to drift rightward and anteriorly (Fig. 6.20B). After a period of time, the mean T vector will lie 180° away from the mean QRS vector. A vector representing the ST segment tends to be parallel with the direction of the mean T vector (Fig. 6.20). When the mean QRS vector is directed vertically, the mean T vector tends to rotate more anteriorly until it attains a superior position. The T wave abnormality is probably due to an increase in, and final elimination of, the transmyocardial pressure gradient during the late stage of left ventricular mechanical systole (Fig. 6.21). The ST segment displacement is due to early repolarization forces.

An example of an electrocardiogram exhibiting systolic pressure overload of the left ventricle is shown in Chapter 9.

THE MEAN T VECTOR AND RIGHT VENTRICULAR HYPERTROPHY:

DIASTOLIC PRESSURE OVERLOAD OF THE RIGHT VENTRICLE(30,31) should theoretically produce a mean T vector that is larger than average, and the ST segment vector should be parallel to the mean T vector(30). Actually, the most common cause of diastolic overload of the right ventricle is a secundum atrial septal defect in which a right ventricular conduction defect dominates the electrocardiogram. The T wave abnormality in such a patient is secondary to the QRS abnormality (see the discussion below regarding primary and secondary T wave abnormalities), and the latter dominates the electrocardiogram rather than abnormalities associated with right ventricular diastolic pressure overload.

SYSTOLIC PRESSURE OVERLOAD OF THE RIGHT VENTRICLE (30,31) due to congenital heart disease, such as pulmonary valve stenosis, tetralogy of Fallot, or the Eisenmenger syndrome, produces a mean QRS vector that is directed to the right and anteriorly. Therefore, the mean T vector will be located 150° to 180° away from the mean QRS vector and will be directed leftward and posteriorly (Fig. 6.22). The transmyocardial pressure gradient of the right ventricle is decreased and finally eliminated by the abnormal systolic pressure generated during the late stage of mechanical ventricular systole. This permits the repolarization process to begin in the endocardium of the right ventricle, producing electrical forces that are opposite normal (Fig. 6.23). A right atrial abnormality is often present.

Early in the natural history of right ventricular hypertrophy due to acquired heart disease, such as mitral stenosis or primary pulmonary hypertension, the mean QRS vector tends to have an intermediate or vertical direction; it usually retains a slightly posterior direction. The mean T vector tends to be directed leftward and posteriorly (Fig. 6.22). A left atrial abnormality may be present with mitral stenosis, and a right atrial abnormality may occur with pulmonary hypertension. Later in the course of disease, as more severe right ventricular hypertension develops, the mean QRS vector tends to be directed more to the right and anteriorly, and the mean T vector eventually lies 150° to 180° away from the mean QRS vector, being directed to the left and posteriorly. The mean ST vector tends to be parallel with the mean T vector.

An example of an electrocardiogram exhibiting systolic overload of the right ventricle is shown in Chapter 9.

THE T WAVE ABNORMALITY OF PERICARDITIS:

As noted earlier, the pericardium itself produces no electrical forces; the electrocardiographic abnormalities produced by pericarditis are due to epicardial damage(4). The mean ST segment vector in pericarditis points toward the centroid of the area of epicardial damage (Fig. 6.14), and because pericarditis is usually generalized, the centroid of epicardial damage is near the cardiac apex. Accordingly, the mean ST vector is relatively parallel with the mean QRS vector. It may be directed a little anterior to the mean QRS vector. The mean QRS vector is directed slightly posteriorly because the conduction system of the left ventricle directs the electrical forces posteriorly whereas the ST segment vector due to pericarditis is directed toward the anatomic left ventricular apex.

Pericarditis also produces abnormalities in the T wave (Fig. 6.15). Early in the disease process, the mean T vector may simply become shorter; later, as the mean ST vector diminishes in size, the mean T vector may tend to point away from the centroid of the epicardial disease process. At times the electrocardiogram may return to normal, or near normal, before the T wave abnormality develops. Even later, the electrocardiogram may become normal or show small but normally directed T waves, or a mean T vector that is directed 60° to 90° away from the mean QRS vector. The residual abnormalities undoubtedly account for some of the unexplained benign T wave abnormalities seen years after a viral infection, because it is likely that unrecognized benign pericarditis occurs with many viral diseases.

The generalized epicardial damage associated with pericarditis delays the normal repolarization process, so that it begins in the endocardium. This produces a mean T vector that is opposite normal. The T wave tends to be inverted in all bipolar leads and lead aVF, and upright in leads aVR and aVL. It is much easier, and conceptually more accurate, to visualize the mean ST segment vector as being relatively parallel with, and the mean T vector as being opposite, the mean QRS vector.

The epicardial injury and ischemia associated with myocardial infarction are localized to a segment of the left ventricle. The mean ST vector points toward the area of epicardial injury, and the mean T vector points away from the area of epicardial ischemia.

Diagramming the ST and T vectors is more sensible and more accurate than memorizing the changes in each of the leads.

Chapter 10 provides examples of electrocardiograms showing the abnormalities of pericarditis.

T Wave Abnormalities Due to Myocardial Ischemia: Myocardial ischemia secondary to inadequate coronary artery blood flow may produce an alteration in the direction of the mean T vector(12). Localized epicardial myocardial ischemia delays repolarization, which normally begins in the epicardium, so that it begins in the endocardial area (Fig. 6.24). This causes the mean T vector to be directed away from the area of epicardial ischemia. For example, the mean T vector tends to point away from an area of *localized inferior epicardial ischemia*; inverted T waves appear in leads II, III, and aVF. The T wave may become larger in lead V1 if the inferior ischemia is located posteriorly as well as inferiorly. The mean T vector may be directed away from an area of *localized anterior epicardial ischemia*; this produces inverted T waves in leads V1, V2, and V3. Because localized epicardial ischemia may develop in many different areas of the left ventricular myocardium, *it is simpler to diagram the direction of the mean T vector*, thereby identifying the location of the epicardial ischemia that caused it (Fig. 6.25), than to memorize the characteristics of the multitude of T wave abnormalities that appear in the electrocardiogram. In such cases, the mean T vector is usually more than 60° away from the mean QRS vector unless the dead area due to the infarct is sufficiently large to alter the direction of the mean QRS vector. This is referred to as an abnormal QRS-T angle(15). The many causes of wide QRS-T angles other than myocardial hypoxia will be discussed subsequently.

The mean T vector points toward an area of *endocardial ischemia*. As a rule, this type of ischemia is generalized, and therefore the mean T vector tends to be parallel with the mean QRS vector. In this condition, the ischemia causes a further delay in the repolarization of the endocardial area, and this creates an exaggeration of the normal condition caused by the transmyocardial pressure gradient.

SECONDARY AND PRIMARY T WAVE CHANGES

Whenever the sequence of depolarization is altered, the sequence of repolarization will also be altered(32). The T wave "abnormality" occurring under such circumstances is called a *secondary T wave "abnormality"* because there is nothing wrong with the repolarization process; the T wave is actually normal for the abnormal QRS complex it follows.

Consider the extent to which the T wave appears abnormal when it follows a premature ventricular depolarization. The T wave is actually normal for that QRS complex; the sequence of repolarization is altered because the sequence of depolarization is abnormal. When there is uncomplicated left or right bundle branch block, the T waves that accompany the QRS complexes will be different from those that follow a QRS complex of normal appearance. They are, however, normal for the particular QRS complexes they follow.

A *primary T wave abnormality* is due to an alteration of the repolarization process that is independent of any abnormality of the QRS complex. The QRS complexes may be normal and the T waves abnormal, or the QRS complexes may be abnormal and the T waves abnormal for some reason other than the abnormality expected from an altered depolarization process. For example, a secondary T wave abnormality is expected in patients with left bundle branch block, but there may also be other additional primary causes of a repolarization abnormality. The abnormality resulting from these additional changes would be labeled a primary T wave abnormality.

The problem facing the clinician is to separate the secondary from the primary T wave abnormalities. This is sometimes accomplished by using the concept of the *ventricular gradient*.

THE VENTRICULAR GRADIENT

It is important to understand the odd sounding term "ventricular gradient." Frank Wilson and his associates recognized the relationship between the sequence and direction of the depolarization process and the sequence and direction of the repolarization process(33) and realized that the sequence of depolarization controlled the sequence of repolarization that followed it. The concept of the ventricular gradient was designed to emphasize this relationship.

The ventricular gradient is a measure of the extent to which the sequence of repolarization follows the sequence of depolarization. This can be computed by diagramming the direction and magnitude of the mean QRS and the mean T vector (Fig. 5.17A). A parallelogram is then constructed, using the mean QRS vector and mean T vector to form the other two sides of the parallelogram. A diagonal line is then drawn from the origin of the vectors to the distant angle of the parallelogram. The diagonal line is called the ventricular gradient.

Normally, the terminus of the diagonal line falls in the left lower quadrant of the hexaxial reference system (Fig. 5.17). The frontal plane direction of the gradient is usually quite easy to construct, but it is more difficult to determine its anterior or posterior direction.

Ordinarily, the normality of a T wave can be determined by identifying a normal or near-normal mean QRS vector and then determining the relationship between it and the mean T vector. In the normal adult, the QRS-T angle should be 45° to 60°, and the mean T vector should be to the left of a vertical mean QRS vector, on either side of an intermediate mean QRS vector, inferior to a horizontal QRS vector, and anterior to a mean QRS vector.

When, however, the QRS complex is bizarre, as it is with left or right bundle branch block, and the T wave is also bizarre, it is useful to diagram the ventricular gradient (Fig. 6.26). The ventricular gradient is normal in uncomplicated bundle branch block but may be abnormal in some patients with a bundle branch block complicated by a primary T wave abnormality. It points away from the area of heart muscle in which there is an abnormal delay in repolarization. This type of abnormality may be due to ischemia related to coronary disease or some other abnormal myocardial process.

Examples of electrocardiograms showing bundle branch block and abnormal ventricular gradients are shown in Chapter 8.

FIGURE 6.19
Diastolic pressure overload of the left ventricle.

A. Normal direction and magnitude of the mean QRS and mean T vectors. **B.** Diastolic pressure overload of the left ventricle. The duration of the QRS complex is 0.10 second or less. Note the slight change in direction of the mean QRS vector to the left. Note, too, that this vector is larger than shown in part A. The mean T vector is also slightly larger. A new mean ST segment vector is now present and is relatively parallel with the mean T vector.

FIGURE 6.20
Systolic pressure overload of the left ventricle.

A. Normal mean QRS and T vectors. **B.** The duration of the QRS complex is 0.10 second or less. When the mean QRS vector is in a vertical position, the mean T vector will gradually become more and more anteriorly directed until it becomes reversed; at that point it is opposite the mean QRS vector. The mean T vector becomes directed superiorly and anteriorly. Note that the mean QRS vector in part B is larger than it is

in part A. A mean ST vector develops and follows the mean T vector as the latter gradually moves 180° away from the mean QRS vector. **C.** When the mean QRS and T vectors are directed to the left (horizontal position), the mean T vector will gradually be directed more and more inferiorly and rightwardly. It also becomes directed more anteriorly, eventually ending up opposite the mean QRS vector. A mean ST vector develops and follows the mean T vector as the latter gradually moves 180° away from the mean QRS vector.

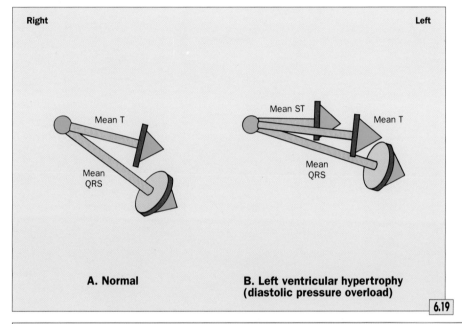

A. Normal

B. Left ventricular hypertrophy (diastolic pressure overload)

6.19

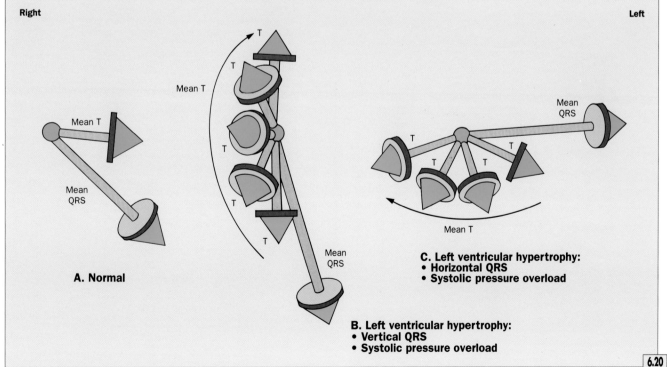

A. Normal

B. Left ventricular hypertrophy:
• Vertical QRS
• Systolic pressure overload

C. Left ventricular hypertrophy:
• Horizontal QRS
• Systolic pressure overload

6.20

FIGURE 6.21
Hypothetical explanation for the electro-cardiographic abnormalities caused by systolic pressure overload of the left ventricle.

A. The hypothetical cell. The wave of depolarization spreads from right to left, producing an upright QRS deflection. The repolarization process spreads from right to left but produces a downward QRS deflection. **B**. Hypothetical cell cooled on the right side. The wave of depolarization spreads from right to left, producing an upright QRS deflection. The repolarization process spreads from left to right because the cell is cooled on the right side; this produces an upright deflection. **C**. A seg-ment of the left ventricle of a normal adult. The transmyocardial pressure is greater in the endocardial area than in the epicardial area (note that the dark grey color fades to light grey, signifying the characteristics of the transmyocardial pressure gradient).

The wave of depolarization spreads from endocardium to epicardium,

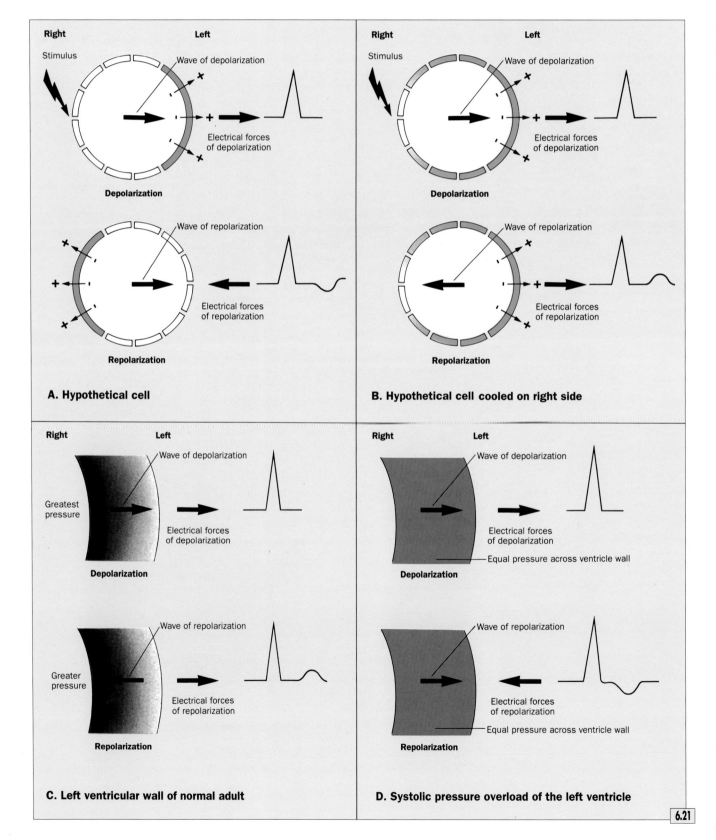

A. Hypothetical cell

B. Hypothetical cell cooled on right side

C. Left ventricular wall of normal adult

D. Systolic pressure overload of the left ventricle

(Figure 6.21 continued.)
producing an upright QRS deflection. The wave of repolarization spreads from epicardium to endocardium, as it does in the cooled hypothetical cell, producing an upright T wave. **D.** Systolic pressure overload of the left ventricle. The muscle is thicker than that shown in part C. The transmyocardial pressure is so great that a significant transmyocardial gradient does not exist. (Note that the dark grey color involves the entire thickness of the left ventricle.) The wave of depolarization occurs from the endocardium to the epicardium, producing an upright QRS deflection. The wave of repolarization spreads

from the endocardium to the epicardium, producing a downward QRS deflection.

FIGURE 6.22

The difference between the electrocardiographic abnormalities produced by congenital heart disease, such as pulmonary valve stenosis (A), and those produced by the early stages of acquired disease, such as mitral stenosis (B).

A. The duration of the QRS complex is 0.10 second or less. The mean QRS vector is directed to the right and anteriorly, and the ST and T vectors are directed opposite the mean QRS vec-

tor. This type of abnormality occurs with congenital disease, such as pulmonary valve stenosis, or advanced acquired disease, such as mitral stenosis with moderately severe pulmonary hypertension. A right atrial abnormality may be apparent in patients with right ventricular hypertension. **B.** The duration of the QRS complex is 0.10 second or less, and the mean QRS vector is located vertically and posteriorly. The mean T vector may be directed to the left and slightly posteriorly. This type of mean QRS vector is often caused by acquired disease. A left atrial abnormality as shown here suggests an early stage of mitral stenosis.

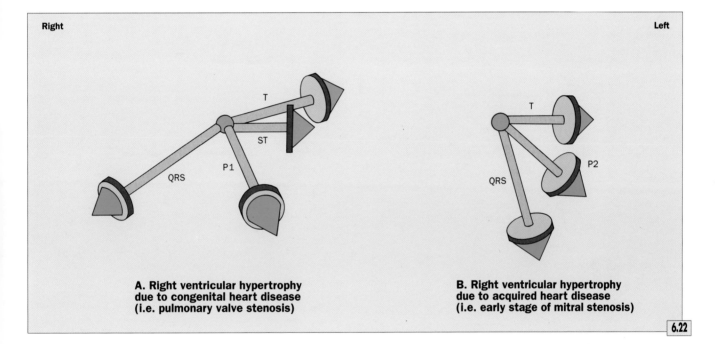

A. Right ventricular hypertrophy due to congenital heart disease (i.e. pulmonary valve stenosis)

B. Right ventricular hypertrophy due to acquired heart disease (i.e. early stage of mitral stenosis)

6.22

FIGURE 6.23

Hypothetical explanation for the electrocardiographic abnormalities caused by systolic pressure overload of the right ventricle.

A. Electrical forces and QRS and T deflections of a hypothetical cell that has been stimulated on the left side. **B.** Electrical forces and QRS and T deflections produced when a hypothetical cell has been cooled but also stimulated on the left side. **C.** Normal depolarization and repolarization of the ventricular wall of a normal adult. The endocardial systolic pressure is greatest in the endocardial area as compared to the epicardial area. Both the QRS complex and T wave are upright. **D.** Systolic pressure overload of the right ventricle. The systolic pressure is so great that there is no significant difference between the endocardial and epicardial pressure. The QRS vector will be directed to the right and the mean T vector will be directed to the left.

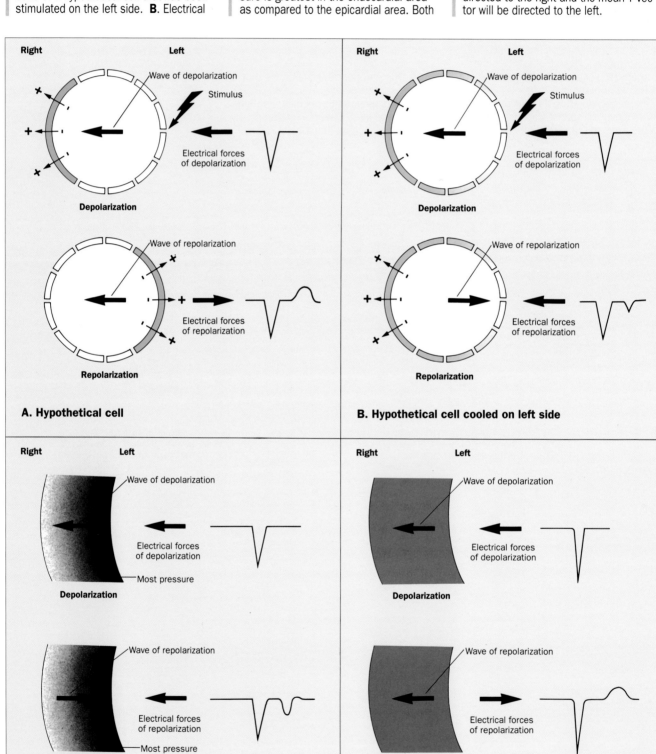

A. Hypothetical cell

B. Hypothetical cell cooled on left side

C. Right ventricular wall of normal adult

D. Systolic pressure overload of the right ventricle

6.23

FIGURE 6.24

The mechanism responsible for the T wave abnormality of epicardial ischemia.

A. A hypothetical cell that has been cooled on the right side: note that both the QRS and T waves are upright.
B. Segment of normal left ventricular myocardium showing the transmyocardial pressure gradient. This causes the repolarization process to begin in the epicardi-

um and progress to the endocardium, producing an upright T wave when the QRS wave is upright. **C**. The effect of epicardial ischemia is to delay the repolarization process in the epicardium (note blue color which represents ischemia). When this occurs, repolarization begins in the endocardium but produces electrical forces in the opposite direction. This results in an inverted

T wave when the QRS wave is upright.

FIGURE 6.25

The direction of the mean T vector due to localized epicardial ischemia of the left ventricle. Area 1: superior-lateral ischemia; Area 2: lateral ischemia; Area 3: inferior ischemia; Area 4: anterior ischemia; Area 5: true posterior ischemia.

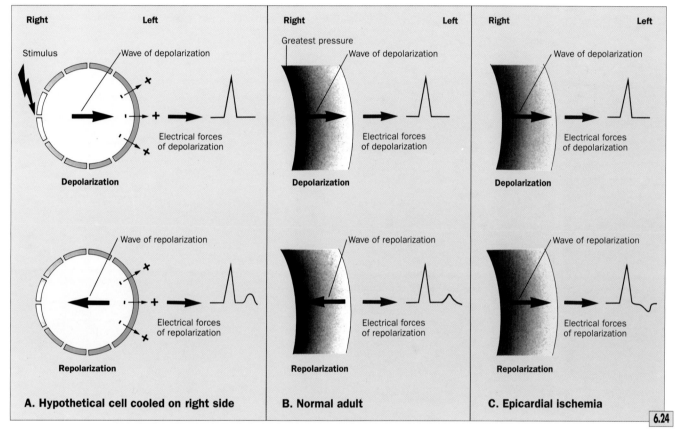

A. Hypothetical cell cooled on right side   B. Normal adult   C. Epicardial ischemia

6.24

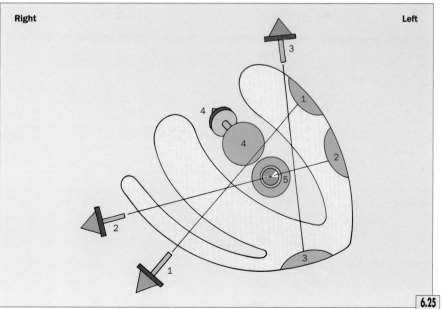

6.25

FIGURE 6.26

The identification of a primary T wave abnormality in patients with right and left bundle branch block.

A. Normal mean QRS and T vectors. Note the normal ventricular gradient (VG). **B**. Uncomplicated right bundle branch block. Note that the ventricular gradient (VG) is normal. There is a secondary T wave abnormality. **C**. Complicated* right bundle branch block due to a primary T wave abnormality. Note that the ventricular gradient (VG) is abnormal. **D**. Uncomplicated left bundle branch block. Note the normal ventricular gradient (VG). This is a secondary T wave abnormality. Note that the ventricular gradient (VG) is abnormal. **E**. Complicated* left bundle branch block due to a primary T wave abnormality. Note the abnormal ventricular gradient (VG).

*Complicated right bundle branch block is said to be present when there is an abnormal mean initial 0.04-second QRS vector; the QRS duration is greater than 0.12 second; the mean QRS vector is more rightward than +120°; the direction of the mean ST vector is not parallel with that of the mean T vector; or a primary T wave abnormality is identified by an abnormal ventricular gradient. Complicated left bundle branch block is said to be present when the QRS duration is greater than 0.12 second; the mean QRS vector is directed more than -30° to the left; the mean ST vector is not parallel with the mean T vector; or a primary T wave abnormality is identified by an abnormal ventricular gradient.

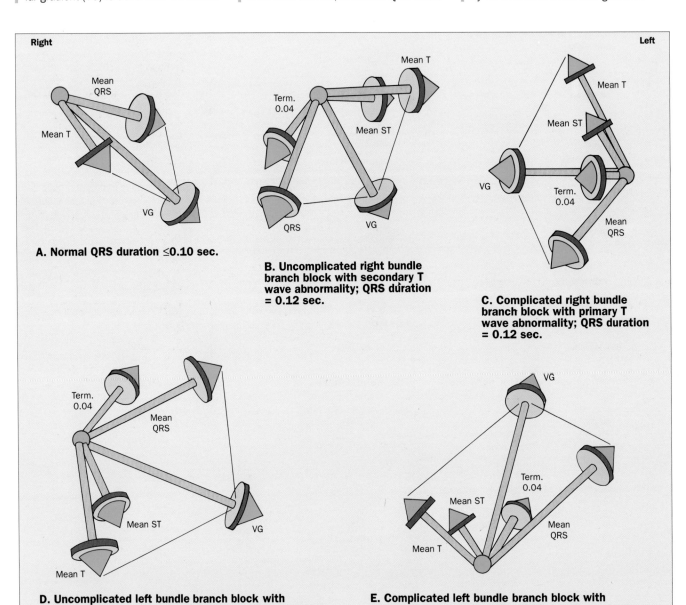

A. Normal QRS duration ≤0.10 sec.

B. Uncomplicated right bundle branch block with secondary T wave abnormality; QRS duration = 0.12 sec.

C. Complicated right bundle branch block with primary T wave abnormality; QRS duration = 0.12 sec.

D. Uncomplicated left bundle branch block with secondary T wave abnormality; QRS duration = 0.12 sec.

E. Complicated left bundle branch block with primary T wave abnormality; QRS duration = 0.12 sec.

6.26

DIGITALIS MEDICATION

Excessive digitalis medication can produce almost any type of cardiac dysrhythmia, including ventricular dysrhythmias, atrial dysrhythmias, and varying degrees of atrioventricular block. Except for ventricular dysrhythmia, however, digitalis medication does not produce any abnormality of the QRS complex because the depolarization process is not altered. The repolarization process, however, is altered considerably. Electrical systole is shortened, and this is reflected in the electrocardiogram as a short QT interval, often as short as 0.32 second.

The QT interval becomes shorter because the ST segment becomes shorter; the duration of the QRS complex does not change. The repolarization process begins very early, probably before the depolarization process has been completed. It is useful to consider the ST segment displacement due to digitalis as an *early T wave* and the usual T wave as a *late T wave*, because both are due to the repolarization process. Digitalis medication seems to facilitate the repolarization process so that it begins in the endocardium rather than the epicardium (Fig. 6.27). In other words, it seems to eliminate the effect of the transmyocardial pressure gradient that may be

responsible for the spread of repolarization from the epicardium to the endocardium in the normal subject(12). The early T wave is influenced by this mechanism more than the late T wave. Accordingly, with this medication, the early repolarization process spreads from the endocardium to the epicardium, producing electrical forces that are opposite the normal direction. As this occurs, the late T wave gradually becomes smaller, to the point at which it may no longer be visible. As long as it can be seen, it is directed as it was prior to the administration of the medication (Fig. 6.28). This is because digitalis affects all of the ventricular muscle rather than part of it. Were the latter the case, the direction of the mean T vector would change. Oddly, digitalis may cause the U wave to become prominent. Ordinarily, a prominent U wave tends to follow a large T wave, but in patients receiving digitalis, the prominent U wave follows a small T wave.

A diagrammatic metaphor demonstrating the effect of digitalis on the electrocardiogram is shown in Figure 6.29.

Hypercalcemia may produce abnormalities of the ST segment, T wave, and QT interval that are identical to the abnormalities produced by digitalis.

FIGURE 6.27
The mechanism responsible for the electrocardiographic abnormalities caused by digitalis medication.

A. Depolarization and repolarization process of the normal ventricular muscle. **B.** The effect of digitalis medication on the repolarization process of the ventricular muscle. Digitalis eliminates the transmyocardial pressure gradient, causing the repolarization process to begin in the endocardium rather than the epicardium. The repolarization process also begins earlier than normal, producing a short QT interval. As shown in the figure at the lower right, the early forces of repolarization produce a downward displacement of the ST segment and a small T wave. The displacement of the ST segment is called the "early T" and the small residual T wave is called the "late T" wave.

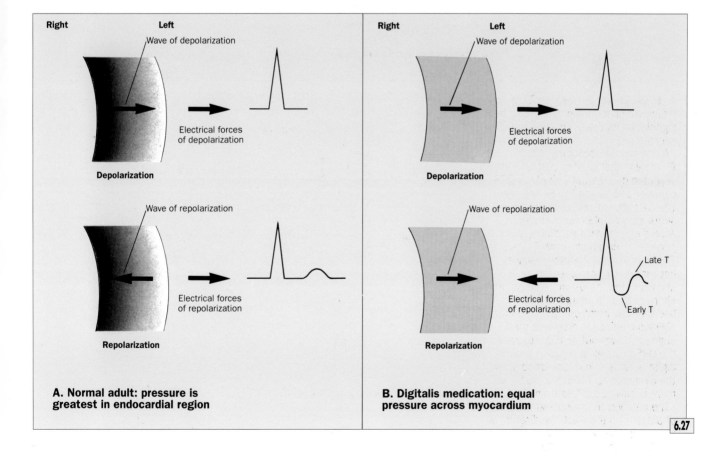

A. Normal adult: pressure is greatest in endocardial region

B. Digitalis medication: equal pressure across myocardium

6.27

F I G U R E   6 . 2 8
The effect of digitalis on the electrocardiogram.
   A. Normal mean QRS and T vectors.
   B. Early effect of digitalis. The PR interval may be longer than it was prior to the

administration of digitalis. Note that the QT interval is shorter than in part A. The "late T" wave is smaller, but its direction is unchanged. The direction of the "early T" wave is opposite that of the "late T" wave. The direction of the

QRS complex has not changed. **C.** More advanced digitalis effect. The PR interval may be prolonged. The QT interval is short. The "early T" wave dominates the tracing, and the "late T" wave is smaller than in B.

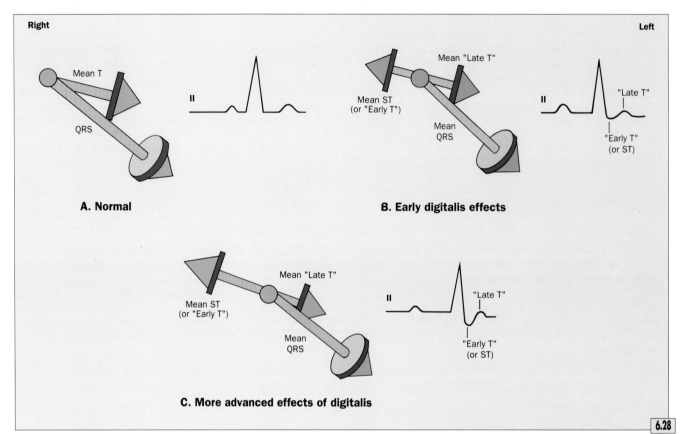

A. Normal

B. Early digitalis effects

C. More advanced effects of digitalis

F I G U R E   6 . 2 9
A diagrammatic metaphor showing how digitalis alters the QT interval and ST segment.
   A. Normal electrocardiogram.
   B. Imagine that a pill of digitalis rolls down the descending limb of the QRS complex and strikes the ST segment. The ST segment will sag; this represents early repolarization forces. Accordingly, this displacement of the ST segment is called an "early T" wave. The "late T" wave becomes smaller because it is incorporated in the ST segment, and the QT interval becomes shorter. **C.** This figure is presented because it is commonly believed that digitalis medication displaces the ST segment downward. In this illustration, the QRS complex is negative and the digitalis pill is thrown upward to strike the ST segment. Therefore the ST segment is elevated in this example.
   The only way to understand the effect of digitalis on the electrocardiogram is to diagram the vectors shown in Figure 6.28. Whether the ST segment is depressed or elevated simply depends on the relationship of the lead axes to

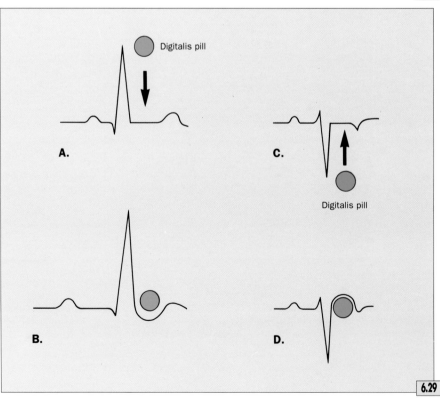

AFTERPOTENTIAL

There are two types of afterpotential: a depolarization afterpotential and a repolarization afterpotential.

DEPOLARIZATION AFTERPOTENTIAL

The technique of signal averaging has made it possible to identify electrical activity following the QRS complex(34). A normal record is shown in Figure. 5.19 and an abnormal record in Figure. 6.30. Such electrical activity is associated with an increased likelihood of ventricular arrhythmias.

REPOLARIZATION AFTERPOTENTIAL

The U wave is produced by repolarization forces that occur after the T wave has been written(13). A U wave may be recorded in the electrocardiogram of normal adults, but it is rarely taller than 0.5 mm. The U wave is usually tallest in those leads in which the T wave is largest. An inverted U wave is abnormal when the preceding T wave is upright. A tall U wave, greater than 2 mm, is abnormal. Prominent U waves occur with hypokalemia, hypomagnesemia, and left ventricular hypertrophy. The U wave may become larger after digitalis, representing an exception to the usual rule that a prominent U wave follows a large T wave. With digitalis, a large U wave may follow a small T wave. The U wave may become inverted in patients with coronary disease or left ventricular hypertrophy.

(Figure 6.29 continued.)
the mean, spatially oriented ST and T vectors.

Hypercalcemia may produce the ST and T wave abnormalities and a short QT interval similar to those produced by digitalis.

FIGURE 6.30
An abnormal signal-averaged electrocardiogram showing a late ventricular potential.

The QRS duration is prolonged to 184 ms, and the voltage content in the last 40 ms is reduced at 3 uV. Normally, the voltage content of the last 40 ms of the filtered QRS should exceed 25 uV. (Illustration provided by Dr. Paul Walter of Emory University.)

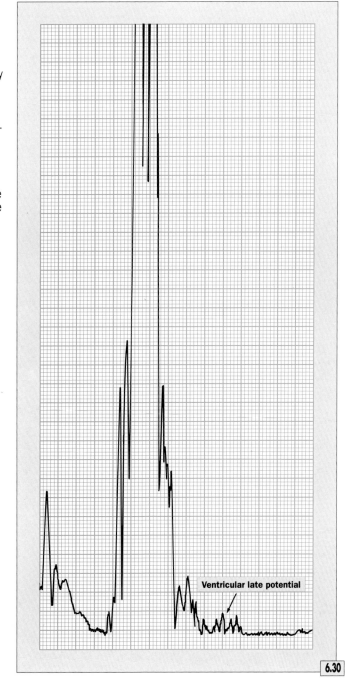

Ventricular late potential

6.30

REFERENCES

1. Wilson FN, Rosenbaum FF, Johnston FD: Interpretation of the ventricular complex of the electrocardiogram. *Adv Intern Med* 1947; 2:1.

2. Wolff L, Parkinson J, White PD: Bundle branch block with short PR interval in healthy young people prone to paroxysmal tachycardia. *Am Heart J* 1930; 5:685.

3. Morris JJ, Estes EH Jr, Whalen RE, et al: P wave analysis in valvular heart disease. *Circulation* 1964; 29:242.

4. Spodick DH: Diagnostic electrocardiographic sequences in acute pericarditis: Significance of PR segment and PR vector changes. *Circulation* 1973; 48:575.

5. Romano C, Gemme G, Pongiglione R: Aritmie cardiache rare dell' eta' pediatrica. II. Accessi sincopali per fibrillazione ventricolane passossistica. *Clin Pediatr* 1963; 45:656.

5a. Ward OC: A new familial cardiac syndrome in children. *J Irish Med Assoc* 1964; 54:103.

6. Jervell A, Lange-Nielsen F: Congenital deaf-mutism, functional heart disease with prolongation of the QT interval, and sudden death. *Am Heart J* 1957; 54(1):59.

7. Fisch C: Electrolytes and the heart, in Hurst JW (ed): *The Heart*, 6th ed. New York: McGraw-Hill, 1986, p. 1466.

8. Bronsky D, Dubin A, Kushner DS, Waldstein SS: Calcium and the electrocardiogram. III. The relationship of the intervals of the electrocardiogram to the level of serum calcium. *Am J Cardiol* 1961; 7:840.

9. Dodge H, Grant R, Seavey P: Effects of induced hyperkalemia on the electrocardiogram. *Am Heart J* 1953; 45:725.

10. Surawicz B, Lepeschkin E: Electrocardiographic pattern of hypopotassemia. *Circulation* 1953; 8:801.

11. Burch GE, Meyers R, Abildskov JA: A new electrocardiographic pattern observed in cerebrovascular accidents. *Circulation* 1954; 9:719.

12. Grant RP, Estes EH Jr: *Spatial Vector Electrocardiography: Clinical Electrocardiographic Interpretation.* New York: Blakiston, 1951.

13. Lepeschkin E: Physiologic basis of the U wave, in Schlant RC, Hurst JW (eds): *Advances in Electrocardiography,* Vol. 2, New York: Grune & Stratton, 1972, p. 353.

14. Jin L, Weisse AB, Hernandez F, et al: Significance of electrocardiographic isolated abnormal terminal P wave force (left atrial abnormality): An echocardiographic and clinical correlation. *Arch Intern Med* 1988; 148(7):1545.

15. Grant RP: *Clinical Electrocardiography: The Spatial Vector Approach.* New York: McGraw-Hill, 1957, p. 49.

16. Romhilt DW, Bove KE, Norris RJ, et al: A critical appraisal of the electrocardiographic criteria for the diagnosis of left ventricular hypertrophy. *Circulation* 1969; 40:185.

17. Romhilt DW, Estes EH: Point-score system for the ECG diagnosis of left ventricular hypertrophy. *Am Heart J* 1968; 75:752.

18. Odom H II, Davis JL, Dinh HA, et al: QRS voltage measurements in autopsied men free of cardiopulmonary disease: A basis for evaluating total QRS voltage as an index of left ventricular hypertrophy. *Am J Cardiol* 1986; 58:801.

19. Siegel RJ, Roberts WC: Electrocardiographic observations in severe aortic valve stenosis: Correlative necropsy study to clinical, hemodynamic, and ECG variables demonstrating relation of 12-lead QRS amplitude to peak systolic transaortic pressure gradient. *Am Heart J* 1982; 103:210.

20. Roberts WC, Day PJ: Electrocardiographic observations in clinically isolated, pure, chronic, severe aortic regurgitation: Analysis of 30 necropsy patients aged 19 to 65 years. *Am J Cardiol* 1985; 55:432.

21. Ouzts H, Clements SD Jr, Hurst JW: Electrical alternans associated with supraventricular tachycardia. *South Med J* 1980; 73:822.

22. McGinn S, White PD: Acute cor pulmonale resulting from pulmonary embolism. *JAMA* 1935; 104:1473.

23. de Luna AB, Carrio I, Subirana MT, et al: Electrophysiological mechanisms of the S1 S11 S111 electrocardiographic morphology. *J Electrocardiol* 1987; 20(1):38.

24. Rosenbaum MB, Elizari MV, Lazzari JO, et al: The differential electrocardiographic manifestations of hemiblocks, bilateral bundle branch block, and trifascicular blocks, in Schlant RC and Hurst JW (eds), *Advances in Electrocardiography,* Vol. 1. New York: Grune & Stratton, p. 145.

25. Clements SD Jr, Hurst JW: Diagnostic value of electrocardiographic abnormalities observed in subjects accidentally exposed to cold. *Am J Cardiol* 1972; 29:889.

26. Lev M: Anatomic basis for atrioventricular block. *Am J Med* 1964; 37:742.

27. Lenegre J: Etiology and pathology of bilateral bundle branch block in relation to complete heart block. *Progr Cardiovasc Dis* 1964; 6:409.

28. First SA, Bayley RH: Peri-infarction block. *Circulation* 1950; 2:31.

29. Holland RP, Brooks H: TQ-ST segment mapping: Critical review and analysis of current concepts. *Am J Cardiol* 1977; 40:110.

30. C Cabrera E, Monroy JR: Systolic and diastolic loading of the heart I: Physiologic and clinical data. *Am Heart J* 1952; 43:661.

31. C Cabrera E, Monroy JR: Systolic and diastolic loading of the heart II: Electrocardiographic data. *Am Heart J* 1952; 43:669.

32. Kossmann CE: The primary "T" wave of the electrocardiogram, in Hurst JW (ed): *Update IV: The Heart.* New York: McGraw-Hill, 1981, p. 71.

33. Wilson FN, MacLeod AG, Barker PS, Johnston FD: The determination and the significance of the areas of the ventricular deflections of the electrocardiogram. *Am Heart J* 1934; 10:46.

34. Breithhardt G, Borggrefe M, Pathophysiological mechanism and clinical significance of ventricular late potentialsy *Eur Heart J* 1986; 7:364.

FIGURE CREDITS

Figure 6.16 From Holland RP, Brooks H: TQ-ST segment mapping; Critical view and analysis of current concepts. *Am J Cardiol* 1977; 40:113.

PART

IMPORTANT FEATURES AND EXAMPLES OF ABNORMAL ATRIAL AND VENTRICULAR ELECTROCARDIOGRAMS

THREE

CHAPTER SEVEN

Atrial Abnormalities and their Relationship to Ventricular Abnormalities

Abnormalities of the atria may be reflected in abnormalities of the P waves, and abnormalities of the P waves may be clues to abnormalities of the ventricles and QRS complexes. The depolarization and repolarization of the atria are discussed in Chapter 4. The abnormal P wave vectors characteristic of right (P1) and left (P2) atrial abnormalities are discussed below. P wave abnormalities may be caused by intrinsic disease of the atria (a localized conduction defect), atrial enlargement, or atrial hypertrophy. So far, it has not been possible to separate one cause from another. Accordingly, we will refer to such abnormalities as atrial abnormalities without specifying their precise nature.

RIGHT ATRIAL ABNORMALITY

The electrocardiographic characteristics of a right atrial abnormality are listed in Table 7.1, and examples of such an abnormality are shown in Figs 7.1 and 7.2.

There are no other abnormalities that resemble these; the problem is to distinguish P waves that are characteristic of a right atrial abnormality from normal P waves.

The ventricular abnormalities responsible for right atrial abnormality are Ebstein's anomaly, tricuspid atresia or stenosis, right ventricular hypertension due to mitral stenosis; left ventricular disease with elevated left ventricular diastolic pressure and pulmonary hypertension; pulmonary emboli; Eisenmenger's syndrome; primary pulmonary hypertension, pulmonary valve stenosis, the tetralogy of Fallot, and chronic obstructive lung disease.

LEFT ATRIAL ABNORMALITY

The electrocardiographic characteristics of a left atrial abnormality are listed in Table 7.2. An example is shown in Figure 7.3.

There are two problems in identifying left atrial abnormalities electrocardiographically. The first is to distinguish the P wave abnormalities that are characteristic of a left atrial disorder from normal P waves. The second occurs because localized atrial disease, undoubtedly interfering with atrial conduction, may simulate left atrial abnormalities caused by the disorders listed below; there is no way to distinguish them with certainty.

The cardiac abnormalities often associated with a left atrial abnormality are rheumatic mitral stenosis, congenital mitral atresia, left atrial myxoma, mitral regurgitation from any cause, left ventricular disease with an elevated left ventricular diastolic pressure due to aortic regurgitation of any cause, aortic stenosis, and cardiomyopathy.

COMBINED RIGHT AND LEFT ATRIAL ABNORMALITIES

The electrocardiographic characteristics of combined right and left atrial abnormalities are listed in Table 7.3. Examples of abnormalities involving both the right and left atria are shown in Figures 7.4 and 7.5.

The problem is to separate the P wave abnormalities that are characterized as right and left atrial abnormalities from normal P waves.

The cardiac abnormalities often associated with right and left atrial abnormalities are rheumatic mitral stenosis with pulmonary hypertension, mitral regurgitation from any cause plus pulmonary hypertension, Eisenmenger's syndrome due to patent ductus arteriosus or ventricular septal defect, cardiomyopathy, and severe heart disease with aortic valve disease, with or without mitral valve disease, plus pulmonary hypertension.

A WORD OF CAUTION

Many unusual and peculiar P waves will be encountered. They are peculiar because they do not exhibit the abnormalities listed in Tables 7.1, 7.2, and 7.3. For the present no more can be said. Some peculiar, but not definitely abnormal, P waves may be due to localized defects in the depolarization of the atria that have nothing to do with ventricular disease.

TABLE 7.1 CHARACTERISTICS OF A RIGHT ATRIAL ABNORMALITY

- The P wave amplitude in adults is greater than 2.5 mm. The increase in amplitude of the P wave is usually noted in leads II or V1, but may be seen in other leads. The duration of the P wave is 0.12 second or less.

- The P wave is usually not notched.

- The mean P vector (Pm) is directed inferiorly about +70° to +90°, and slightly anteriorly.

- The mean P vector for the first half of the P wave (P1) is often directed to the right of, and is always anterior to the mean P vector (Pm). The amplitude of the first half of the P wave (P1) is responsible for the increase in amplitude of the mean P wave (Pm) vector.

- The mean P vector for the second half of the P wave (P2) is usually smaller than the mean vector representing P1, and is directed to the left of and posterior to the mean P vector (Pm).

- The abnormal P waves in a case of right atrial abnormality may change from one electrocardiogram to the next, especially when they are caused by chronic pulmonary disease.

FIGURE 7.1

This electrocardiogram was recorded from a 36-year-old female with Ebstein's anomaly of the tricuspid valve. The PR interval is 0.22 second; the QRS duration is 0.13 second; and the QT interval is 0.36 second.

P waves: The amplitude of the P wave measured in lead II is 2.25 mm. In lead V2, it is 4 mm and its duration is 0.08 second. The direction of Pm is at +45°, and slightly anterior. P1 is at +50°, directed slightly anteriorly. P2 is at +30°, almost parallel with the frontal plane. When the amplitude of P2 is multiplied by its duration in V1, the product is -0.08 mm/sec. The shape, duration, and amplitude of the P waves, plus the direction of the P1 vector, indicate a right atrial abnormality. The measurement of -0.08 mm/sec for the second half of the P wave in V1 does not indicate a left atrial abnormality in this patient. The depolarization of the huge, abnormal right atrium produces the abnormality of the P wave (P2) in lead V1; the electrical forces are initially directed anteriorly and then posteriorly on their way to the left atrium. First degree atrioventricular block and a right atrial abnormality are present.

QRS complex: The mean QRS vector is directed +110° to the right and slightly anteriorly. The mean initial 0.04 second QRS vector is directed +80° inferiorly, and slightly posteriorly (note Q waves in leads aVL, V1, and V2). This is likely to be abnormal: the initial QRS forces are posterior to the subsequent forces, producing the Q waves followed by R and S waves in lead V2. The mean terminal 0.04-second QRS vector is directed +120° inferiorly, and flush with the frontal plane. (Note that the last 0.04 second of the QRS complex in lead aVR is almost isoelectric, whereas the initial portion of the complex is negative; the terminal QRS forces are directed more to the right than are the initial ones). The QRS duration and the direction of the mean QRS and mean terminal 0.04-second QRS vectors indicate a variety of right bundle branch block.

T waves: The mean T vector is directed -60° to the left and slightly posteriorly. The ventricular gradient is not definitely abnormal. The T wave abnormalities are of the secondary type.

A. The frontal plane projections for the mean P, P1, P2, mean QRS, the initial 0.04-second QRS, the terminal 0.04-second QRS, and T vectors. **B.** The spatial orientation of the mean P vector. Note the course of the transitional pathway on the chest. **C.** The spatial orientation of the mean P1 vector. Note the course of the transitional pathway on the chest. **D.** The spatial orientation of the mean P2 vector. Note the transitional pathway.

Summary: This electrocardiogram shows first-degree atrioventricular block, a right atrial abnormality, right bundle branch block, an abnormal mean initial 0.04-second QRS vector, and a secondary T wave abnormality. The P wave abnormality of the magnitude shown here, plus right bundle branch block, has a predictive value of almost 100 percent in indicating Ebstein's anomaly of the tricuspid valve. The abnormal mean initial 0.04-second QRS vector produces abnormal Q waves. In another setting, myocardial infarction should be considered, but with the abnormal P waves and right bundle branch block, the QRS abnormality here is more likely the "pseudo-infarction" of Ebstein's anomaly.

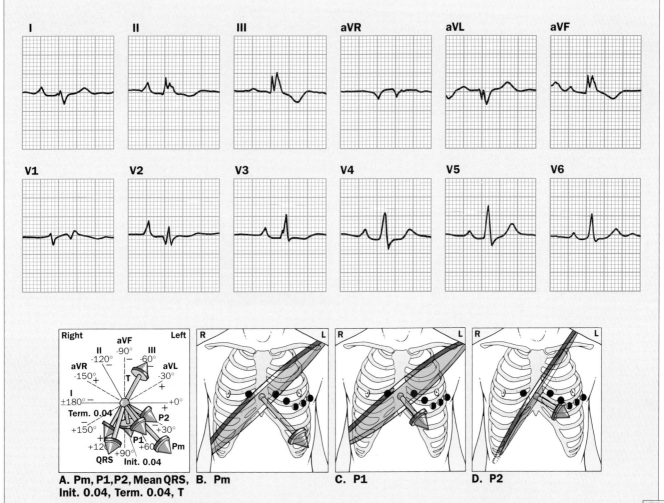

A. Pm, P1, P2, Mean QRS, Init. 0.04, Term. 0.04, T   B. Pm   C. P1   D. P2

7.1

FIGURE 7.2
This electrocardiogram was recorded from a 72-year old man with atherosclerotic coronary heart disease and obstructive lung disease. The PR interval is 0.16 second, the QRS duration is 0.09 second, and the QT interval is 0.28 second.

P waves: The amplitude of the P wave measured in lead II is 3.25 mm and its duration is 0.08 second. The mean P vector (Pm) is directed vertically at about +80°, and slightly anteriorly. Note the depressed PQ and ST segments, produced by the Ta wave. There

is definite evidence of right atrial abnormality.

QRS complex: The QRS magnitude is normal; the total QRS amplitude is 135 mm. The mean initial 0.02 second QRS vector is directed slightly to the left, superiorly, and anteriorly. The

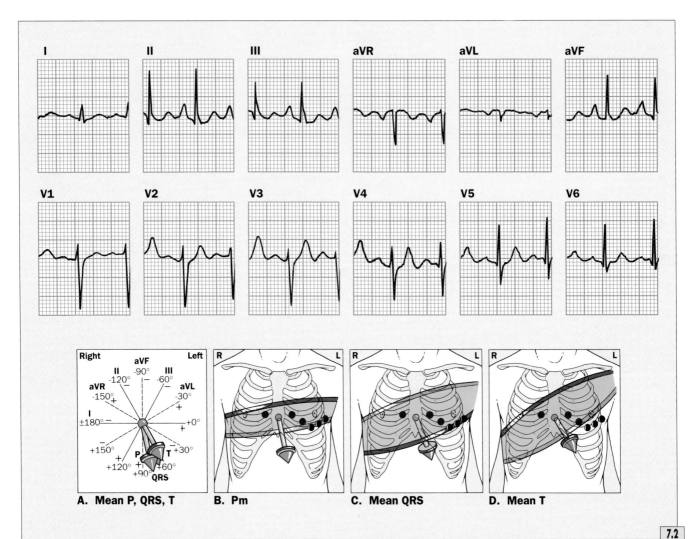

A. Mean P, QRS, T   **B. Pm**   **C. Mean QRS**   **D. Mean T**

7.2

TABLE 7.2 CHARACTERISTICS OF A LEFT ATRIAL ABNORMALITY

- The duration of the P wave is usually greater than 0.12 second. This is usually detected in leads II and V1.

- The P wave is usually notched at the halfway mark.

- The mean P vector (Pm) is usually directed about +30° to +70° inferiorly, and parallel with the frontal plane or slightly posteriorly.

- The P1 vector is normal.

- The mean P vector for the second half of the P wave (P2) is superior and posterior to the mean P vector (Pm).

- The duration and magnitude of the second half of the P wave in lead V1 is crucial to the identification of a left atrial abnormality. This is likely to be present when the duration of the second half of the P wave (measured in fractions of a second) multiplied by its amplitude (measured in millimeters), is greater than 0.03 mm/sec. The predictive value of the measurement increases as the product increases.

(Figure 7.2 continued.)
mean QRS vector is directed vertically about +70°, and about 60° posteriorly.

T wave: The mean T vector is directed at +65° to the left and anteriorly; the QRS-T angle is about 75°.

A. The frontal plane projections of the mean P (Pm), QRS, and T wave vectors. **B.** The spatial orientation of the mean P vector (Pm). Note the course of the transitional pathway on the chest. **C.** The spatial orientation of the mean QRS vector. Note the course of the transitional pathway on the chest. **D.** The spatial orientation of the mean T vector. Note the course of the transitional pathway on the chest.

Summary: A right atrial abnormality associated with a posteriorly directed vertical mean QRS vector should lead the clinician to search for acquired diseases, such as cor pulmonale, as a cause for these electrocardiographic abnormalities.

FIGURE 7.3

This electrocardiogram was recorded from a 34-year-old woman with mitral stenosis due to rheumatic heart disease. The PR interval is 0.21 second; the QRS duration is about 0.09 second; and the QT interval is 0.42 second.

P wave: The amplitude of the P wave measures 2.25 mm in lead II, and the duration of the wave is 0.11 to 0.12 second. It is notched at about the halfway mark. The mean P vector (Pm) is directed inferiorly (+70°) and posteriorly. The mean vector for right atrial depolarization (P1) is directed inferiorly and slightly posteriorly and that of left atrial depolarization (P2) is directed inferiorly and posteriorly. The product produced by multiplying the second half of the P wave by its amplitude as measured in lead V1 is 0.065 mm/sec. The P wave duration of 0.11 to 0.12 second, plus the abnormality of the second half of the P wave in lead V1 (with the product of duration multiplied by amplitude exceeding -0.03 mm/sec) indicates a left atrial abnormality. The Ta wave is seen in lead II where it displaces the PQ segment downward. First-degree atrioventricular block is present.

QRS complex: The mean QRS vector is directed inferiorly by about +70°, and moderately posteriorly. Although the mean QRS vector is directed normally, there is the possibility of its being directed abnormally when it is considered along with the abnormal P2.

T wave: The mean T vector is directed at +35° and posteriorly; this is abnormal. The direction of the mean T vector suggests a delay in repolarization of

(Figure 7.3 continued.)
the right ventricle.

A. The frontal plane projections for the mean P, QRS, and T vectors.
B. The spatial orientation of the mean P vector (Pm). Note the course of the transitional pathway on the chest.
C. The spatial orientation of the mean P1 vector. Note the course of the transitional pathway on the chest. **D.** The spatial orientation of the mean P2 vector. Note the course of the transitional pathway on the chest. **E.** The spatial orientation of the mean QRS

vector. Note the course of the transitional pathway on the chest. **F.** The spatial orientation of the mean T vector, showing the course of the transitional pathway on the chest.

Summary: The abnormalities are first degree atrioventricular block, a definite left atrial abnormality, a mean QRS vector directed inferiorly (+70°) and posteriorly, and a mean T vector that is directed away from the right ventricle. The predictive value of this cluster of abnormalities for mitral stenosis approaches 100 percent.

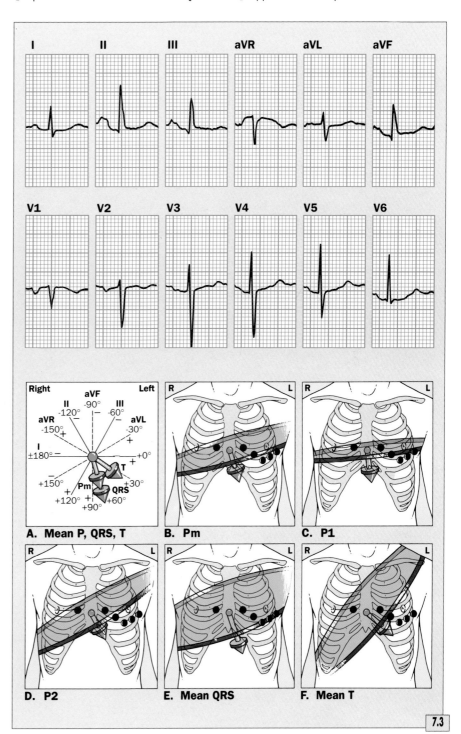

A. Mean P, QRS, T   B. Pm   C. P1

D. P2   E. Mean QRS   F. Mean T

7.3

F I G U R E   7 . 4

Combined right and left atrial abnormalities. This electrocardiogram was recorded from a 49-year-old man with severe aortic regurgitation. The PR interval is 0.155 second; the QRS duration is 0.08 second; and the QT interval is 0.34 second.

P waves: The amplitude of the P wave in lead II is 2.75 mm and its duration is 0.09 second. The mean P vector (Pm) is directed inferiorly (+62°), and abnormally posteriorly. The product of the duration of the second half of the P wave (0.05 second) multiplied by the amplitude (l.5 mm) in lead V1 is -.075 mm/sec. The increased amplitude of the P waves and their duration of 0.09 second, signify a right atrial abnormality, while the definitely abnormal P wave in lead V1 indicates a left atrial abnormality. A small Ta wave is seen during the PQ segment in lead II.

QRS complex: The duration of the QRS complex is normal (0.08 second). The mean QRS vector is directed inferiorly (+65°) and markedly posteriorly. The 12-lead total QRS amplitude is more than 237 mm (note that the QRS amplitude is probably even greater than this because it overruns the edge of the electrocardiographic paper in leads V2, V3, V5, and V6), and this increase is indicative of left ventricular hypertrophy.

T wave: The mean T vector is directed inferiorly (about +90°) and markedly anteriorly. The QRS-T angle is abnormal (about 150°), and characteristic of early systolic pressure overload of the left ventricle. This occurs with severe or longstanding left ventriclar diastolic pressure overload. The T wave is abnormal and represents left ventricular hypertrophy. The T wave vector will gradually become increasingly anteriorly directed, finally assuming a direction opposite that of the mean QRS vector.

A. The frontal plane projections of the mean P (Pm), QRS, and T vectors.
B. The spatial orientation of the mean P vector (Pm). Note the course of the transitional pathway on the chest.
C. The spatial orientation of the mean QRS vector. Note the transitional pathway on the chest. **D.** The spatial orientation of the mean T vector. Note the transitional pathway on the chest.

Summary: There is evidence of a right atrial abnormality (a P wave duration 0.09 second and amplitude of 2.75 mm) as well as a left atrial abnormality (the duration of the second half of the P wave multiplied by its amplitude equals 0.075 mm/sec) in lead V1. The total 12-lead QRS amplitude with a normal QRS duration indicates left ventricular hypertrophy. The mean T vector is abnormal, being directed 150° away from the mean QRS vector; this indicates an early stage of systolic pressure

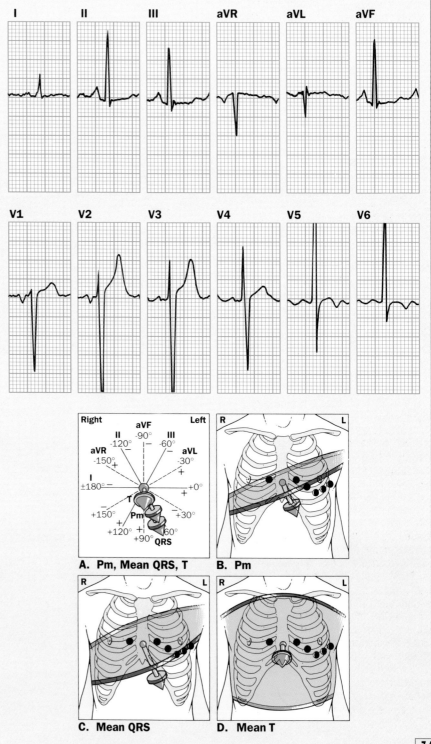

TABLE 7.3 CHARACTERISTICS OF RIGHT AND LEFT ATRIAL ABNORMALITIES

- The electrocardiographic abnormalities are a combination of right and left atrial abnormalities listed in Tables 7.1 and 7.2.
- The amplitude of the P waves is often greater than 2.5 mm.
- The duration of the P waves is greater than 0.12 second as noted in leads II and V1.
- The amplitude of the first half of the P wave (P1) in lead V1 may be 2.5 mm.
- The second half of the P wave in lead V1 is abnormal; the duration of the second half of the P wave multiplied by its amplitude gives a product that is greater than 0.03 mm/sec.

A. Pm, Mean QRS, T   **B. Pm**

C. Mean QRS   **D. Mean T**

(Figure 7.4 continued.)
overload of the left ventricle. The patient had aortic regurgitation, which produced diastolic pressure overload of the left ventricle. This figure illustrates how a late stage of diastolic pressure overload of the left ventricle blends into an early stage of systolic pressure overload of the left ventricle. The ECG in this patient could be due to aortic stenosis, a late phase of aortic regurgitation, or the late stage of mitral regurgitation. In any of these conditions, heart failure is likely, because the right atrial abnormality is related to an increase in pulmonary artery pressure which can be caused by advanced disease.

FIGURE 7.5
Combined right and left atrial abnormalities. This electrocardiogram was recorded from a 25-year-old man with dilated cardiomyopathy. He had severe heart failure and was waiting for cardiac transplantation. The PR interval is 0.24 second; the QRS duration is 0.10 second; and the QT interval is 0.32 second. The ventricular rate is 109 depolarizations per minute.

P waves: The amplitude of the P wave in lead II is 3 mm and its duration is 0.10 second. The mean P vector (Pm) is directed inferiorly (+45°) and posteriorly. The duration of the second half of the P wave (Pm) in lead V1 is 0.04 second, and when this is multiplied by the P2 wave amplitude which is 2.5 mm, the product is -0.10 mm/sec; this indicates the presence of a left atrial abnormality. There is evidence of a right atrial abnormality, in that the P waves in lead II have an amplitude of 3 mm and a duration of 0.10 second.

QRS complex: The duration of the QRS complex is 0.10 second. The mean QRS vector is directed inferiorly (+110°) and posteriorly. The 12-lead total QRS amplitude is more than 228 mm (the deflections are recorded below the grid marks on the paper in leads V2, V3, and V4).

T waves: The mean T vector is directed superiorly (-90°) and markedly anteriorly. The QRS-T angle is almost 180°. The T wave abnormality is characteristic of systolic pressure overload of the left ventricle.

A. The frontal plane projection of the mean P (Pm), QRS, and T vectors.
B. The spatial orientation of the mean P vector (Pm). Note the course of the transitional pathway on the chest.
C. The spatial orientation of the mean QRS vector. Note the transitional pathway on the chest. **D.** The spatial orientation of the mean T vector. Note the

(Figure 7.5 continued.)
transitional pathway on the chest.
Summary: Analysis of the P waves indicates the presence of both right and left atrial abnormalities. The mean QRS vector is directed inferiorly (+110°) and posteriorly suggesting either hypertrophy of the right and left ventricles or left ventricular hypertrophy plus left posterior-inferior division block. The

T wave abnormality indicates systolic pressure overload of the left ventricle. There are biatrial abnormalities and biventricular hypertrophy. Whereas these abnormalities could be due to a combination of anatomic and physiologic factors, in this case, they are due to dilated cardiomyopathy which produced severe heart failure and pulmonary hypertension.

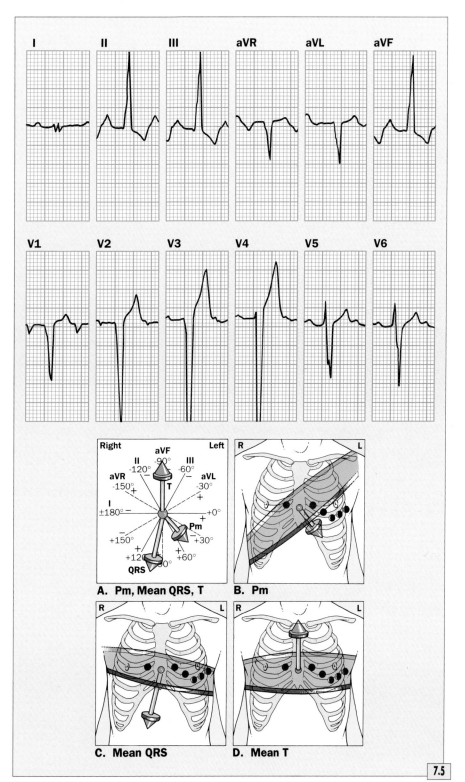

A. Pm, Mean QRS, T
B. Pm
C. Mean QRS
D. Mean T

Ventricular Conduction Defects and Pre-excitation of the Ventricles

In order to understand the abnormalities of the ventricular conduction system it is necessary to review the normal and abnormal anatomy of the ventricles, the left and right bundle branch conduction systems, anomalous conduction pathways, and normal and abnormal ventricular depolarization and repolarization (see Chapters 5 and 6). A conduction defect usually *slows* conduction and delays the depolarization of a portion of the ventricles.

The delta wave of the Wolf-Parkinson-White syndrome, an early QRS abnormality, is usually considered to be a conduction abnormality. However, it is actually due to *early* activation of a still relatively refractory part of the normal ventricle.

While one can consider many abnormalities of the QRS complex as being due to altered conduction within the ventricular muscle, this discussion is limited to alterations of the conduction system itself, and to alteration of the conduction system plus myocyte damage. For example, the sequence of depolarization responsible for the abnormal Q waves of myocardial infarction could be considered a conduction defect, but it occurs because myocytes have been removed (see Chapter 10).

QRS complexes of greater than 0.12 second duration are often associated with damage to the ventricular myocytes in conjunction with conduction system abnormalities; the combination, however, is viewed as a conduction defect. At times, therefore, abnormalities of the conduction system itself overlap with, and are superimposed on, abnormalities produced by damage to the myocytes.

Left or right ventricular hypertrophy alone rarely produces a QRS duration of greater than 0.10 second. Therefore, when the duration is greater than 0.10 seconds, it is proper to consider a conduction system abnormality in addition to ventricular hypertrophy. When, however, the QRS duration is 0.10 second, it is necessary to distinguish between a primary conduction defect and left or right ventricular hypertrophy, based on the direction of the initial and terminal QRS forces.

Although the QRS duration is usually 0.10 second or longer when there is a conduction defect, certain types of defects may be present even when the QRS duration is less than 0.10 second. These are recognized by identifying an abnormal direction of the terminal QRS electrical forces.

VENTRICULAR CONDUCTION DEFECTS WITH QRS DURATIONS OF 0.12 SECOND OR LESS

RIGHT VENTRICULAR CONDUCTION DELAY

The electrocardiographic characteristics of right ventricular conduction delay are listed in Table 8.1, and the electrocardiographic abnormalities that must be differentiated from those characteristic of the right ventricular conduction delay are listed in Table 8.2. Examples are shown in Figures 8.1 and 8.2.

In some of these cases, no other cardiac abnormalities may be identified. The conduction defect may be congenital, with failure of some of the fibers of the right bundle to develop normally. An atrial septal defect may be present. Acute pulmonary embolism may produce a right ventricular conduction delay, and slight right ventricular hypertrophy, such as that caused by mild pulmonary valve stenosis, may also be associated with right ventricular conduction delay in the electrocardiogram.

S1, S2, S3 VENTRICULAR CONDUCTION DEFECT

The electrocardiographic characteristics of the S1, S2, S3 type of ventricular conduction defect are listed in Table 8.3 and the abnormalities that must be differentiated from them are listed in Table 8.4. Examples are shown in Figures 8.3 and 8.4.

Our knowledge of the causes of the S1, S2, S3 type of ventricular conduction defect is incomplete. It occurs when no additional heart disease can be found, as a normal variant possibly due to an absence of Purkinje fibers in a portion of the right ventricle. It is also found in acquired disease such as chronic obstructive lung disease and emphysema, pulmonary embolism, acute severe lung disease, and hypertrophic cardiomyopathy.

LEFT VENTRICULAR CONDUCTION DELAY

The electrocardiographic characteristics of left ventricular conduction delay are listed in Table 8.5, and the abnormalities that must be differentiated from them are listed in Table 8.6. An example is shown in Figure 8.5.

Left ventricular conduction delay may occur in the absence of any recognizable heart disease, or it may be due to disease of the left ventricular conduction system of unknown cause. Theoretically, it could be caused by any condition known to cause left bundle branch block. The difference is that the duration of the QRS complex associated with left ventricular conduction delay is 0.10 to 0.11 second, whereas in left bundle branch block it is 0.12 second or more. Although left ventricular hypertrophy is often present in patients with a left ventricular conduction delay, the direction of the mean initial 0.04-second QRS vector is similar to that of left bundle branch block, rather than that of left ventricular hypertrophy. No Q waves are present in leads I and V6, and the R wave is either small or absent in lead V1, in a left ventricular conduction delay. Small Q waves plus other signs of left ventricular hypertrophy are usually present in leads I and V6 in cases of left ventricular hypertrophy.

LEFT ANTERIOR-SUPERIOR DIVISION BLOCK

The electrocardiographic characteristics of left anterior-superior division block are listed in Table 8.7, and the abnormalities that must be distinguished from it are shown in Table 8.8. Examples are shown in Figures 8.6 and 8.7.

Additional heart disease may not be identified in patients with left anterior-superior division block, though it can be due to primary conduction system disease of unknown cause, and may be associated with cardiomyopathy of any cause, including ischemic cardiomyopathy. It may be associated with left ventricular hypertrophy secondary to severe aortic valve disease, mitral valve regurgitation or hypertension, and may be caused by myocardial infarction. At times it may also be related to cardiac surgery or hyperkalemia.

LEFT POSTERIOR-INFERIOR DIVISION BLOCK

The electrocardiographic characteristics of left posterior-inferior division block are listed in Table 8.9. A number of abnormalities must be differentiated from those that typify left posterior-inferior block (Table 8.10). An example of the condition is shown in Figure 8.8. It is not possible to make these differentiations without access to a previously recorded electrocardiogram.

The etiology of left posterior-inferior division block may be difficult to establish, and no additional heart disease may be found. The condition may be caused by myocardial infarction, primary disease of the conduction system (of unknown origin), or cardiomyopathy of any cause, including ischemic cardiomyopathy. It may occur in patients with advanced valve disease, those who have had cardiac surgery, and those with hyperkalemia. The posterior-inferior division is less vulnerable to damage than other parts of the conduction system. This explains why pure posterior-inferior division block is so rare, and why left posterior-inferior block is more often associated with right bundle branch block.

Note: As stated in several places in this book, the model presented here is a clinically useful approximation of the real situation within the heart. At times, the explanation moves beyond the known evidence. When this occurs, every effort has been made to extend the facts in a logical manner.

FIGURE 8.1

This electrocardiogram, showing right ventricular conduction delay, was recorded from a 14-year-old adolescent girl who had a secundum type of atrial sep-

tal defect. A two-dimensional echocardiogram revealed a large left-to-right shunt, paradoxical septal motion, and a dilated right atrium and right ventricle.

The heart rate is 87 complexes per

minute and the rhythm is normal. The PR interval is 0.15 second and the QRS duration is 0.09 second. The duration of the QT interval is 0.32 second.

(Figure 8.1 continued on page 8.4.)

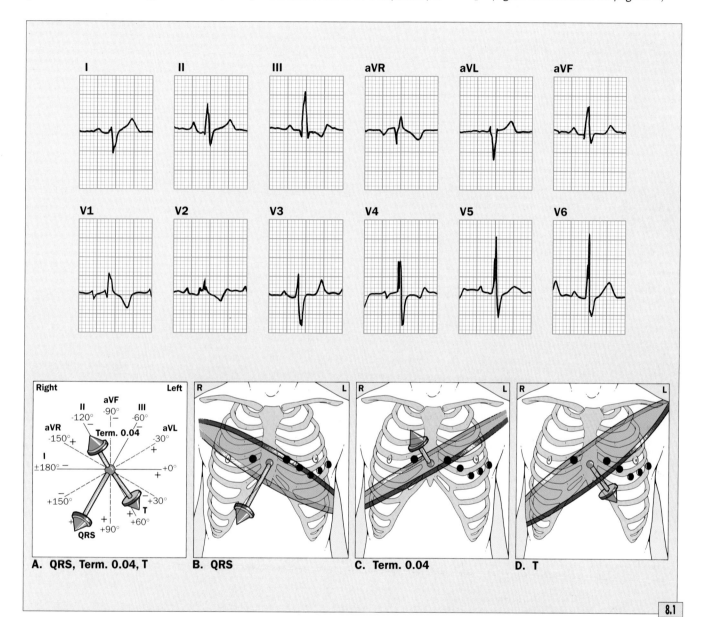

A. QRS, Term. 0.04, T   B. QRS   C. Term. 0.04   D. T

TABLE 8.1 ELECTROCARDIOGRAPHIC CHARACTERISTICS OF RIGHT VENTRICULAR CONDUCTION DELAY

- The QRS duration may be 0.08 second in children. It is usually 0.09 or 0.10 second in adults, but is never more than 0.11 second.

- The mean QRS vector is usually directed anteriorly, vertically, to the right or in the intermediate zone.

- The initial mean 0.04-second QRS vector is normally directed.

- The terminal mean 0.04-second QRS vector is directed to the right and anteriorly, producing a prominent secondary R wave in lead V1.

TABLE 8.2 ELECTROCARDIOGRAPHIC ABNORMALITIES THAT MUST BE DIFFERENTIATED FROM THOSE OF RIGHT VENTRICULAR CONDUCTION DELAY

- A QRS complex duration of 0.12 second or more, indicating right bundle branch block. The duration of the QRS complex in right ventricular conduction delay is never more than 0.11 second. It is usually 0.09 to 0.10 second in adults and less than this in children.

- A mean terminal 0.04-second QRS vector directed to the right, superiorly and posteriorly. This is associated with the S1, S2, S3 type of conduction disturbance. The mean terminal 0.04-second QRS vector associated with right ventricular conduction delay is directed to the right and anteriorly.

(Figure 8.1 continued.)

P Waves: The height of the P wave in lead II is 2.25 mm, suggestive of right atrial abnormality.

QRS complexes: The mean QRS vector is abnormally directed at about +120° vertically, and about 20° anteriorly. The mean terminal 0.04-second QRS vector is superiorly directed about -120° and about 10° anteriorly, indicating that the last portion of the heart to undergo depolarization is located to the right and anteriorly.

T Waves: The mean T vector is directed about +52° inferiorly and about 20° to 30° posteriorly.

A. The frontal plane projections of the mean QRS, the mean terminal 0.04-second QRS, and mean T vectors. **B.** The spatial orientation of the mean QRS vector. The transitional pathway is only an approximation in this patient. The resultant QRS complex is positive in leads V1 and V2, and approaches transitional in leads V3, V4, V5, and V6. The transitional pathway in this patient undoubtedly undulates. **C.** The spatial

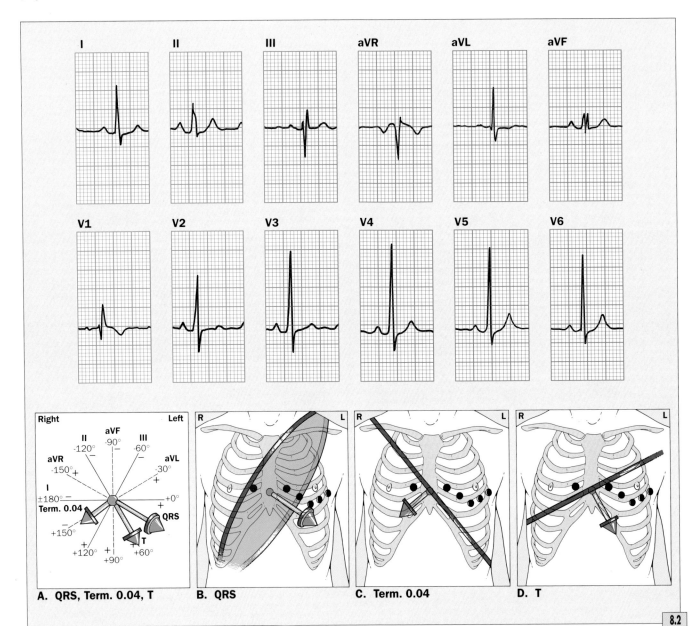

A. QRS, Term. 0.04, T   B. QRS   C. Term. 0.04   D. T

8.2

(Figure 8.1 continued.)
orientaion of the mean terminal 0.04-second QRS vector. **D.** The spatial orientation of the mean T vector.

Summary: This type of electrocardiogram occurs with diastolic pressure overload of the right ventricle. It is commonly caused by a secundum type of atrial septal defect, occuring in at least 90 percent of patients with such a defect. As time passes, the electrocardiogram may change to that characteristic of right bundle branch block. The electrocardiographic abnormality may persist after the defect has been surgically corrected.

F I G U R E 8 . 2
This electrocardiogram, showing right ventricular conduction delay, was recorded from a young man with moderate pulmonary valve regurgitation secondary to a Brock procedure for congenital pulmonary valve stenosis.

The heart rate is 82 complexes per minute and the rhythm is normal. The duration of the PR interval is 0.18 second. The duration of the QRS complex is 0.08 second and that of the QT interval is 0.31 second.

P waves: The P waves are normal and the Ta wave is prominent.

QRS complexes: The mean QRS vector is directed +30° inferiorly and 20° anteriorly. Its frontal plane projection is normal but its anterior direction is abnormal. The mean terminal 0.04-second QRS vector is parallel with and directed at +145° in the frontal plane. It is directed toward the right ventricle. The R waves are large in leads V1 and V2, suggesting right ventricular hypertrophy.

T waves: The mean T vector is directed vertically at about +60°, and parallel with the frontal plane.

A. The frontal plane projections of the mean QRS, mean terminal 0.04-second QRS, and mean T vectors. **B.** The spatial orientation of the mean QRS vector. **C.** The spatial orientation of the mean initial 0.04-second QRS vector. **D.** The spatial orientation of the mean T vector.

Summary: This tracing is shown to point out that it is not uncommon for pulmonary valve stenosis, which should produce systolic pressure overload of the right ventricle, to cause a right ventricular conduction delay. This can occur even when there is no pulmonary valve regurgitation. The increased size of the R waves in leads V1 and V2 suggests right ventricular hypertrophy, but the mean QRS vector is not directed to the right.

TABLE 8.3 ELECTROCARDIOGRAPHIC CHARACTERISTICS OF THE S1, S2, S3 VENTRICULAR CONDUCTION DEFECT

- The duration of the QRS complex is normal.
- The terminal mean 0.04-second QRS vector is directed to the right, superiorly, and posteriorly.
- The mean T vector is usually large and normally directed. Accordingly, the ventricular gradient is usually normal even though the size of mean QRS vector is small.

TABLE 8.4 ELECTROCARDIOGRAPHIC ABNORMALITIES THAT MUST BE DIFFERENTIATED FROM THOSE OF THE S1, S2, S3 TYPE OF CONDUCTION DEFECT

- A QRS duration of 0.12 second or more, as in right bundle branch block. In The S1, S2, S3 type of conduction defects, the duration of the QRS complex is less than 0.10 second and the mean terminal 0.04-second QRS vector is directed to the right, superiorly, and posteriorly.
- A terminal 0.04-second QRS vector which is directed to the right, inferiorly and anteriorly, as in a right ventricular conduction delay. It is directed to the right, superiorly, and posteriorly when there is an S1, S2, S3 type of conduction delay.
- The large but normally directed T wave vector associated with the S1, S2, S3 type of conduction defect might be mistaken for the T wave of hyperkalemia. Careful inspection, however, reveals that the ascending limb of the T wave is more slanted than the descending limb when the S1, S2, S3 pattern is present. In hyperkalemia, the ascending and descending limbs are equally slanted.

FIGURE 8.3

This electrocardiogram, illustrating the S1, S2, S3 type of tracing, was recorded from a normal 31-year-old man.

The heart rhythm is normal, and the heart rate is about 85 complexes per minute. The PR interval is 0.20 second and the QRS duration is 0.08 second. The QT interval is 0.34 second.

P waves: The P waves are normal.

QRS complexes: The mean QRS vector is directed +50° inferiorly and 10° to 15° posteriorly. The mean initial 0.04-second QRS vector is directed +70° inferiorly and about 90° anteriorly. The mean terminal 0.04-second QRS vector is directed -90°

superiorly and about 90° posteriorly. There is no S wave in lead I because the terminal QRS vector is perpendicular to lead I; if it were directed -95° superiorly, it would have recorded an S wave.

T wave: The T wave is large. The mean T vector is directed +60° inferiorly and 10° to 15° anteriorly.

A. The frontal plane projections of the mean QRS, mean initial 0.04-second QRS, mean terminal 0.04-second QRS, and mean T vectors. **B.** The spatial orientation of the mean QRS vector. **C.** The spatial orientation of the mean initial 0.04-second QRS vector. **D.** The spatial orientation of the mean terminal 0.04-

second QRS vector. **E.** The spatial orientation of the mean T vector.

Summary: Whereas the S1, S2, S3 pattern is usually seen in patients with no other heart disease, it can be recorded from patients with emphysema and, rarely, in patients with idiopathic ventricular hypertrophy (see Fig. 8.4). In the normal person, it is believed to be due to an absence of Purkinje fibers in a portion of the outflow tract of the right ventricle. The depolarization wave spreads from this area in a posterior direction. (Reproduced with permission from the publisher and author; see Figure Credits.)

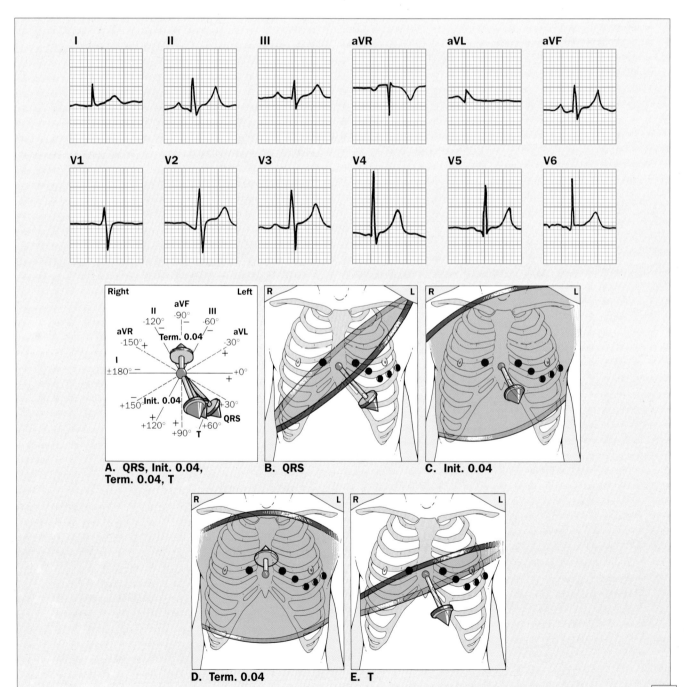

A. QRS, Init. 0.04, Term. 0.04, T

B. QRS

C. Init. 0.04

D. Term. 0.04

E. T

FIGURE 8.4

This electrocardiogram, showing an S1, S2, S3 pattern, was recorded from a 28-year-old woman with idiopathic hypertrophic subaortic stenosis. The aortic gradient in the left ventricular outflow tract was 60 mm Hg by echo-Doppler ultrasonography.

The heart rate is 65 complexes per minute, and the rhythm is normal. The PR interval is 0.16 second. The QRS duration is 0.08 second and the QT interval is 0.40 second. The U waves are prominent.

P waves: The P waves are normal.

QRS complex: The mean QRS vector is directed -118° superiorly and about 90° posteriorly. It is grossly abnormal: the mean initial 0.04-second QRS

vector is directed about -160° to the left and about 40° anteriorly; the mean terminal 0.04-second QRS vector is directed -155° to the left and about 90° posteriorly. The terminal QRS forces produce S waves in leads I, II, and III.

T waves: The mean T vector is directed about +70° inferiorly and 10° posteriorly.

A. The frontal plane projections of the mean QRS, the mean initial 0.04-second QRS, mean terminal 0.04-second QRS, and mean T vector. **B.** The spatial orientation of the mean QRS vector. **C.** The spatial orientation of the mean initial 0.04-second QRS vector. **D.** The spatial orientation of the mean terminal 0.04-second QRS vector. **E.** The spatial orientation of the mean T vector.

Summary: In this unusual electrocardiogram, the initial QRS force abnormality could be mistaken for the abnormal Q waves of myocardial infarction. As described in Chapter 11, idiopathic hypertrophic subaortic stenosis may produce the electrocardiographic signs of pseudoinfarction. The terminal 0.04-second QRS vector produces the S1, S2, S3 pattern. The wave of depolarization responsible for the terminal QRS forces probably begins in the outflow tract of the right ventricle, and is directed to the right and posteriorly. The S1, S2, S3 pattern commonly occurs when there is no other evidence of heart disease; this example indicates that it may also occur as a result of severe heart disease.

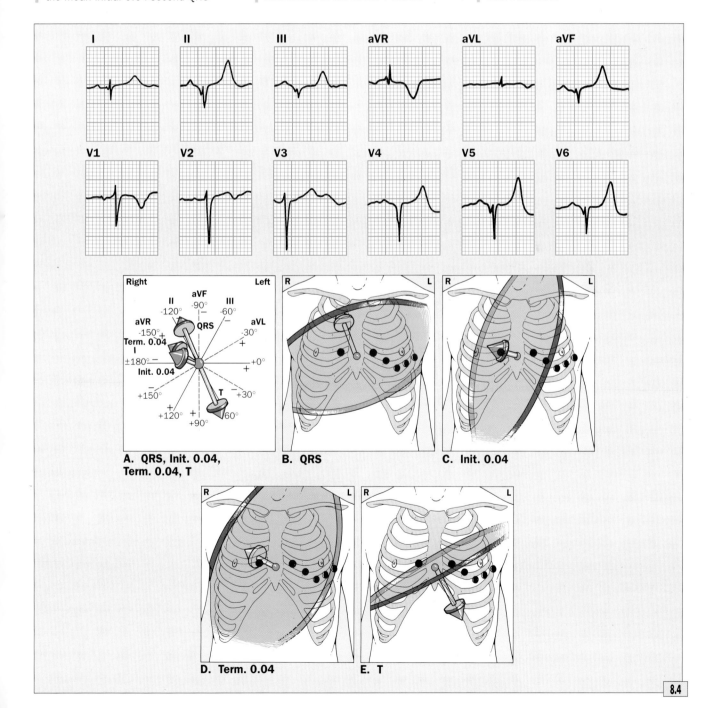

A. QRS, Init. 0.04, Term. 0.04, T

B. QRS

C. Init. 0.04

D. Term. 0.04

E. T

8.4

FIGURE 8.5

This electrocardiogram, showing a left ventricular conduction defect, was recorded from a 62-year-old man who had angina pectoris and near syncope secondary to calcific aortic stenosis and coronary atherosclerosis. The electrocardiogram was made after replacement of the aortic valve, coronary bypass surgery, and coronary angioplasty.

The rhythm is normal and the heart rate is 74 complexes per minute. The duration of the PR interval is 0.17 second. The duration of the QRS complex is 0.08 second in leads I, aVR,V4 and V5. It is 0.10 second in leads II, aVL,V1, V2, and V3, and 0.12 second in leads III and aVF. One gets the distinct impression that the QRS duration is less than 0.12 second as one would expect to see in left bundle branch block.

P waves: The P waves are normal.

QRS complex: The mean QRS vector is directed at +20° and about 45° posteriorly. The mean terminal 0.04-second QRS vector is directed to +50° and 45° posteriorly. There are no Q waves in leads I and V6, and there is a very small R wave in lead V1. This is characteristic of left bundle branch block, but the QRS duration in this tracing is shorter than usual in left bundle branch block.

ST segment: The mean ST vector is directed -160° to the right and about 25° anteriorly.

T waves: The mean T vector is directed +165° to the right and 45° anteriorly.

A. The frontal plane projections of the mean QRS, mean terminal 0.04-second QRS, mean ST, and mean T vectors.

B. The spatial orientation of the mean QRS vector. **C.** The spatial orientation of the mean terminal 0.04-second QRS vector. **D.** The spatial orientation of the mean ST vector.**E.** The spatial orientation of the mean T vector.

Summary: It is difficult to be certain about the duration of the QRS complex in this tracing. It is clearly greater than 0.10 second and cannot be explained as being due to left ventricular hypertrophy alone. If it is less than 0.12 second, it represents a left ventricular conduction defect because of the absent Q waves in leads I and V6 and small R wave in lead V1 as occur with left bundle branch block. The directions of the mean ST and T vectors in this electrocardiogram suggest systolic overload of the left ventricle in addition to a left ventricular conduction defect.

TABLE 8.5 ELECTROCARDIOGRAPHIC CHARACTERISTICS OF LEFT VENTRICULAR CONDUCTION DELAY

- The duration of the QRS complex is 0.10 to 0.11 second; it is always less than 0.12 second.

- The mean QRS vector is directed to the left and posteriorly; it is never directed as much as 30° to the left.

- The initial mean 0.04-second QRS vector is directed to the left and posteriorly; it may inscribe a small R wave or no R wave in lead V1, but does not inscribe a Q wave in leads I and V6.

- The terminal mean 0.04-second QRS vector is directed to the left and posteriorly.

- This defect simulates uncomplicated left bundle branch block, but the QRS duration is not sufficiently prolonged to meet the criteria for this condition.

TABLE 8.6 ELECTROCARDIOGRAPHIC ABNORMALITIES THAT MUST BE DIFFERENTIATED FROM THOSE OF LEFT VENTRICULAR CONDUCTION DELAY

- The duration of the QRS complex is 0.12 second or greater, indicating left bundle branch block. It is less than 0.12 second when there is left ventricular conduction delay. Otherwise, the two conditions are similar in that Q waves are not present in leads I and V6, and either no R wave or a small R wave is present in lead V1.

- Mean QRS vector directed as far as -30° to the left, and posteriorly as in left anterior-superior division block. When there is left ventricular conduction delay, this vector is directed posteriorly and to the left, but not as far as -30°.

- The duration of the QRS complex may be 0.10 second when there is left ventricular hypertrophy, and in these cases, the mean initial 0.04-second QRS vector is usually directed so that it inscribes a Q wave in leads I and V6. It does not do so when there is left ventricular conduction delay.

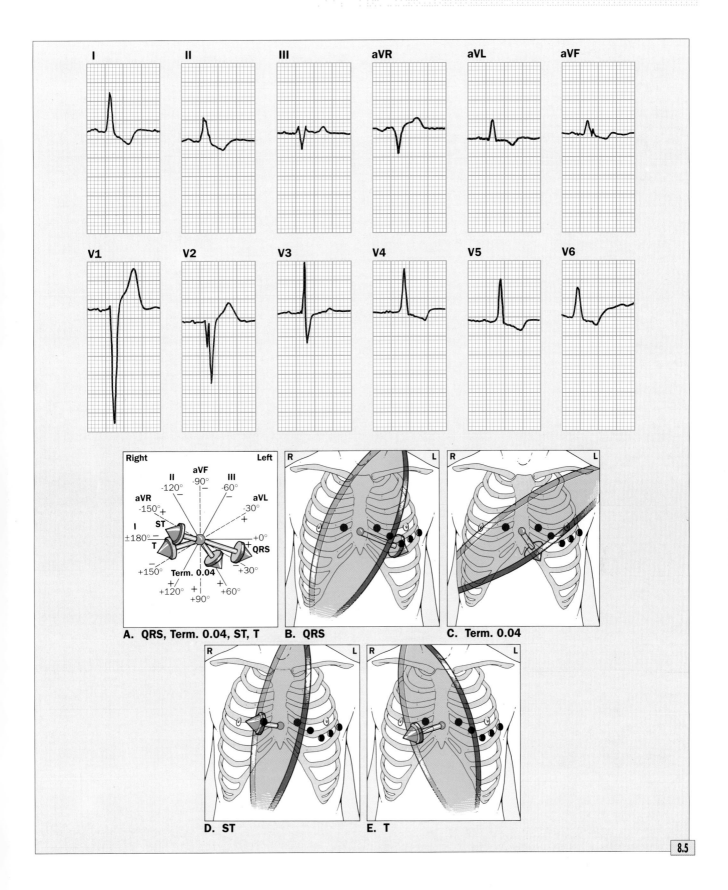

A. QRS, Term. 0.04, ST, T   B. QRS   C. Term. 0.04

D. ST   E. T

FIGURE 8.6

This electrocardiogram, showing left anterior-superior division block, was recorded from a 40-year-old woman following the removal of a myxomatous mitral valve for severe mitral regurgitation. Early in life, this patient had bacterial endocarditis on a patent ductus arteriosus, as well as a septic embolus to her brain. She survived with antibotic therapy and the patent ductus was treated surgically. As years passed, she developed increasing mitral regurgitation, atrial fibrillation, and increasing heart failure. Digoxin was continued after her mitral valve replacement. The electrocardiogram was approximately the same before and after the mitral valve surgery.

Sinus tachycardia is present and the heart rate is 102 complexes per minute. The duration of the PR interval is 0.20 second. The duration of the QRS complex is 0.09 second and that of the QT interval is 0.32 second.

P waves: The P waves are abnormal because they are 0.12 mm wide and 2.5 mm high in leads V2 and V3. P2 is directed at +60°, and parallel with the frontal plane. P2 measures -0.05 mm/sec in lead V1. These features signify a left atrial abnormality.

QRS complex: The mean QRS vector is directed -65° superiorly and about 30° to 40° posteriorly. The mean terminal 0.04-second QRS vector is directed -58° superiorly and 60° posteriorly. When the QRS duration is 0.10 sec, this degree of leftward deviation of the mean QRS and mean terminal 0.04-second QRS vectors indicates the presence of left anterior-superior division block.

T waves: The mean T vector is directed about +85° inferiorly and about 10°

anteriorly. This is due to left ventricular systolic pressure overload from long-standing, advanced diastolic overload of the left ventricle (see Chapter 6).

A. The frontal plane projections of the mean QRS, mean terminal 0.04-second QRS, and mean T vectors. **B.** The spatial orientation of the mean QRS vector. **C.** The spatial orientation of the mean terminal 0.04-second QRS vector. **D.** The spatial orientation of the mean T vector.

Summary: This electrocardiogram shows a left atrial abnormality, left anterior-superior division block, and left ventricular systolic pressure overload (see Chapter 6). In this patient, these abnormalities are due to severe mitral regurgitation from myxomatous mitral valve disease. Left anterior-superior division block can be due to many different causes (see page 8.2). It is

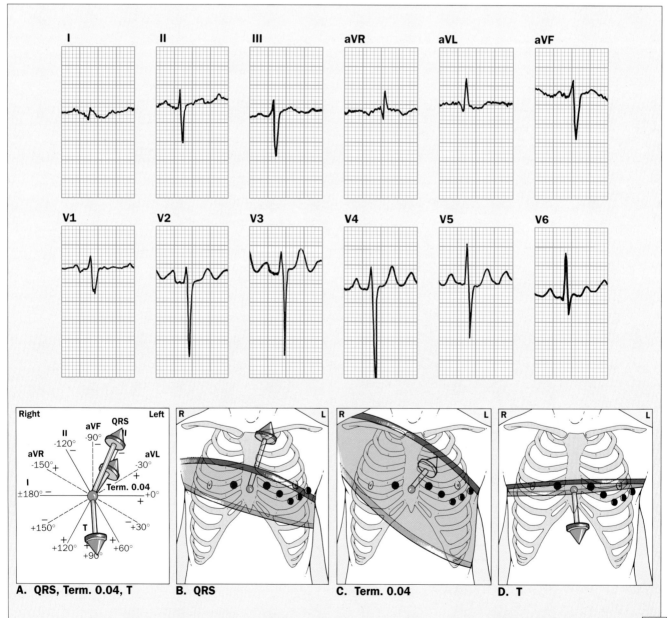

A. QRS, Term. 0.04, T   B. QRS   C. Term. 0.04   D. T

8.6

(Figure 8.6 continued.)
necessary to exclude other causes of such a marked left axis deviation of the mean QRS vector, such as extensive inferior myocardial infarction. Other electrocardiographic clues to an inferior infarction, however, are commonly present. Note that there is no clue to inferior infarction in this patient's electrocardiogram.

FIGURE 8.7

This electrocardiogram, showing left anterior-superior division block, was recorded from a 73-year-old woman who had a prior episode that could have been a myocardial infarction. She accepted a thallium scan but would not accept coronary arteriography. The thallium scan revealed a reperfusion defect indicating ischemia

and a questionable scar in the distribution of the right coronary artery.

The rhythm is normal, and the heart rate is 86 complexes per minute. The duration of the PR interval is 0.13 second, the duration of the QRS complex is 0.10 second and that of the QT interval is 0.32 second.

P waves: The P waves are normal.

QRS complex: The mean QRS vector is directed about -70° superiorly, and about 30° posteriorly. The mean terminal 0.04-second QRS vector is directed superiorly at about -85°, and about 85° posteriorly. When the QRS duration is 0.10 second, this degree of leftward deviation of these vectors signifies left anterior-superior division block. Anterior infarction cannot be identified with certainty in this tracing merely because there is poor "R wave

progression" in leads V1, V2, V3, and V4, which can be due to the posterior direction of the initial QRS forces that accompany a leftward, posteriorly directed QRS loop (see Chapter 6). On the other hand, an anterior infarction cannot be excluded, since this abnormality may be the only electrocardiographic clue to an infarction.

T waves: The mean T vector is directed +80° inferiorly and about 10° to 15° anteriorly. The QRS-T angle is about 150°. The T wave abnormality occurred after the patient experienced her possible myocardial infarction.

A. The frontal plane projections of the mean QRS, mean terminal 0.04-second QRS, and mean T vectors. **B.** The spatial orientation of the mean QRS vector. **C.** The spatial orientation of the mean
(Figure 8.7 continued on page 8.13.)

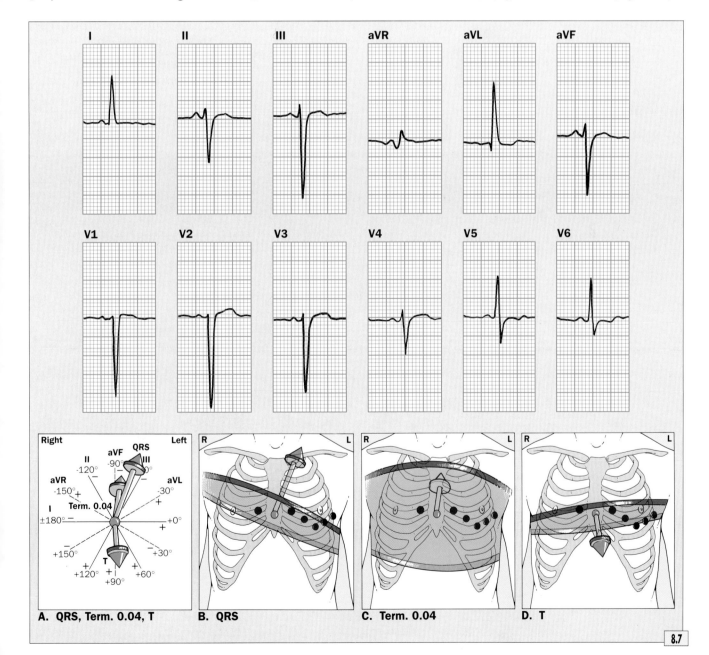

A. QRS, Term. 0.04, T   B. QRS   C. Term. 0.04   D. T

TABLE 8.7 ELECTROCARDIOGRAPHIC CHARACTERISTICS OF LEFT ANTERIOR-SUPERIOR DIVISION BLOCK

- The QRS duration is 0.09 to 0.11 second; it is usually 0.10 second.
- The mean QRS vector is directed -30° or more to the left.
- Inferior infarction and pre-excitation of the ventricles are excluded as causes for abnormal leftward deviation of the mean QRS vector.
- The terminal mean 0.04-second QRS vector is directed superiorly and posteriorly. It may be directed superiorly, slightly to the right, and posteriorly.

TABLE 8.8 ELECTROCARDIOGRAPHIC ABNORMALITIES THAT MUST BE DIFFERENTIATED FROM THOSE OF LEFT ANTERIOR-SUPERIOR DIVISION BLOCK

- In left anterior-superior division block, the duration of the QRS complex is 0.10 second. In left ventricular hypertrophy, it may reach this magnitude but usually does not.
- The mean QRS vector may be directed to the left when there is left ventricular hypertrophy, but does not reach -30°, as it does with left anterior-superior division block.
- The mean QRS vector of left ventricular conduction delay is not directed -30° or more to the left, as it is in left anterior-superior division block.
- A QRS complex duration of 0.12 second or more, as in left bundle branch block. It is 0.10 second when there is left anterior-superior block.
- Initial 0.04-second QRS vector in left ventricular conduction delay does not inscribe a Q wave in leads I and V6; it usually does so when there is left anterior-superior division block. This feature distinguishes one condition from the other, and signifies that the septum is depolarized normally during left anterior-superior division block but abnormally in left ventricular conduction delay.
- An inferior myocardial infarction that removes sufficient myocardium from the affected area to cause the mean QRS vector to be directed more than -30° to the left. Other signs of infarction will serve to identify the true cause of the left axis deviation of the mean QRS vector.

TABLE 8.9 ELECTROCARDIOGRAPHIC CHARACTERISTICS OF LEFT POSTERIOR-INFERIOR DIVISION BLOCK

- The QRS duration is 0.9 to 0.11 second; it is usually 0.10 second.
- The mean QRS vector is directed about +120° to the right and slightly posteriorly.*
- A previous electrocardiogram that does not show the mean QRS vector directed to the right. Without this, it is impossible to identify this block.
- Anterolateral infarction, right ventricular hypertrophy, acute and chronic cor pulmonale, and emphysema can be excluded by other clinical methods.

*It is not possible to assign a precise number of degrees to the rightward direction of the mean QRS axis in order to identify the presence of left posterior-inferior division block. Some authors state that it should be +110° to the right and I have used +120° in this book.

TABLE 8.10 ELECTROCARDIOGRAPHIC ABNORMALITIES THAT MUST BE DIFFERENTIATED FROM THOSE OF LEFT POSTERIOR-INFERIOR DIVISION BLOCK

- The tall, thin normal adult may have a mean QRS vector that is directed vertically and posteriorly. On rare occasions it may be directed as much as +110° to +120° to the right. It may be impossible to distinguish this finding from the abnormality due to a posterior-inferior conduction defect.
- Myocardial infarction of the anterolateral ventricular wall may produce a QRS complex duration of 0.10 second, and a mean QRS vector direction of +120° to the right and posteriorly*. These are the salient features of right posterior-inferior division block. Other evidence of infarction (i.e., abnormal ST and T vectors) may be present, to distinguish it.
- The duration of the mean QRS complex is 0.12 second or more, as in right bundle branch block, with the mean QRS vector directed to the right and anteriorly.
- Right ventricular hypertrophy may produce a mean QRS vector that is directed to the right and anteriorly, but this may not arise early in its natural history when due to acquired disease in the adult. Accordingly, the electrocardiographic abnormalities due to acquired right ventricular hypertrophy are difficult to distinguish from those due to posterior-inferior conduction block. Additional clinical data are needed to distinguish the two.
- It is usually necessary to compare a current electrocardiogram with a previously recorded one to identify left inferior-posterior division block. Its appearance on the current electrocardiogram distinguishes this condition from right ventricular hypertrophy.

*Some authors state that posterior-inferior division block causes the mean QRS axis to be directed about +110° to the right. I have used the figure of +120° in an effort to separate it from the rare normal that can be as much as +110°.

(Figure 8.7 continued.)
terminal 0.04-second QRS vector.
D. The spatial orientation of the mean T vector.

Summary: The presumptive cause of the abnormal left axis deviation of the mean QRS (-70°) and terminal 0.04-second QRS vectors in this patient is atherosclerotic coronary heart disease. The history, plus an abnormal reperfusion defect on thallium scan, support the diagnosis. In addition to these findings, the T wave abnormality occurred after the episode that suggested infarction.

FIGURE 8.8

This electrocardiogram, showing septal infarction and possible left posterior-inferior division block, was recorded from a 70-year-old woman who had a clinical diagnosis of atherosclerotic heart disease.

The rhythm is normal and the heart rate is 80 complexes per minute. The duration of the PR interval is 0.20 second, the duration of the QRS complex is 0.09 second and that of the QT interval is 0.34 second.

P waves: The P waves are difficult to identify; they are prominent in leads V1, V2, and V3.

QRS complex: The mean QRS vector is directed +135° inferiorly and about 15° to 20° posteriorly. The initial mean 0.04-second QRS vector, not plotted here, is directed about -20° to the left and about 30° posteriorly. The mean terminal 0.04-second QRS vector is directed +145° inferiorly and about 10° posteriorly.

T waves: The mean T vector is directed -5° to the left and about 15° posteriorly.

A. The frontal plane projections of the mean QRS, mean terminal 0.04-second QRS, and mean T vectors. **B.** The spatial orientation of the mean QRS vector. **C.** The spatial orientation of the mean terminal 0.04-second QRS vector. **D.** The spatial orientation of the mean T vector.

Summary: The direction of the initial QRS forces suggests an inferior-septal infarction. The marked right axis deviation of the mean QRS vector suggests left posterior-inferior block. When conduction in the left posterior-inferior division is blocked, the depolarization of

the left ventricle is guided by the intact left anterior-superior division; this may create a vector that is directed to the right. Other causes of marked right axis deviation of the mean QRS vector, such as right ventricular hypertrophy, pulmonary embolism, and extensive anteriolateral myocardial infarction, must be excluded. The QRS duration of 0.09 second rather than 0.12 second excludes right bundle branch block. The mean terminal 0.04-second QRS vector is usually directed to the right and posteriorly in left posterior-inferior division block, rather than anteriorly, as it usually is in right ventricular conduction delay. It is impossible to be certain about the identification of left posterior-inferior division block without comparing its electrocardiogram with a previous tracing that does not show the characteristic abnormalities. Left posterior-inferior division block is rare because this part of the conduction system is less vulnerable to damage than the other parts. This is why left posterior-inferior block is more often seen in association with right bundle branch block.

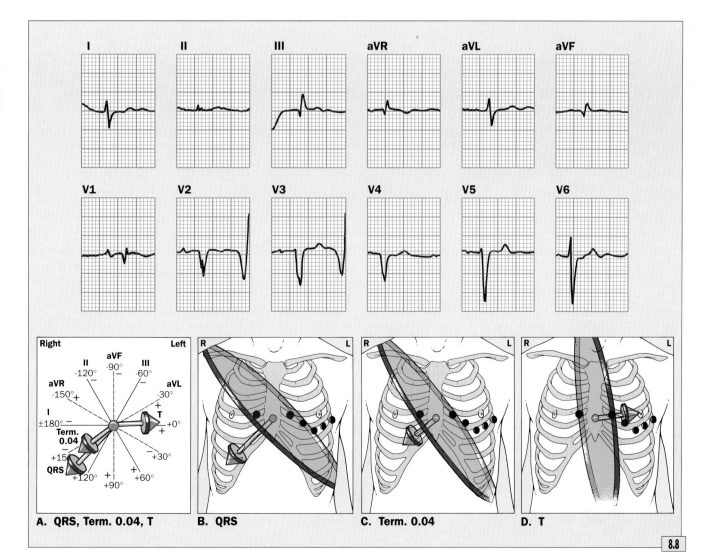

A. QRS, Term. 0.04, T   B. QRS   C. Term. 0.04   D. T

8.8

VENTRICULAR CONDUCTION DEFECTS WITH QRS DURATION 0.12 SECOND OR MORE

UNCOMPLICATED LEFT BUNDLE BRANCH BLOCK

The electrocardiographic characteristics of uncomplicated left bundle branch block are listed in Table 8.11. The electrocardiographic abnormalities that must be differentiated from these are listed in Table 8.12. Examples of this condition are shown in Figures 8.9 through 8.11.

Left bundle branch block may occur in the absence of any additional recognizable heart disease. The likelihood of additional cardiac disease is, however, greater when uncomplicated right bundle branch block exists. Futhermore, while coronary disease may produce left bundle branch block, the conduction defect occurs commonly in the absence of such disease. Left bundle branch block alone, without evidence of coronary or any other disease, causes an anterior reperfusion defect in the thallium scan. Accordingly, an error can be made by assuming that left bundle branch block plus an anterior myocardial perfusion defect as seen in a thallium scan is due to coronary disease.

Left bundle branch block may be caused by dilated cardiomyopathy of any cause, including ischemic cardiomyopathy, neuromuscular disease, collagen disease, neoplastic disease, radiation fibrosis, or drug toxicity. The conduction defect may be caused by Lev's disease (disease of the conduction system caused by impingement from without) or Lenagre's disease (a primary disease of the conduction system). It may be caused by severe aortic stenosis, aortic regurgitation, or mitral regurgitation of any cause, and severe left ventricular hypertrophy of any origin may eventually lead to its development. The block may also be the result of cardiac surgery or hyperkalemia.

COMPLICATED LEFT BUNDLE BRANCH BLOCK

LEFT BUNDLE BRANCH BLOCK PLUS LEFT ANTERIOR-SUPERIOR DIVISION BLOCK: The electrocardiographic characteristics of left bundle branch block plus left anterior-superior division block are listed in Table 8.13. The electrocardiographic abnormalities that must be differentiated from it are listed in Table 8.14. Examples of this complex condition are shown in Figures 8.12 and 8.13.

The causes of uncomplicated left bundle branch block are discussed above. These must be considered whenever there is left bundle branch block plus left anterior-superior division block. If such a combination is identified, it is appropriate to consider conditions that produce more diffuse involvement of the left conduction system and left ventricular myocytes. This combination defect may be due to Lev's disease, Lenagre's disease, dilated cardiomyopathy including ischemic cardiomyopathy, acute myocardial infarction due to coronary disease, advanced left ventricular hypertrophy and disease due to severe aortic valve or mitral regurgitation. It may also be a result of cardiac surgery or hyperkalemia.

LEFT BUNDLE BRANCH BLOCK AND PRIMARY ST AND T WAVE ABNORMALITIES: The electrocardiographic characteristics of left bundle branch block plus primary ST and T wave abnormalities are listed in Table 8.15, and the electrocardiographic abnormalities that must be differentiated from those seen in this condition are highlighted in Table 8.16. An example is shown in Figure 8.14.

Uncomplicated left bundle branch block produces secondary ST and T wave abnormalities. Primary ST and T wave abnormalities, in addition to secondary ST and T wave abnormalities, can be caused by an additional disease process; the most common is coronary disease with its associated myocardial ischemia, myocardial injury, and infarction, but other causes of myocardial disease, as well as cardiac surgery, may also be responsible.

UNCOMPLICATED RIGHT BUNDLE BRANCH BLOCK

The electrocardiographic characteristics of uncomplicated right bundle branch block are listed in Table 8.17, and abnormalities that must be differentiated from those of uncomplicated right bundle branch block are shown in Table 8.18. An example of the condition is shown in Figure 8.15.

Uncomplicated right bundle branch block may occur in the absence of any additional, recognizable heart disease. Whereas acute and chronic coronary disease may produce it, the isolated abnormality is not sufficient evidence for a diagnosis of coronary disease. Right bundle branch block can be caused by dilated cardiomyopathy of any cause, including ischemic cardiomyopathy, neuromuscular disease, collagen disease, neoplastic disease, radiation fibrosis, and drug toxicity. The conduction defect may also be caused by Lev's disease, Lenagre's disease, or severe valve disease. Even calcific aortic stenosis or aortic regurgitation can produce the conduction defect, as can an atrial septal defect. Other congenital defects that produce severe right ventricular hypertrophy may produce right bundle branch block, and acute pulmonary embolism may be responsible for its sudden development. Additionally, right bundle branch block may result from cor pulmonale related to obstructive lung disease or pulmonary emphysema, and from cardiac surgery or hyperkalemia.

COMPLICATED RIGHT BUNDLE BRANCH BLOCK

RIGHT BUNDLE BRANCH BLOCK PLUS LEFT ANTERIOR-SUPERIOR DIVISION BLOCK: The electrocardiographic characteristics of right bundle branch block plus left anterior-superior division block are listed in Table 8.19. Examples of it are shown in Figures 8.16 and 8.17.

The electrocardiographic abnormalities of right bundle branch block plus left anterior-superior division block are so unusual they approach uniqueness. There is no electrocardiographic differential diagnosis. It is not possible to distinguish between primary disease of the conduction system and disease of the myocardium with secondary conduction system involvement.

Right bundle branch block plus left anterior-superior division block may be caused by coronary disease and myocardial infarction; primary disease of the conduction system, including Lev's disease and Lenagre's disease; cardiomyopathy of any cause, including ischemic cardiomyopathy; and advanced left and right ventricular hypertrophy due to aortic valve disease or mitral regurgitation. In children, the most common cause is an ostium primum type of atrial septal defect, or one of the variations of an atrioventricular canal. Right bundle branch block plus left anterior-superior division block may be the result of cardiac surgery or hyperkalemia.

RIGHT BUNDLE BRANCH BLOCK PLUS LEFT POSTERIOR-INFERIOR DIVISION BLOCK: Left posterior-inferior division block occurs commonly in association with right bundle branch block, and the electrocardiographic characteristics of the combined conduction defects are listed in Table 8.20. The electrocardiographic abnormalities that must be differentiated from the combined block are listed in Table 8.21. Examples of the condition are shown in Figures 8.18 and 8.19.

It is appropriate to consider diseases that involve the right and left conduction systems and right and left ventricles when, in addition to right bundle branch block, there is evidence of associated left posterior-inferior division block. This combination of conduction defects may be due to coronary disease, Lev's disease, Lenagre's disease, dilated cardiomyopathy of any cause, including ischemic cardiomyopathy, advanced heart disease due to severe valve disease, and cor pulmonale and emphysema. Right bundle branch block plus left posterior-inferior division block may also be the result of cardiac surgery or hyperkalemia.

RIGHT BUNDLE BRANCH BLOCK PLUS PRIMARY ST OR T WAVE ABNORMALITIES: The electrocardiographic characteristics of right bundle branch block plus primary ST or T wave abnormalities are listed in Table 8.22. The electrocardiographic abnormalities that must be differentiated from these combined defects are listed in Table 8.23. Sample electrocardiograms are shown in Figures 8.20 and 8.21.

The causes of right bundle branch block are listed on page 8.14. Whenever primary ST and T wave abnormalities are present in addition to right bundle branch block, it is proper to consider associated myocardial infarction, especially when the ST and T wave abnormalities develop acutely. Cardiomyopathy, especially hypertrophic cardiomyopathy, may also be responsible for the primary ST and T wave abnormalities. Right bundle branch block plus primary ST and T wave abnormalities may be the result of cardiac surgery.

QRS CONDUCTION DEFECT DUE TO EXPOSURE TO COLD

THE OSBORN WAVE: The electrocardiographic abnormalities due to cold exposure are listed in Table 8.24. The electrocardiographic abnormalities associated with exposure to severe cold are virtually unique; for practical purposes, no other condition produces them (Table 8.25). An example of such a QRS conduction defect (the Osborn wave) is shown in Figure 8.22.

The electrocardiographic manifestations described here occur in individuals exposed to severe cold as the result of excess alcohol consumption, accident or inadequate heat in their environment. These abnormalities may occasionally occur when hypothermia is used in addition to anesthesia for prolonged surgical procedures. They rarely occur as the result of hypothermia associated with coronary bypass surgery. The precise cause of the Osborn wave is unknown; perhaps the depolarization of the basilar portion of the left ventricle is delayed because that area of the heart is cooled more than the remainder of the heart. The effect of hypothemia on the brain, and its relationship to the QRS, ST, and T waves, has not been adequately studied.

TABLE 8.11 ELECTROCARDIOGRAPHIC CHARACTERISTICS OF UNCOMPLICATED LEFT BUNDLE BRANCH BLOCK

- The mean QRS vector is directed to the left and posteriorly. When left bundle branch block occurs, this vector shifts about 30° to the left of its previous direction. It is never directed more than -30° to the left. The QRS duration is 0.12 second.

- The mean initial 0.04-second QRS vector is directed to the left and posteriorly; therefore, a small R wave (or the absence of an R wave) may be seen in lead V1, and no Q waves are seen in leads I and V6.

- The mean terminal 0.04-second QRS vector is directed to the left and posteriorly.

- Secondary ST and T wave abnormalities are present. The mean ST and T vectors tend to be directed opposite the mean QRS vector. The ventricular gradient is normally directed.

- The electrocardiographic abnormalities of uncomplicated left bundle branch block may obscure the QRS abnormalities of myocardial infarction. The presence of uncomplicated left bundle branch block makes it difficult to identify left ventricular hypertrophy.

TABLE 8.12 ELECTROCARDIOGRAPHIC ABNORMALITIES THAT MUST BE DIFFERENTIATED FROM THOSE OF UNCOMPLICATED LEFT BUNDLE BRANCH BLOCK

- Complicated left bundle branch block, associated with a QRS duration of greater than 0.12 second. In this condition, the mean QRS vector is directed more then -30° to the left, the mean ST and T vectors may not be opposite the mean QRS vector, or the ventricular gradient is abnormal.

- The electrocardiographic abnormalities of left ventricular conduction delay may simulate those of left bundle branch block, but the duration of the QRS complex is less than 0.12 second.

- The electrocardiographic abnormalities of left ventricular hypertrophy may simulate those of left bundle branch block except

that in the former, the mean initial 0.04-second QRS vector is directed so that it inscribes a Q wave in leads I and V6; it does not do so when there is left bundle branch block. The duration of the QRS complex does not reach 0.12 second when there is left ventricular hypertrophy.

- The electrocardigraphic abnormalities of pre-excitation of the ventricles, which occurs in patients with the Wolff-Parkinson-White syndrome, may simulate those of left bundle branch block. The short PR interval and delta waves seen with pre-excitation of the ventricles are clues to this diagnosis, since they do not occur with left bundle branch block.

F I G U R E 8 . 9

This electrocardiogram, showing left bundle branch block, was recorded from a 67-year-old woman. She gave a history of having hypertension for five years, and complained of chest discomfort and dyspnea on effort. Cardiac catheterization revealed mild aortic regurgita-tion,

no gradient across the aortic valve, and normal coronary arteries.

The rhythm is normal and the heart rate is 65 complexes per minute. The duration of the PR interval is 0.20 second, the duration of the QRS complex is 0.12 second and that of the QT interval is 0.42 second.

P waves: The P waves are normal.

QRS complex: The mean QRS vector is directed about -15° to the left and about 50° to 60° posteriorly. The mean terminal 0.04-second QRS vector is directed about -30° to the left and 85° posteriorly.

ST segment: The mean ST segment

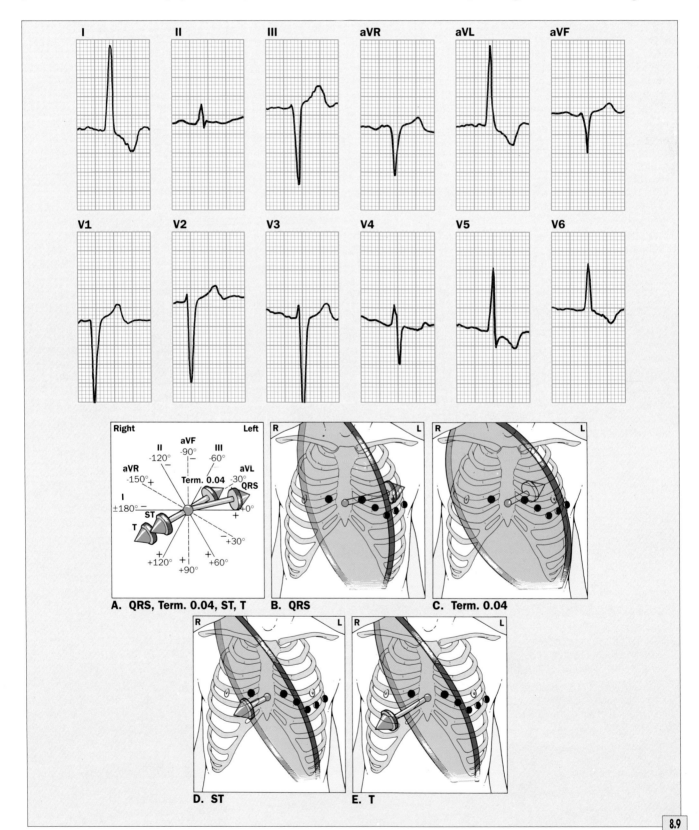

A. QRS, Term. 0.04, ST, T   B. QRS   C. Term. 0.04

D. ST   E. T

(Figure 8.9 continued.)
vector is directed +150° to the right and 30° anteriorly; it is relatively parallel with the mean T vector and opposite the mean QRS vector.

T waves: The mean T vector is directed +150° to the right and 30° anteriorly; it is relatively parallel with the mean ST vector and opposite the mean QRS vector.

A. The frontal plane projections of the mean QRS, mean terminal 0.04-second QRS, mean ST, and mean T vectors. **B.** The spatial orientation of the mean QRS vector. **C.** The spatial orientation of the mean terminal 0.04-second QRS vector. **D.** The spatial orientation of the mean ST vector. **E.** The spatial orientation of the mean T vector.

Summary: This electrocardiogram shows the characteristics of left bundle branch block. The cause of the left bun-

dle branch block in this patient is not known. Her coronary arteries were normal at coronary arteriography, and there was only slight aortic regurgitation.

FIGURE 8.10
This electrocardiogram, showing left bundle branch block, was recorded from a 40-year-old man without other evidence of heart disease. He did not have a coronary arteriogram.

The heart rhythm is normal and the heart rate is 70 complexes per minute. The duration of the PR interval is 0.16 second, the duration of the QRS complex is 0.12 second, and that of the QT interval is 0.40 second.

P waves: The P waves are normal.

QRS complex: The mean QRS vector is directed at +12° and 45° to 50° posteriorly. The mean terminal 0.04-second

QRS vector is directed -20° to the left and 30° posteriorly. There are no Q waves in leads I and V6, and there is a small R wave in lead V1.

T waves: The mean T vector is directed vertically at about +30, and anteriorly to an undetermined degree. It is probably directed about 45° to 60° anteriorly because the T wave in lead V1 is little larger than that in lead V6.

A. The frontal plane projections of the mean QRS, mean terminal 0.04-second QRS, and mean T vectors. **B.** The spatial orientation of the mean QRS vector. **C.** The spatial orientation of the mean terminal 0.04-second QRS vector. **D.** The spatial orientation of the mean T vector.

Summary: This electrocardiogram illustrates all of the features of left
(Figure 8.10 continued on page 8.18.)

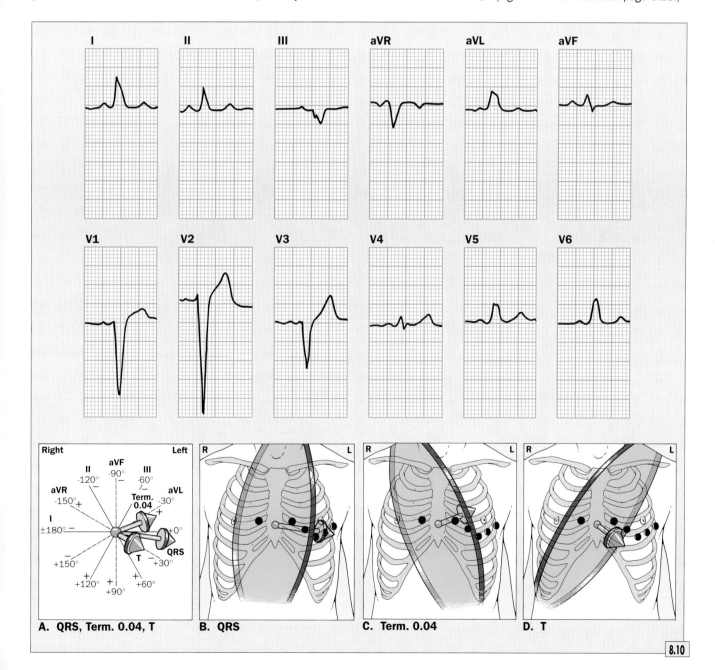

A. QRS, Term. 0.04, T   B. QRS   C. Term. 0.04   D. T

(Figure 8.10 continued.)
bundle branch block, including a QRS duration of 0.12 second, a mean QRS and mean terminal 0.04 second QRS vector directed to the left and posteriorly, the absence of Q waves in leads I and V6, and a small R wave in lead V1. The mean T vector has an unusual ori-

entation, being directed moderately anteriorly, so that the QRS-T angle is 90 to 100°. It is not opposite to the mean QRS as is usual. The cause of the left bundle branch block in this patient is not known. (Reproduced with permission from the publisher and author; see Figure Credits.)

FIGURE 8.11

This electrocardiogram, recorded from a middle-aged woman, shows uncomplicated left bundle branch block. The presence of this abnormality stimulated a request for a thallium scan, the positive features of which led to the performance of a coronary arteriogram. The

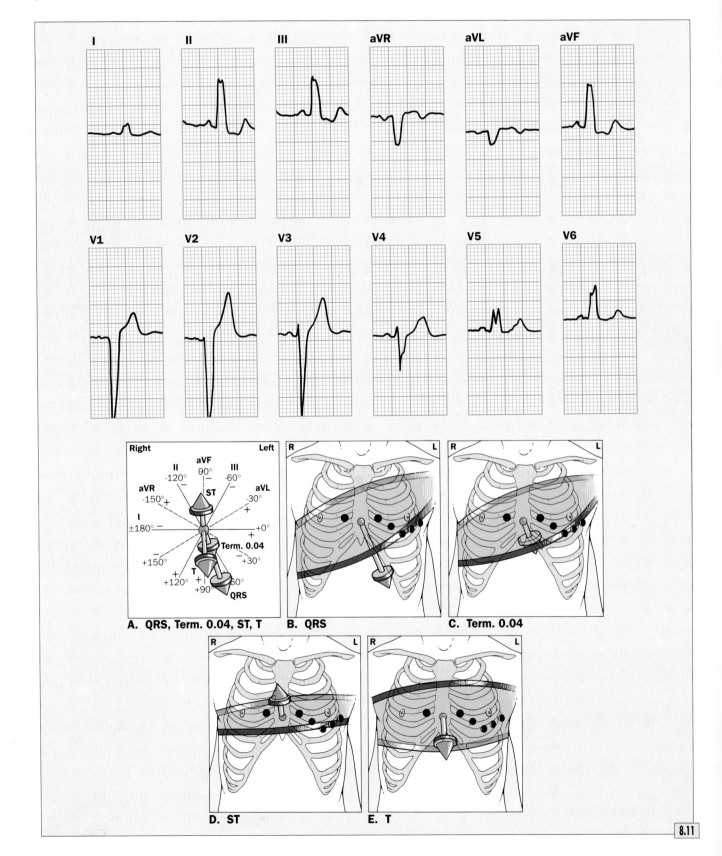

(Figure 8.11 continued.)
thallium scan showed pseudo-ischemia, and the coronary arteriogram was normal. It was soon learned that the abnormal sequence of myocardial activation produced by left bundle branch block causes a false-positive thallium scan.

The heart rhythm is normal, and the heart rate is 90 complexes per minute. The PR interval is 0.14 second, the QRS duration is 0.12 second, and the QT interval is 0.40 second.

P waves: The P waves are normal.

QRS complex: The mean QRS vector is directed about +70° vertically, and about 45° posteriorly. The terminal 0.04-second QRS vector is directed about +70° vertically and about 45° posteriorly. These abnormalities signify the presence of left bundle branch block.

ST segment: The mean ST segment vector is directed about -95° superiorly and about 35° anteriorly.

T waves: The mean T vector is directed about +85° vertically, and anteriorly. It is not possible to establish exactly how far anteriorly the mean T vector is directed, but because the T wave is larger in lead V1 than in lead V6, the mean T vector must be directed at least 60° anteriorly.

A. The frontal plane projections of the mean QRS, mean terminal 0.04-second QRS, mean ST, and mean T vectors.

B. The spatial orientation of the mean QRS vector. **C.** The spatial orientation of the mean terminal 0.04-second QRS vector. **D.** The spatial orientation of the mean ST vector. **E.** The spatial orientation of the mean T vector.

Summary: The electrocardiogram shows left bundle branch block, but it is atypical because the mean T vector is not directed opposite the mean QRS vector; however, the ventricular gradient appears to be normal. The thallium scan shows antero-septal and inferior ischemia, but the coronary arteriogram was normal. The findings in this case show that left bundle branch block is clearly able to produce a false–positive reperfusion defect in the thallium scan.

TABLE 8.13 ELECTROCARDIOGRAPHIC CHARACTERISTICS OF LEFT BUNDLE BRANCH BLOCK PLUS LEFT ANTERIOR-SUPERIOR DIVISION BLOCK

- The QRS duration is 0.12 second or more.

- The mean QRS vector is directed -30° or more to the left and posteriorly.

- The initial mean 0.04-second QRS vector is directed to the left and posteriorly. The R wave is absent or small in lead V1 and there are no Q waves in leads I and V6.

- The terminal mean 0.04-second QRS vector is directed to the left, superiorly, and posteriorly. It may even be directed to the right, superiorly, and posteriorly.

- Secondary ST and T wave abnormalities are present. The mean ST and T vectors are directed opposite the mean QRS vector.

- The electrocardiographic manifestations of left bundle branch block plus left anterior-superior division block may obscure the abnormalities of myocardial infarction or left ventricular hypertrophy.

TABLE 8.14 ELECTROCARDIOGRAPHIC ABNORMALITIES THAT MUST BE DIFFERENTIATED FROM THOSE OF LEFT BUNDLE BRANCH BLOCK PLUS LEFT ANTERIOR-SUPERIOR DIVISION BLOCK

- Uncomplicated left bundle branch block is excluded because the mean QRS vector is directed -30° or more to the left; this indicates a conduction defect that is more distal than the left bundle branch. The wave of depolarization spreads from the right side of the septum to the left, and enters the posterior-inferior division without difficulty, but because of a conduction defect or myocyte damage in the anterior-superior division, it has difficulty entering the areas of myocardium ordinarily served by the anterior-superior division. It does so, however, and may produce a wave of depolarization that is opposite normal.

- The possibility of isolated left anterior-superior division block is eliminated when the duration of the QRS complex is discovered to be 0.12 second or greater.

- Isolated left ventricular hypertrophy does not exhibit a QRS duration of 0.12 second, and the mean QRS vector is not directed beyond -30° to the left.

FIGURE 8.12

This electrocardiogram, showing left bundle branch block and left anterior-superior division block, was recorded from a 70-year-old man with arteriographically proven atherosclerotic coronary heart disease.

The rhythm is normal and the heart rate is 63 complexes per minute. The duration of the PR interval is 0.28 second, the duration of the QRS complex is 0.12 second in leads II and aVL, and the duration of QT interval is 0.36 second.

P waves: The duration of the P wave in lead II is 0.12 second and the second half of the P wave in lead V1 measures -0.05 mm/sec. These findings indicate a left atrial abnormality.

QRS complex: The mean QRS vector is directed -60° to the left and about 45° posteriorly. The mean terminal 0.04-second QRS vector is directed -95° superiorly and 80° posteriorly.

T waves: The mean T vector is directed at +90°, and 20° anteriorly.

A. The frontal plane projections of the mean QRS, mean terminal 0.04-second QRS, and mean T vectors. **B.** The spatial orientation of the mean QRS vector.
C. The spatial orientation of the mean terminal 0.04-second QRS vector.
D. The spatial orientation of the mean T vector.

Summary: It is difficult to determine the exact duration of the QRS complex in this electrocardiogram. It is definitely 0.12 second in leads II, III, aVR, and aVL. The mean QRS vector is directed -70° to the left. In uncomplicated left bundle branch block, the shift is not this extreme. It is likely that when depolarization spreads from the right side of the septum into the left ventricle, it enters areas ordinarily served by the left posterior-inferior division, creating a vector that is directed leftward and posteriorly. Furthermore, the wave of depolarization spreads in a retrograde manner into the area of muscle ordinarily served by the left anterior-superior division, directing this vector leftward rather than inferiorly and anteriorly, as it does normally. The altered depolarization occurs when the conduction in the left common bundle branch is blocked, and there is additional conduction blockage in the proximal por-

tion of the left anterior-superior division system. The conduction defect in this patient is most likely due to coronary artery disease.

FIGURE 8.13

This electrocardiogram, showing left bundle branch block and left anterior-superior division block, was recorded from an 81-year-old man with severe calcific aortic valve stenosis. The patient complained of chest discomfort. He had undergone cardiac catheterization. The pressure gradient across the aortic valve was 86 mm Hg and the coronary arteries were normal.

Atrial fibrillation is present, and the ventricular rate is 96 complexes per minute. The duration of the QRS complex is 0.13 second and the duration of the QT interval is 0.38 second.

QRS complex: The direction of the mean QRS vector is -70° to the left and 10° to 15° posteriorly. There are no Q waves in leads I and V6, and there is no R wave in lead V1. The mean terminal 0.04-second QRS vector is directed -110° superiorly and 80° posteriorly. The mean QRS vector and mean terminal

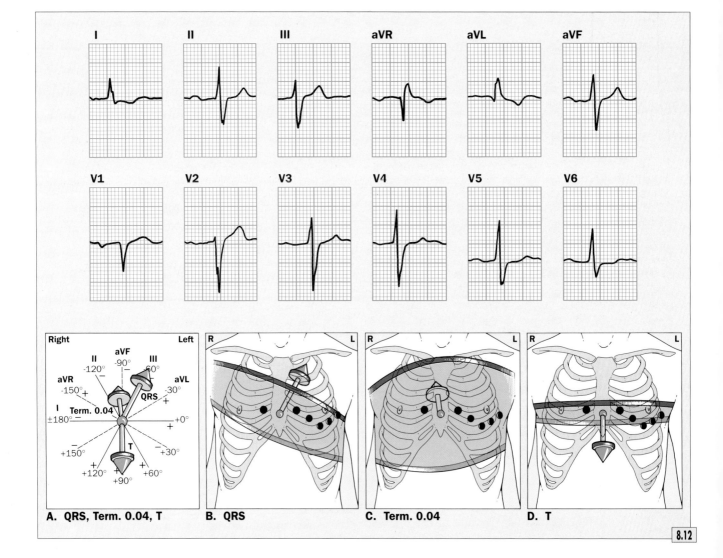

A. QRS, Term. 0.04, T   **B. QRS**   **C. Term. 0.04**   **D. T**

8.12

(Figure 8.13 continued.)
0.04-second QRS vector are directed farther to the left than when there is uncomplicated left bundle branch block.

T waves: The mean T vector is directed at +95° and about 80° anteriorly.

A. The frontal plane projections of the mean QRS, mean terminal 0.04-second QRS, and mean T vectors. **B.** The spatial orientation of the mean QRS vector. **C.** The spatial orientation of the mean terminal 0.04-second QRS vector. **D.** The spatial orientation of the mean T vector.

Summary: The electrocardiographic abnormalities characteristic of left bundle branch block are present in this electrocardiogram. The mean QRS vector is, however, directed more leftward

than it should be in uncomplicated left bundle branch block. This occurs because there may be a block of conduction in the proximal portion of the left anterior-superior division as well as in the left common bundle. The electrical impulse passes down the right bundle branch and the wave of depolarization passes from right to left through the septum into the left ventricle. Having done so, it enters the area served by the left posterior-inferior division, producing leftward and posterior electrical forces. Because the proximal portion of the left anterior-superior division is damaged, the depolarization process spreads in a retrograde manner in the myocardium served by this portion of the conduction system, pro-

ducing electrical forces that are directed leftward, superiorly, and posteriorly.

Note the size of the QRS voltage. This may be due to left ventricular hypertrophy. One must be cautious, however, in using QRS voltage to identify left ventricular hypertrophy in a patient with left bundle branch block. At times, unopposed electrical forces occurring during the QRS cycle may produce an increase in QRS voltage when there is no left ventricular hypertrophy. This patient undoubtedly had sclerosis and even calcification of parts of the cardiac skeleton in association with aortic stenosis. This can damage the conduction system and produce ventricular conduction abnormalities and complete heart block.

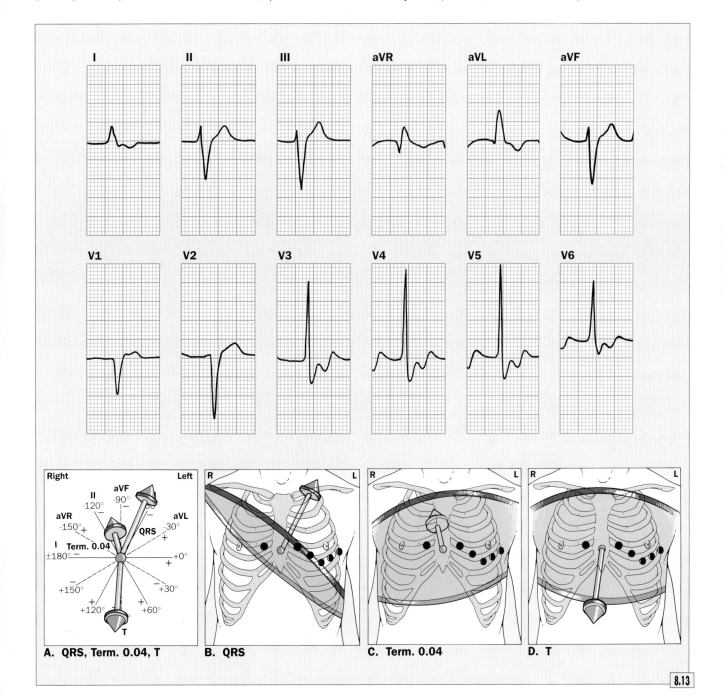

A. QRS, Term. 0.04, T   **B. QRS**   **C. Term. 0.04**   **D. T**

8.13

F I G U R E   8 . 1 4

This electrocardiogram, showing left bundle branch block plus a primary T wave abnormality, was recorded from an 83-year-old woman with severe asymmetrical septal hypertrophy. An echo-Doppler study revealed a peak instantaneous gradient across the aortic outflow tract of 66 mm Hg, mild mitral regurgitation, mild tricuspid regurgitation, and a trace of aortic regurgitation.

The rhythm is normal and the heart rate is 78 complexes per minute. The duration of the PR interval is 0.16 second, the duration of the QRS complex is 0.12 second, and that of the QT interval is 0.38 second.

P waves: The P waves are normal.

QRS complex: The mean QRS vector is directed -18° to the left and 45° to 50° posteriorly. The mean terminal 0.04-second QRS vector is directed -60° to the left and about 20° posteriorly. There are no Q waves in leads I and V6, and no R wave in lead V1. These abnormalities are characteristic of left bundle branch block.

T waves: The mean T vector is directed at -170°, and 45° anteriorly. The ventricular gradient is abnormal because it is directed superiorly.

A. The frontal plane projections of the mean QRS, mean terminal 0.04-second QRS, and mean T vectors. **B.** The spatial orientation of the mean QRS vector. **C.** The spatial orientation of the mean terminal 0.04-second QRS vector. **D.** The spatial orientation of the mean T vector.

Summary: The electrocardiographic abnormalities indicating left bundle branch block are straightforward. The mean T wave vector should be directed opposite the mean QRS vector. In addition to this, the computed ventricular gradient should lie in the area between 0 and +90° in the frontal plane when the T wave abnormality is secondary to the altered sequence of depolarization caused by the left bundle branch block. In the electrocardiogram shown here, the T wave shows a primary abnormality because the ventricular gradient is directed superiorly. This indicates that the repolarization process is altered because of an inferior myocardial abnormality; the T wave abnormality is not simply due to the altered repolarization that always follows the abnormal depolarization associated with left bundle branch block. In this patient, the primary T wave abnormality could be due to a localized myocardial abnormality associated with idiopathic hypertrophy or myocardial ischemia. She did not have a coronary arteriogram.

TABLE 8.15 ELECTROCARDIOGRAPHIC CHARACTERISTICS OF LEFT BUNDLE BRANCH BLOCK PLUS PRIMARY ST AND T WAVE ABNORMALITIES

- The QRS abnormalities of uncomplicated left bundle branch block or left bundle branch block plus left anterior-superior division block are present.

- The duration of the QRS is 0.12 second or more.

- The mean T wave vector is usually directed opposite the mean QRS vector produced by left bundle branch block or left bundle branch block plus left anterior-superior division block (secondary T wave abnormality). Whenever there is a primary T wave abnormality as well, the mean T vector may not be opposite the mean QRS vector. The ventricular gradient, when it can be calculated, is abnormal. When a primary T wave abnormality is present, one should deduce the existence of a primary repolarization abnormality within the myocardium.

- When the mean ST vector does not parallel a secondary mean T vector, a primary ST wave abnormality is considered to exist, and it is proper to consider the presence of epicardial injury. The mean ST vector parallels the mean T vector in uncomplicated left bundle branch block or in left bundle branch block plus left anterior-superior division block. This is a secondary ST wave abnormality.

TABLE 8.16 ELECTROCARDIOGRAPHIC ABNORMALITIES THAT MUST BE DIFFERENTIATED FROM THOSE OF LEFT BUNDLE BRANCH BLOCK PLUS PRIMARY ST AND T WAVE ABNORMALITIES

- A mean QRS vector directed less than -30° to the left, and a QRS complex duration of 0.12 second, as in uncomplicated left bundle branch block. The ST and T vectors associated with this condition are directed opposite the mean QRS vector, and the ventricular gradient is normal. When this is not the case, an abnormality of the ST and T vectors is assumed, and the ventricular gradient, when it can be calculated, is abnormally directed. It is sometimes difficult to determine the exact direction of the mean ST or T vectors and to calculate the ventricular gradient; this limits the use of the analysis of the ST and T vectors.

- A mean ST vector (when it can be determined) pointing toward an area of epicardial myocardial injury, rather than opposite the direction of the mean QRS vector; this suggests epicardial injury associated with myocardial infarction.

- A mean T vector and ventricular gradient (when they can calculated) directed away from an area of epicardial myocardial ischemia, as is associated with myocardial infarction or other myocardial causes of an abnormality of repolarization.

- Many primary ST and T wave abnormalities are undoubtedly masked by the enormous secondary abnormalities produced by the large ST and T vectors associated with left bundle branch block.

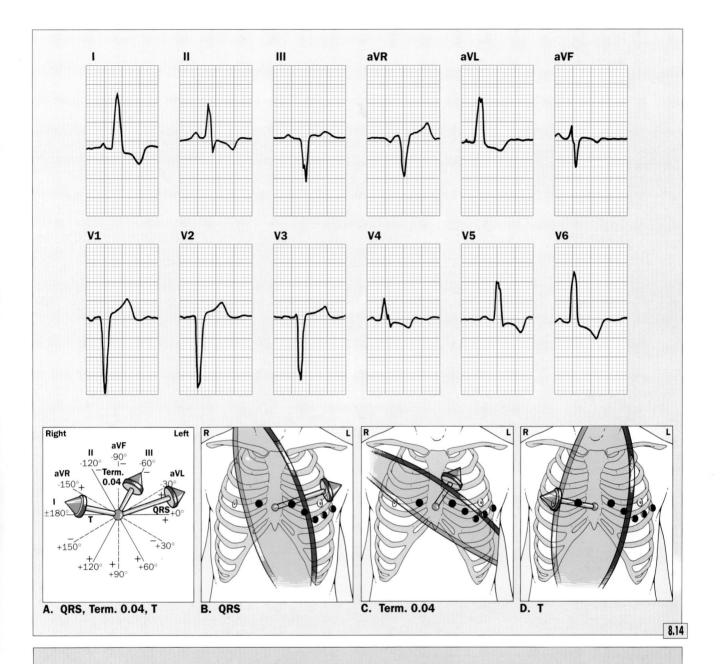

A. QRS, Term. 0.04, T   B. QRS   C. Term. 0.04   D. T

8.14

TABLE 8.17 ELECTROCARDIOGRAPHIC CHARACTERISTICS OF UNCOMPLICATED RIGHT BUNDLE BRANCH BLOCK

- The duration of the QRS complex is 0.12 second.

- The mean QRS vector is directed to the right, inferiorly, and anteriorly. It shifts about 30° to the right of a previously normally directed mean QRS vector. It is rarely directed more than +120° to the right.

- The mean initial 0.04-second QRS vector is normally directed.

- The mean terminal 0.04-second QRS vector is directed to the right and anteriorly.

- Secondary ST and T wave abnormalities are present. The mean ST and T vectors are directed opposite the mean QRS vector. The ventricular gradient is normal.

- The electrocardiographic abnormalities of uncomplicated right bundle branch block do not obscure the signs of myocardial infarction or left ventricular hypertrophy.

FIGURE 8.15

This electrocardiogram, showing uncomplicated right bundle branch block, was recorded routinely from a 44-year-old man with no cardiac symptoms prior to surgery for a right renal tumor.

The rhythm is normal and the heart rate is 90 complexes per minute. The duration of the PR interval is 0.12 second. The duration of the QRS complex is 0.12 second and the duration of the QT interval is 0.36 second.

P waves: The P waves are normal.

QRS complexes: The mean QRS vector is directed +108° inferiorly and parallel with the frontal plane. The direction of the mean terminal 0.04-second QRS vector is -155°, also parallel with the frontal plane. These abnormalities are characteristic of right bundle branch block.

T waves: The mean T vector is directed about +35° inferiorly and parallel with the frontal plane. The ventricular gradient is normally directed.

A. The frontal plane projections of the mean QRS, mean terminal 0.04-second QRS, and mean T vectors. **B.** The spatial orientation of the mean QRS vector.

C. The spatial orientation of the mean terminal 0.04-second QRS vector.

D. The spatial orientation of the mean T vector.

Summary: This electrocardiogram has all of the characteristics of uncomplicated right bundle branch block. Given the direction of the mean QRS vector, it is not necessary to be concerned about the possibility of associated left posterior-inferior division block, as is the case in Figure 8.20. The cause of the conduction defect in this patient was unknown, and coronary arteriography

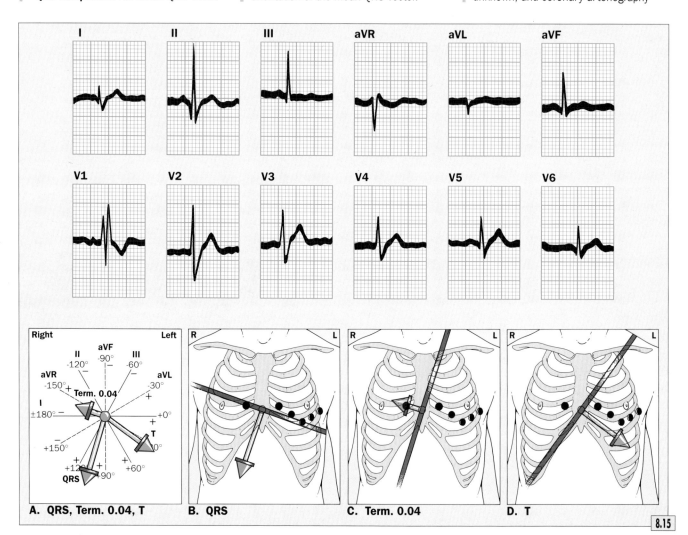

A. QRS, Term. 0.04, T   B. QRS   C. Term. 0.04   D. T

8.15

TABLE 8.18 ELECTROCARDIOGRAPHIC ABNORMALITIES THAT MUST BE DIFFERENTIATED FROM THOSE OF UNCOMPLICATED RIGHT BUNDLE BRANCH BLOCK

- A QRS duration of 0.12 second, which distinguishes right bundle branch block from right ventricular conduction delay, the S1, S2, S3 pattern, or right posterior-inferior division block, in which the QRS duration is never more than 0.10 second. When the duration is greater than 0.12 second, it is proper to consider myocyte damage or an additional defect within the conduction system.

- Right ventricular hypertrophy, that may produce a mean QRS vector directed to the right and anteriorly. However, in this condition, the QRS duration is less than 0.12 second, usually being

about 0.10 second. When the QRS duration is 0.12 second, both right ventricular hypertrophy and right bundle branch block may be present in the same electrocardiogram, thus presenting a problem.

- A mean QRS vector that is directed to the right and anteriorly, as may be produced in myocardial infarction. Other signs of infarction, such as an abnormal initial QRS vector and abnormal ST and T vectors, indicate its presence. The problem is that both infarction and right bundle branch block may be present in the same electrocardiogram.

(Figure 8.15 continued.)
was not possible when this tracing was recorded. (Reproduced with permission from the publisher and author; see Figure Credits.)

FIGURE 8.16

This electrocardiogram, showing the triad of first-degree heart block, right bundle branch block, and left anterior-superior division block, was recorded from a 79-year-old man with atherosclerotic coronary heart disease. The patient had coronary bypass surgery for high-grade obstruction of the left anterior descending, diagonal, circumflex, and right coronary arteries. He gave a history of two

myocardial infarctions, and a cororary arteriogram was performed after the second. Six months later he had a syncopal episode. He showed evidence of ventricular standstill on telemetry, and a pacemaker was inserted.

The rhythm is normal and the heart rate is 67 complexes per minute. The duration of the PR interval is 0.22 second, signifying first-degree atrioventricular conduction block. The QRS duration is 0.12 second and the QT interval is 0.38 second.

P waves: The second half of the P wave in lead V1 measures -0.04 mm/sec, suggesting a left atrial abnormality.

QRS complex: The mean QRS vector is

directed about -85° superiorly and is parallel with the frontal plane. This orientation produces a QRS complex that is positive in lead V1, resembling that of right bundle branch block. The mean terminal 0.04-second QRS vector is directed -145° superiorly and is parallel with the frontal plane. The directions of these two vectors indicate the presence of left anterior-superior division block. The terminal QRS forces of right bundle branch block are directed to the right and anteriorly, and the terminal QRS forces resulting from left anterior-superior division block are directed to the left and posteriorly since they are controlled by the intact left

(Figure 8.16 continued on page 8.26.)

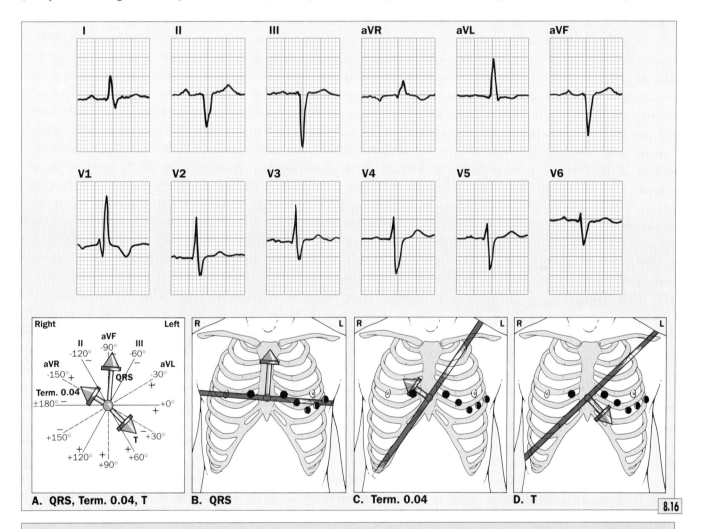

A. QRS, Term. 0.04, T   B. QRS   C. Term. 0.04   D. T   8.16

TABLE 8.19 ELECTROCARDIOGRAPHIC CHARACTERISTICS OF RIGHT BUNDLE BRANCH BLOCK AND LEFT ANTERIOR-SUPERIOR DIVISION BLOCK

- The duration of the QRS complex is 0.12 second or more; it is often greater than 0.12 second.

- The mean QRS vector is directed -30° or more to the left, anteriorly or parallel with the frontal plane. The extremity leads suggest the left bundle branch block and the precordial leads suggest right bundle branch block.

- The terminal mean 0.04-second QRS vector is directed superiorly and anteriorly; it may be directed superiorly, to the right, anteriorly, or parallel with the frontal plane.

- Secondary ST and T wave abnormalities are present. The mean ST and T vectors are directed opposite the mean QRS vector.

(Figure 8.16 continued.)
posterior-inferior division. The summation of these forces produces a mean terminal QRS vector directed far to the right, superiorly, anteriorly, or parallel with the frontal plane. The entire mean QRS vector shifts to the left and anteriorly.

T waves: The mean T vector is directed +45° inferiorly, parallel with the frontal plane. The ventricular gradient is directed superiorly, signifying a primary T wave abnormality, the usual cause of which would be altered repolarization in the epicardial region of the inferior wall of the left ventricle.

A. The frontal plane projections of the mean QRS, mean terminal 0.04-second QRS, and mean T vectors. **B.** The spatial orientation of the mean QRS vector. **C.** The spatial orientation of the mean ter-

minal 0.04-second QRS vector. **D.** The spatial orientation of the mean T vector.

Summary: This patient had proven advanced athersclerotic coronary heart disease. Although this is probably the cause of the three identified conduction abnormalities, the patient might also have two distinct conditions: sclerosis of the cardiac skeleton and coronary atherosclerosis. A QRS duration of 0.12 second and mean QRS vector directed far to the left and either anteriorly or parallel with the frontal plane is almost always due to right bundle branch plus left anterior-superior division block.

FIGURE 8.17

This electrocardiogram, showing right bundle branch block and left anterior-superior division block, was recorded

from a 70-year-old man with atherosclerotic coronary heart disease, aortic sclerosis and slight aortic regurgitation. The patient had class 2 angina pectoris for 3 months prior to coronary arteriography, which revealed 100 percent obstruction of the first and third marginal branches of the circumflex coronary arteries. The proximal and distal left anterior descending arteries and the first marginal all showed 16 percent narrowing. The ejection fraction was 35 percent. There was mild hypokinesis of the antero-basal segment, akinesis of the infero-apical segment, anterior dyskinesis, and apical akinesis. This electrocardiogram was made 10 days after the coronary arteriogram.

The rhythm is normal and the heart rate is about 100 complexes per minute. The duration of the PR interval

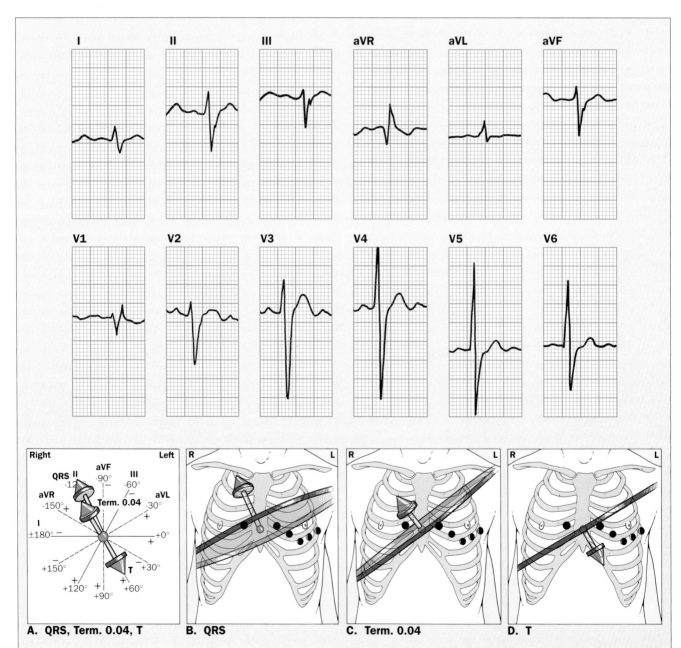

A. QRS, Term. 0.04, T   **B. QRS**   **C. Term. 0.04**   **D. T**

(Figure 8.17 continued.)
is 0.20 second, the duration of the QRS complex is 0.13 second and that of the QT interval is 0.36 second.

P waves: The P waves are normal.

QRS complex: The mean QRS vector is directed -115° superiorly and about 10° posteriorly. The mean terminal 0.04-second QRS vector is directed -123° superiorly and 5° to 10° anteriorly. The QRS complex in lead V1 is characteristic of right bundle branch block, and the direction of the mean QRS vector and mean terminal 0.04-second QRS vector is characteristic of right bundle branch block plus left anterior-superior division block (see discussion of the QRS forces in the legend to Figure 8.16).

T waves: The mean T vector is directed +60° inferiorly and parallel with the frontal plane. The ventricular gradient is directed superiorly and away from an area of altered repolarization in the epi-

cardial region of the inferior portion of the left ventricle. This feature is indicating the presence of a primary T wave abnormality.

A. The frontal plane projections of the mean QRS, mean terminal 0.04-second QRS, and mean T vectors. **B.** The spatial orientation of the mean QRS vector. **C.** The spatial orientation of the mean terminal 0.04-second QRS vector. **D.** The spatial orientation of the mean T vector.

Summary: This patient has atherosclerotic heart disease with evidence of considerable myocardial damage. Presumably, the conduction abnormalities are due to coronary disease, but as discussed in the legend to Figure 8.16, they may be due to sclerosis of the cardiac skeleton. Whenever the duration of the QRS complex is 0.12 second or more, the mean QRS vector is directed far to the left and almost parallel with the frontal plane, and the mean terminal

0.04-second QRS vector is directed superiorly, (occasionally by more than -90°) parallel with the frontal plane or oriented anteriorly, right bundle branch plus left anterior-superior division block is said to exist.

F I G U R E   8 . 1 8
This electrocardiogram, showing right bundle branch block plus left posterior-inferior division block, was recorded from a 60-year-old man with coronary disease. He was admitted to the coronary care unit because of severe chest pain of 12 hours duration.

The rhythm is normal and the heart rate is 102 complexes per minute. The duration of the PR interval is 0.14 second, the duration of the QRS complex is 0.12 second and that of the QT interval is 0.40 second.

P waves: The second half of the
(Figure 8.18 continued on page 8.28.)

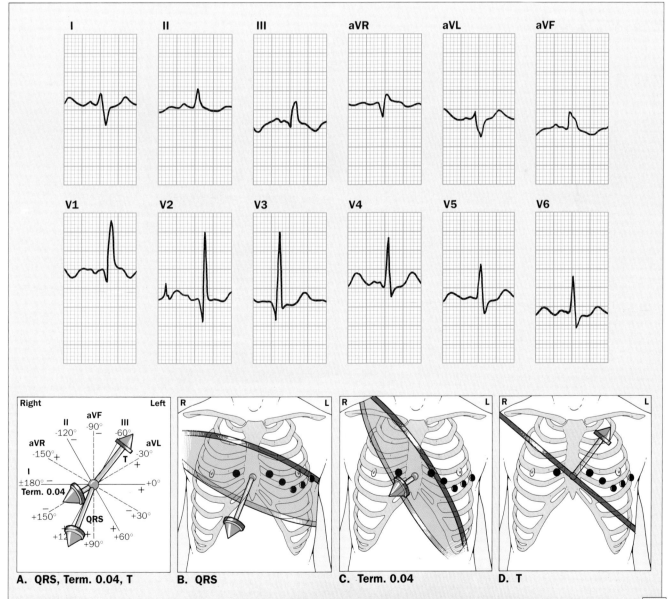

A. QRS, Term. 0.04, T   B. QRS   C. Term. 0.04   D. T

8.18

(Figure 8.18 continued.)
P wave in lead V1 measures -0.03 mm/sec.

QRS complex: The mean QRS vector is directed about +118° inferiorly and about 70° anteriorly. The mean initial 0.04-second QRS vector is not plotted here, but is directed +30° inferiorly and about 45° posteriorly. The mean terminal 0.04-second QRS vector is directed about +150° inferiorly and about 30° anteriorly. These vector orientations suggest right bundle branch block and left posterior-inferior division block. The initial QRS abnormality indicates the dead zone of an anteroseptal infarction.

T waves: The mean T vector is directed -50° to the left and is parallel with the frontal plane. **A.** The frontal plane projections of the mean QRS, mean terminal 0.04-second QRS, and mean T vectors. **B.** The frontal plane projection of the mean QRS vector. **C.** The spatial orientation of the mean terminal 0.04-second vector. **D.** The spatial orientation of the mean T vector.

Summary: This electrocardiogram shows anteroseptal infarction, right bundle branch block, and possible left posterior-inferior division block. It can be used to raise a question: how far to the right should the mean QRS vector be to indicate the presence of left posterior-inferior division block? The answer is not known. It is known that the mean QRS vector will not shift to the right of its previous position by more than 30° when right bundle branch block develops. Therefore, the direction of the mean QRS vector of right bundle branch block is predetermined by its direction prior to the development of the block. The same is true for left bundle branch block, since the mean QRS vector does not shift more than 30° to the left of its position prior to the block. If a tracing made prior to the right bundle branch block shows a QRS vector that is directed +90° inferiorly, the mean QRS vector after the block will be directed +120°.

Because most electrocardiograms do not exhibit a mean QRS vector of +90° but rather, of +30° to +70°, it is proper to consider left posterior inferior division block whenever the mean QRS vector is directed inferiorly by more than +110°. Left posterior inferior division block is highly likely when the mean QRS vector is directed +120° inferiorly. The predictability of left posterior-inferior division block increases the farther to the right the mean QRS vector is directed. Left posterior-inferior block is probably more common when there is right bundle branch block because the left posterior-inferior division is less vulnerable to injury than the other parts of the conduction system. The terminal 0.04 second vector represents the summation of electrical forces of depolarization guided by the intact left anterior-superior division and those created by the late depolarization of the right ventricle. (Reproduced with permission from the publisher and author; see Figure Credits.)

F I G U R E   8 . 1 9
This electrocardiogram, showing complicated right bundle branch block, was recorded from a 63-year-old hypertensive patient. Left posterior-inferior division block is also likely.

The rhythm is normal and the heart rate is 100 complexes per minute. The duration of the PR interval is 0.12 second, the duration of the QRS complex is 0.12 second and the duration of the QT

TABLE 8.20 ELECTROCARDIOGRAPHIC CHARACTERISTICS OF RIGHT BUNDLE BRANCH BLOCK PLUS LEFT POSTERIOR-INFERIOR DIVISION BLOCK

- The QRS duration is 0.12 second or more; it is often greater than 0.12 second.

- The mean QRS vector is directed more than +120° to the right and anteriorly.

- The terminal mean 0.04-second QRS vector is directed far to the right. It may be directed anteriorly, parallel with the frontal plane, or even posteriorly.

- Secondary ST and T wave abnormalities are present.

- It is difficult to identify this combination of conduction defects unless a previously recorded electrocardiogram shows a mean QRS vector that is directed no more than +90° vertically. Identification requires a previously recorded electrocardiogram that does not show the influence of left posterior-inferior division block.

TABLE 8.21 ELECTROCARDIOGRAPHIC ABNORMALITIES THAT MUST BE DIFFERENTIATED FROM THOSE OF RIGHT BUNDLE BRANCH BLOCK PLUS LEFT POSTERIOR-INFERIOR DIVISION BLOCK

- The identification of right bundle branch block is straightforward; the mean QRS vector is directed inferiorly and to the right, and the QRS complex is 0.12 second or more. The problem is to determine just how far to the right the mean QRS vector must be directed to raise the possibility of posterior-inferior division block; an arbitrary figure of +120° seems to be acceptable. A mean terminal 0.04-second QRS vector directed far to the right and anteriorly, parallel with the frontal plane, or even posteriorly, strongly suggests posterior-inferior division block. This is why the mean QRS vector is directed +120° to the right or more when there is right bundle branch block plus left inferior-posterior division block.

- Right bundle branch block plus lateral myocardial infarction may produce a mean QRS vector and a terminal 0.04-second QRS vector that simulate right bundle branch block plus left posterior-inferior division block. Other electrocardiographic signs of infarction may be present, but they do not preclude the existence of left posterior-inferior division block.

(Figure 8.19 continued.)
interval is 0.32 second.

P waves: The P waves are normal.

QRS complexes: The mean QRS vector is directed +135° to the right and it is parallel with the frontal plane. The mean terminal 0.04-second QRS vector is directed about -180° to the right and is almost parallel with the frontal plane. Generally, such vector orientations indicate right bundle branch block when the QRS duration is 0.12 second. The concern here is that both of the vectors are directed further to the right than is usually the case with right bundle branch block. In this situation, it is proper to consider the coexistence of left posterior-

inferior division block. However, posterior-inferior division conduction block cannot be identified without a previously recorded electrocardiogram showing right bundle branch block but lacking a right-axis QRS vector deviation of this degree.

T waves: The mean T vector is directed vertically at 30° and is parallel with the frontal plane. It tends to point away from the mean QRS vector. The ventricular gradient is normal.

A. The frontal plane projections of the mean QRS, mean initial 0.04-second QRS, and mean T vector. **B.** The spatial orientation of the mean QRS vector. **C.** The spatial orientation of the mean

terminal 0.04-second QRS vector. **D.** The spatial orientation of the mean T vector.

Summary: The abnormalities here, including the duration of the QRS complex (0.12 second), the direction of the mean QRS vector and terminal 0.04-second QRS vector, and the ventricular gradient indicate right bundle branch block. It is probably correct to consider additional left posterior-inferior division block as well. The cause of the conduction defect in this hypertensive patient is unknown; the question cannot always be answered. No coronary arteriogram was performed nor should have been. (Reproduced with permission of the publisher and author; see Figure Credits.)

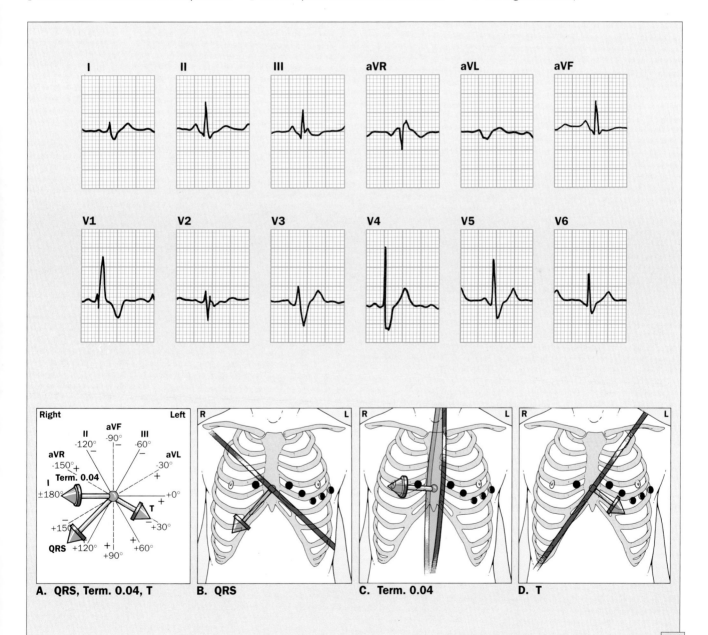

A. QRS, Term. 0.04, T   B. QRS   C. Term. 0.04   D. T

8.19

FIGURE 8.20
This electrocardiogram shows right bundle branch block, left posterior–inferior division block, and a primary T wave abnormality.

The rhythm is normal and the heart rate is 100 complexes per minute. The duration of the PR interval is 0.16 second, that of the QRS complex is 0.12 second, and that of the QT interval is 0.36 second.

P waves: The P waves are normal.

QRS complexes: The mean QRS vector is directed at +165° and is parallel with the frontal plane. The mean terminal 0.04-second QRS vector is directed at +165°, also parallel with the frontal plane. These vectors are characteristic of right bundle branch block plus left posterior-inferior block.

T waves: The mean T vector is directed +178° to the right and about 20° posteriorly. The ventricular gradient is abnormally directed at about +170° to the right, away from an area of altered epicardial repolarization in the antero-lateral and apical regions of the heart.

A. The frontal plane projections of the mean QRS, mean terminal 0.04-second QRS, and mean T vectors. **B.** The spatial orientation of the mean QRS vector. **C.** The spatial orientation of the mean terminal 0.04-second QRS vector.
D. The spatial orientation of the mean T vector.

Summary: This electrocardiogram shows right bundle branch block. The mean QRS vector and the mean terminal 0.04-second QRS vector are directed so far to the right that left posterior-inferior division block is almost certain. The mean T vector is abnormally directed, as is the ventricular gradient, indicating anterolateral and apical epicardial ischemia. (Reproduced with permission from the publisher and author; see Figure Credits.)

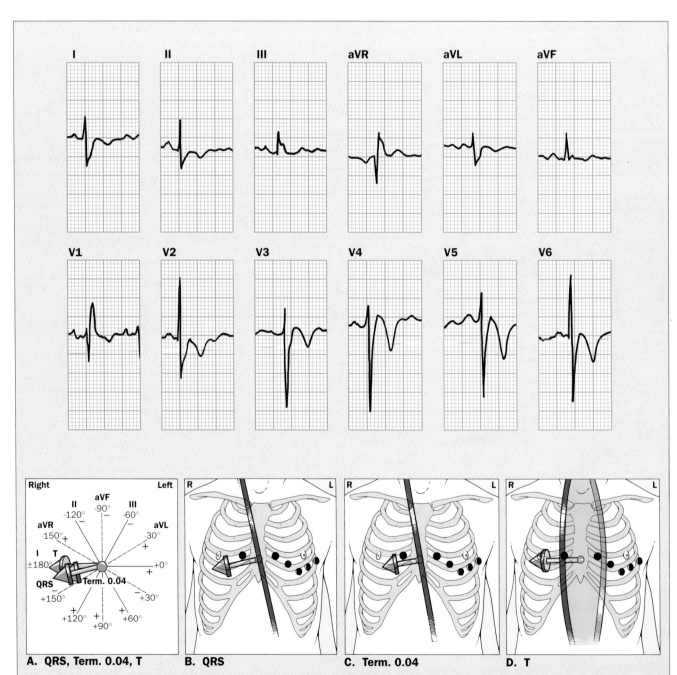

A. QRS, Term. 0.04, T   B. QRS   C. Term. 0.04   D. T

8.20

FIGURE 8.21

This electrocardiogram, showing right bundle branch block and infero-posterior myocardial infarction, was recorded from a 60-year-old patient.

The rhythm is normal and the heart rate is 60 complexes per minute. The duration of the PR interval is 0.16 second, that of the QRS complex is 0.12 second, and that of the QT interval is 0.44 second.

P waves: The second half of the P wave is -0.03 mm/sec in leads V1 and V2, suggesting a left atrial abnormality.

QRS complexes: The mean QRS vector is directed about -75° to the left and about 10° anteriorly. The mean initial 0.04-second QRS vector is directed -70° to the left and at least 30° anteriorly. The mean terminal 0.04-second QRS vector is directed at -155° superiorly and at about 30° anteriorly. The initial QRS force abnormality is consistent with an inferior-posterior dead zone, which is the probable cause of the marked left axis deviation of the mean QRS vector. The mean terminal 0.04-second QRS vector indicates right bundle branch block.

ST segment: The ST segment vector is directed 90° inferiorly and about 20° to 30° posteriorly. It points toward an area of inferior-posterior epicardial injury.

T waves: The mean T vector is directed about -58° to the left, and anteriorly to an uncertain degree. The ventricular gradient is oriented abnormally in a superior direction, and these findings indicate epicardial myocardial ischemia of the inferior-posterior region of the left ventricle.

A. The frontal plane projections of the mean QRS, mean initial and terminal 0.04-second QRS, mean ST vector, and

(Figure 8.21 continued on page 8.32.)

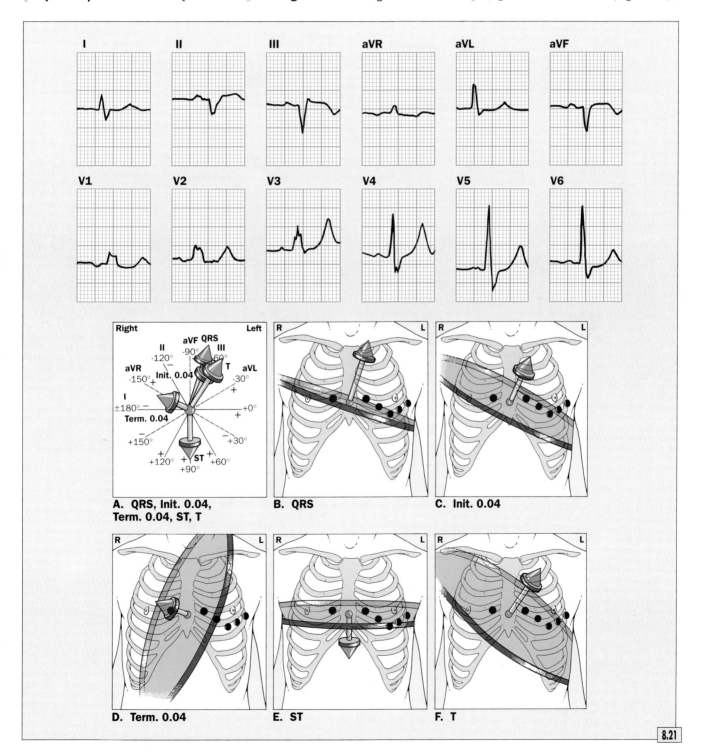

A. QRS, Init. 0.04, Term. 0.04, ST, T

B. QRS

C. Init. 0.04

D. Term. 0.04

E. ST

F. T

8.21

(Figure 8.21 continued.)
mean T vectors. **B.** The spatial orientation of the mean QRS vector. **C.** The spatial orientation of the mean initial 0.04-second QRS vector. **D.** The spatial orientation of the mean terminal 0.04-second QRS vector. **E.** The spatial orientation of the mean ST vector. **F.** The spatial orientation of the mean T vector. **Summary:** The cause of the unusually directed mean terminal 0.04-second QRS vector can only be speculative. It may be due to right bundle branch block and left posterior-inferior division block. The purpose of this illustrative

---

TABLE 8.22 ELECTROCARDIOGRAPHIC CHARACTERISTICS OF RIGHT BUNDLE BRANCH BLOCK PLUS PRIMARY ST AND T WAVE ABNORMALITIES

- The duration of the QRS complex is 0.12 second or more.

- The QRS abnormalities of uncomplicated right bundle branch block, or of right bundle branch block plus left anterior or posterior division block are present.

- The mean T wave vector associated with right bundle branch block, or of right bundle branch block plus left anterior-superior or left posterior-inferior division block is directed opposite the mean QRS vector. This is a secondary T wave abnormality.

- When the T wave vector is not opposite the mean QRS vector, a primary T wave abnormality may be present in addition to the secondary T wave abnormality. In such cases, the ventricular gradient, when it can be calculated, is abnormal.

- The direction of the mean ST segment vector usually parallels that of the mean T vector. This is a secondary ST segment abnormality. When the mean ST segment vector does not parallel the mean T vector, a primary ST segment abnormality is present, and one should deduce that a myocardial abnormality such as myocardial infarction exists in conjunction with the conduction defect.

TABLE 8.23 ELECTROCARDIOGRAPHIC ABNORMALITIES THAT MUST BE DIFFERENTIATED FROM RIGHT BUNDLE BRANCH BLOCK PLUS PRIMARY ST AND T WAVE ABNORMALITIES

- The ST and T vectors associated with uncomplicated right bundle branch block: they are directed opposite the mean QRS vector, which is usually directed inferiorly, to the right, and anteriorly.

- When the ST or T vectors are not directed opposite the mean QRS vector, an abnormality of the ST and T vectors is assumed to be present, and the ventricular gradient, when calculated, is found to be abnormally directed. It is sometimes difficult to determine the exact direction of the mean ST or T vectors and to calculate the ventricular gradient, limiting the use of analysis of the ST and T vectors and the ventricular gradient.

- When the ST segment vector can be calculated, it may point toward an area of epicardial injury rather than away from the mean QRS vector.

- When the mean T vector and ventricular gradient can be calculated, they may be directed away from an area of epicardial ischemia rather than away from the mean QRS vector.

- Many primary ST and T wave abnormalities are undoubtedly masked by the enormous secondary abnormalities produced by the large ST and T vectors associated with right bundle branch block.

TABLE 8.24 THE QRS ABNORMALITIES DUE TO EXPOSURE TO COLD (OSBORN WAVE)

- Sinus bradycardia, atrial fibrillation, or junctional rhythm which may be present when there is moderately severe hypothermia (a body temperature below 26°C).

- QRS duration which may be prolonged to 0.16 second or more.

- An Osborn wave present as the terminal portion of the QRS complex. This wave seems to follow a fairly normal initial QRS contour, and appears to be responsible for the prolongation of the QRS complex. The mean vector representing the Osborn wave seems to be directed to the left and posteriorly.

TABLE 8.25 ELECTROCARDIOGRAPHIC ABNORMALITIES THAT MUST BE DIFFERENTIATED FROM THOSE DUE TO COLD EXPOSURE

- The combination of sinus bradycardia atrial fibrillation or junctional rhythm, a prolonged QRS complex, and an Osborn wave, an artifact due to shivering, is virtually unique. It is, for practical purposes, caused only by prolonged exposure to cold (a body temperature below 26°C).

- On rare occasions, a secondary deflection may be identified in the last portion of the QRS complex when bundle branch block unrelated to hyopthermia is present. The clinical setting usually distinguishes this electrocardiographic abnormality from those due to cold exposure.

(Figure 8.21 continued.)
case is to show a primary ST segment vector. This vector does not parallel the T wave vector, and is caused by inferior-posterior epicardial injury and a primary T wave abnormality due to inferior-posterior epicardial injury. (Reproduced with permission from the publisher and author; see Figure Credits.)

FIGURE 8.22

This electrocardiogram shows the effect of severe hypothermia. The atrial arrhythmia, Osborn wave, and long QT interval are characteristic of this condition. The patient, a 58-year-old man with pyelonephritis, obstructive lung disease, and a previous myocardial infarction, was seen in the emergency clinic. He was moribund, with a rectal temperature of 75°F, having been exposed to extremely low temperatures in a nursing

home. He died 12 hours later.

The heart rhythm shows atrial fibrillation with a ventricular response of 40 complexes per minute. The QRS duration is 0.16 second. The QT interval is 0.72 second (the upper limit of normal for a heart rate of 40 is 0.49 second). The QRS duration is 0.16 second.

QRS complex: The mean QRS vector is directed +60° inferiorly and about 20° posteriorly. The Osborn wave is huge, and when represented as a vector, is directed about +60° inferiorly and about 20° posteriorly. It is characteristic of severe hypothermia.

T wave: The mean T vector is directed about +60° vertically and about 10° to 15° anteriorly. The left precordial T waves do not fit the vector orientation of the right precordial T waves. There are two possible explanations for this: the V3 and V6 electrodes might not be prop-

erly placed, or the transitional pathway for the mean T wave vector may be undulating. Remember that the zero potential pathway as determined by inspecting the precordial leads is a mean pathway.

A. The frontal plane projections of the mean QRS, the mean Osborn wave, and the mean T vectors. **B.** The spatial orientation of the mean QRS vector. **C.** The spatial orientation of a mean vector representing the Osborn wave. **D.** The spatial orientation of the mean T vector.

Summary: The predictive value of these electrocardiographic abnormalities for hypothermia is almost 100 percent. The Osborn wave appears to be due to slowed depolarization of the inferior-posterior-lateral portion of the left ventricle. (Reproduced with permission from the publisher and author; see Figure Credits.)

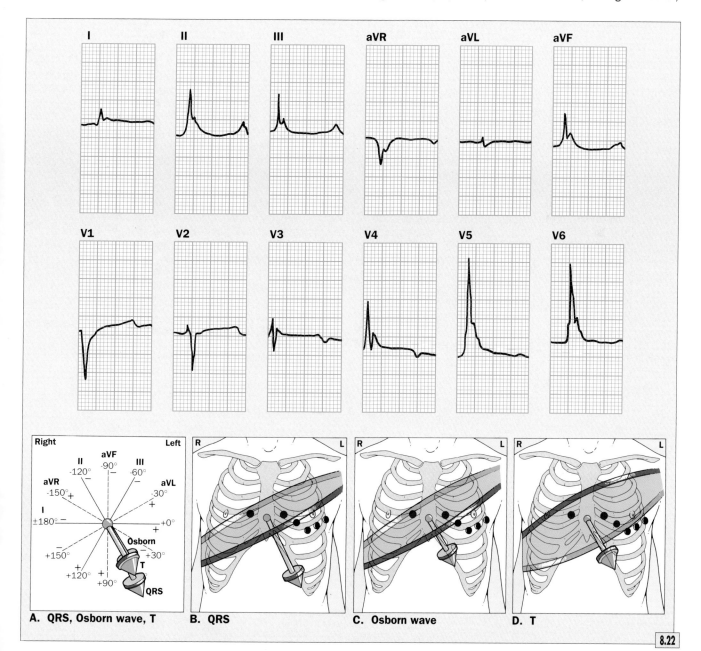

A. QRS, Osborn wave, T   **B. QRS**   **C. Osborn wave**   **D. T**

8.22

VENTRICULAR CONDUCTION DEFECTS ASSOCIATED WITH A QRS DURATION OF 0.14 TO 0.18 SECOND

The electrocardiographic characteristics of the ventricular conduction defects associated with a QRS duration of 0.14 to 0.18 second are listed in Table 8.26. The abnormalities that must be differentiated are listed in Table 8.27. An example is shown in Figure 8.23.

Whenever the QRS duration is 0.14 to 0.18 second, it is wise to consider a severe conduction defect in the right or left bundle branches, or both branches, plus extensive disease of the myocytes. This may occur as a result of coronary artery disease, cardiomyopathy, or advanced left and right ventricular disease due to severe cardiac valve disease. This type of conduction defect may also be the result of cardiac surgery or hyperkalemia.

PRE-EXCITATION OF THE VENTRICLES

I believe that this interesting abnormality is more common than formerly reported. It is due to an accessory conduction pathway that permits the wave of excitation to pass from the atria to the ventricles without the delay that normally occurs in the atrioventricular node. When this happens, the PR interval is short and depolarization of the ventricular myocardium begins abnormally early. Because the ventricular muscle is activated outside of the usual conduction pathway, the depolarization process may produce an unusual slurring of the first portion of the QRS complex. This is called a delta wave. The superior portion of the right side of the ventricular septum is usually depolarized first. This early depolarization produces a short PR interval, the delta wave, and prolongs the duration of the QRS complex. Secondary ST and T wave abnormalities are to be expected.

Many different accessory pathways have been identified. Initially, the electrocardiographic abnormalities produced by the different pathways were divided into types A and B. Later, types C and D were added. Now that many different pathways have been identified, it seems futile to try to identify all of the different types with the 12-lead surface electrocardiogram; electrophysiologic testing is needed to identify the location of an accessory pathway with sufficient reliability to permit surgical treatment. Total surface body mapping has improved to such a degree that, with the use of current techniques, one can identify the location of an accessory pathway.

THE WOLFF-PARKINSON-WHITE SYNDROME: The Wolff-Parkinson-White syndrome consists of the electrocardiographic abnormalities of ventricular pre-excitation, including a short PR interval, a delta wave, and a QRS duration of 0.10 to 0.18 second, plus episodes of atrial tachycardia or atrial fibrillation. The atrial tachyarrhythmia occurs because the wave of excitation passes unimpeded down the accessory conduction pathway, making a retrograde passage into the atria through the normal conduction system.

THE LOWN-GANONG-LEVINE SYNDROME: This syndrome has a short PR interval (0.12 second) and a normal QRS duration without a delta wave, plus episodes of atrial tachyarrhythmia. This is also due to ventricular pre-excitation.

The delta wave associated with ventricular pre-excitation may produce abnormal Q waves that are commonly mistaken to be a result of myocardial infarction.

The accessory pathways responsible for ventricular pre-excitation may be left-sided, right-sided, or septal. Any of these can produce a short PR interval, delta wave, and broad QRS complex. There is also a group of anomalous pathways known as the nodoventricular and fasciculoventricular fibers. They are called Mahaim fibers to honor the investigator who identified them. A diagram illustrating the various anomalous bypass tracts is shown in Figure 8.24. Other accessory pathways that may produce pre-excitation of the ventricles need additional investigation. Although many different anomalous pathways may be responsible for the Lown-Ganong-Levine syndrome (a short PR interval with a normal QRS complex), Brechenmacher discovered an atriofascicular pathway that he considered to be its cause(1).

The electrocardiographic characteristics of pre-excitation of the ventricles are listed in Table 8.28. The electrocardiographic abnormalities that must be differentiated from them are listed in Table 8.29. Examples are shown in Figures 8.25 through 8.27.

This condition usually occurs in the absence of any recognized cardiac disease, and with greater than average prevalence in patients with idiopathic cardiac hypertrophy, atrial septal defects, or Ebstein's anomaly.

COMMON ERRORS IN THE RECOGNOTION OF PRE-EXCITATION OF THE VENTRICLES: The electrocardiographic abnormalities of pre-excitation may simulate those of myocardial infarction. Given this, it must be remembered that true myocardial infarction can occur in middle-aged patients with electrocardiographic abnormalities reflecting pre-excitation.

TABLE 8.26 QRS-COMPLEX DURATION OF 0.14 TO 0.18 SECOND

- A QRS-complex duration of 0.14 to 0.18 second indicates more than isolated left or right bundle block or any combination of conduction defects.

- When the QRS duration is 0.14 to 0.18 second, it is proper to consider diffuse conduction system disease plus extensive damage to the ventricular myocytes.

TABLE 8.27 ABNORMALITIES THAT MUST BE DIFFERENTIATED FROM THOSE CAUSING A QRS-COMPLEX DURATION OF 0.14 TO 0.18 SECOND

- The diagnosis is straightforward; when the duration of the QRS complex is 0.14 to 0.18 second, there is usually a severe conduction abnormality plus extensive disease of the ventricular myocytes.

- Pre-excitation of the ventricles stands as a possible exception to the above rule. It is identified by the short PR interval and delta wave.

FIGURE 8.23

This electrocardiogram, showing a QRS duration of 0.16 second, was recorded from a 73-year-old man with severe dilated cardiomyopathy.

The rhythm is normal and the heart rate is 74 complexes per minute. The duration of the PR interval is 0.24 second, the duration of the QRS complex is 0.19 second and that of the QT interval is 0.40 second.

P waves: The duration of the P wave in lead II is 0.13 second and the last half of the P wave in lead V1 measures -0.03 mm/sec. These features suggest a left atrial abnormality.

QRS complex: The mean QRS vector is directed at +10° vertically in the frontal plane and 85° posteriorly. The mean terminal 0.04-second QRS vector

(Figure 8.23 continued on page 8.36.)

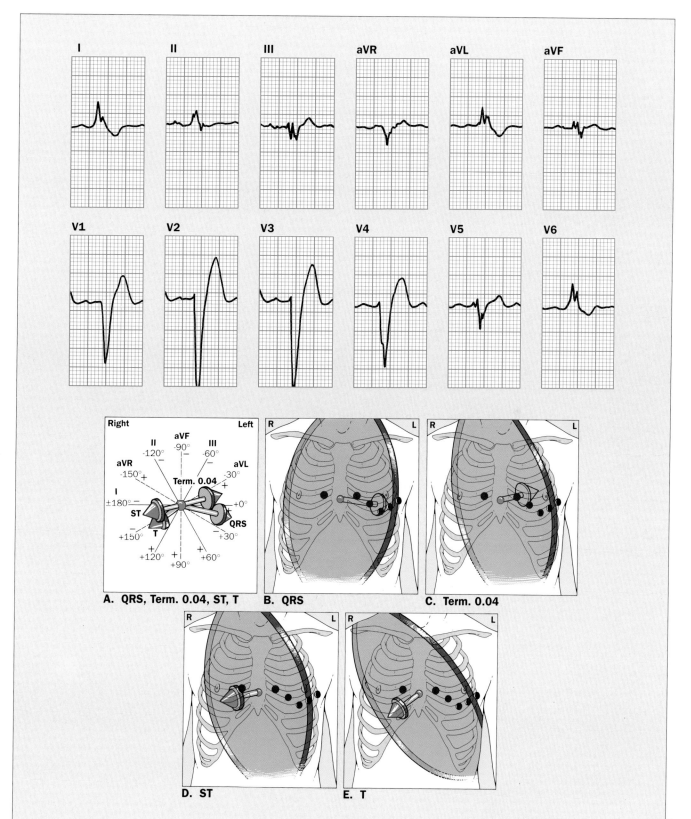

A. QRS, Term. 0.04, ST, T   B. QRS   C. Term. 0.04

D. ST   E. T

(Figure 8.23 continued.)
is directed at -22° and at 85° posteriorly. A QRS duration of 0.16 second signifies left bundle branch block plus extensive myocyte damage.

ST segment: The mean ST vector is directed +165° to the right and 85° anteriorly.

T waves: The mean T vector is directed +148° to the right and 85° anteriorly.

A. The frontal plane projections of the mean QRS, mean terminal 0.04-second QRS, mean ST, and mean T vectors.
B. The spatial orientation of the mean QRS vector. **C.** The spatial orientation of the mean terminal 0.04-second QRS

vector. **D.** The spatial orientation of the mean ST vector. **E.** The spatial orientation of the mean T vector.

Summary: The purpose of this illustrative case is to emphasize the abnormalities responsible for a QRS duration that is greater than 0.16 second. Ventricular conduction defects rarely produce prolongation of the QRS complex to 0.16 second, and when the QRS duration is from 0.16 to 0.20 second, it is highly likely that conduction defects plus extensive myocyte damage are present. The damage is usually due to multiple myocardial infarctions, dilated cardiomyopathy including ischemic car-

diomyopathy, or drug intoxication. An exception is found in some patients with pre-excitation of the ventricles; the QRS duration in these patients ranges from 0.10 to 0.20 second, though the ventricular myocytes are normal.

F I G U R E   8 . 2 4

Illustration of various anatomic bypass tracts capable of producing anomalous atrioventricular conduction (ventricular pre-excitation). The expected electrocardiographic features are noted beneath each of the four diagrams (A through D). (Reproduced with permission from the publisher and author; see Figure Credits.)

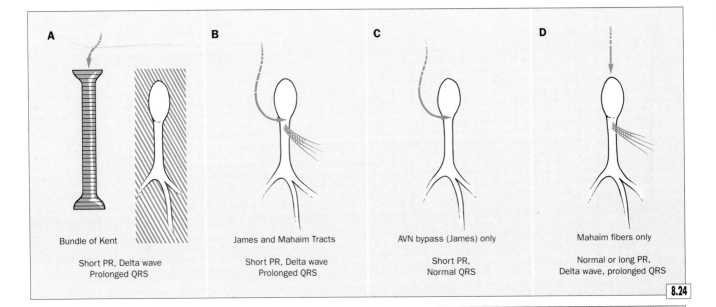

A
Bundle of Kent

Short PR, Delta wave
Prolonged QRS

B
James and Mahaim Tracts

Short PR, Delta wave
Prolonged QRS

C
AVN bypass (James) only

Short PR,
Normal QRS

D
Mahaim fibers only

Normal or long PR,
Delta wave, prolonged QRS

8.24

TABLE 8.28 THE ELECTROCARDIOGRAPHIC CHARACTERISTICS OF PRE-EXCITATION OF THE VENTRICLES

Pre-excitation of the ventricles associated with the Wolff-Parkinson-White syndrome (characteristic electrocardiographic abnormalities plus atrial tachyarrhythmias) is marked by:

- A short PR interval (0.12 second).
- A QRS-complex duration of 0.10 to 0.18 second.
- A characteristic delta wave.
- Secondary ST and T wave abnormalities.
- A mean initial 0.04-second QRS vector that incorporates the

delta wave and is often directed in such a manner as to simulate an inferior or anterior myocardial infarction.

Pre-excitation of the ventricles associated with the Lown-Ganong-Levine syndrome (characteristic electrocardiographic abnormalities plus atrial tachyarrhythmias) is marked by:

- A short PR interval (0.12 second or less).
- A normal QRS-complex duration (0.08 to 0.10 second).
- The absence of a delta wave.

TABLE 8.29 ELECTROCARDIOGRAPHIC ABNORMALITIES THAT MUST BE DIFFERENTIATED FROM THOSE OF PRE-EXCITATION OF THE VENTRICLES

- When all of the features of pre-excitation of the ventricles are present (see Table 8.28), the diagnosis is definite. The abnormalities are unique.

- Any patient with paroxysmal atrial tachyarrhythmia should be observed for pre-excitation of the ventricles.

FIGURE 8.25

This electrocardiogram, showing pre-excitation of the ventricles, was recorded from a 66-year-old man. The rhythm is normal and the heart rate is 55 complexes per minute. The duration of the PR interval is 0.12 second, that of the QRS complex is 0.17 second and that of the QT interval is 0.40 second.

P waves: The P waves are normal. The PR interval, measured in the precordial leads, is 0.12 second.

QRS complex: The mean QRS vector is directed -70° to the left and to an uncertain number of degrees (at least 50°) anteriorly. The initial portion of the QRS complex is slurred, producing the delta wave. A mean vector representing the delta wave is directed -55° to the left and to an uncertain number of degrees anteriorly. The QRS voltage is enormous, but when the QRS complex is abnormally wide, many QRS forces are unopposed, resulting in a large voltage that is not dependent on ventricular thickness.

T waves: The mean T vector is directed +72° inferiorly and 60° posteriorly.

A. The frontal plane projections of the mean QRS vector, mean delta vector, and mean T vectors. **B.** The spatial orientation of the mean QRS vector. **C.** The spatial orientation of a mean vector representing the delta wave. **D.** The spatial orientation of the mean T vector.

Summary: The short PR interval and the prolonged QRS complex with a delta wave are characteristic of pre-excitation of the ventricles. The surface electrocardiogram cannot identify the location of the accessory conduction pathway; electrophyiologic testing is required. This is why the surface electrocardiogram is not useful for categorizing the accessory pathway. The tracing shown here was formerly labeled as Type A; the vector representing the delta wave is directed anteriorly.

Most patients with evidence of pre-excitation of the ventricles have episodes of atrial tachycardia or fibrillation, (the Wolff-Parkinson-White syndrome). Whereas pre-excitation usually occurs in patients without other evidence of heart disease, the physician should search for an atrial septal defect, Ebstein's disease, or hypertrophic cardiomyopathy because pre-excitation is somewhat more common in these conditions. It is not uncommon to make a misdiagnosis of myocardial infarction in these cases because large, abnormal Q waves are often present in the electrocardiogram. Such a misdiagnosis of inferior myocardial infarction could be made on the basis of the electrocardiogram shown here.

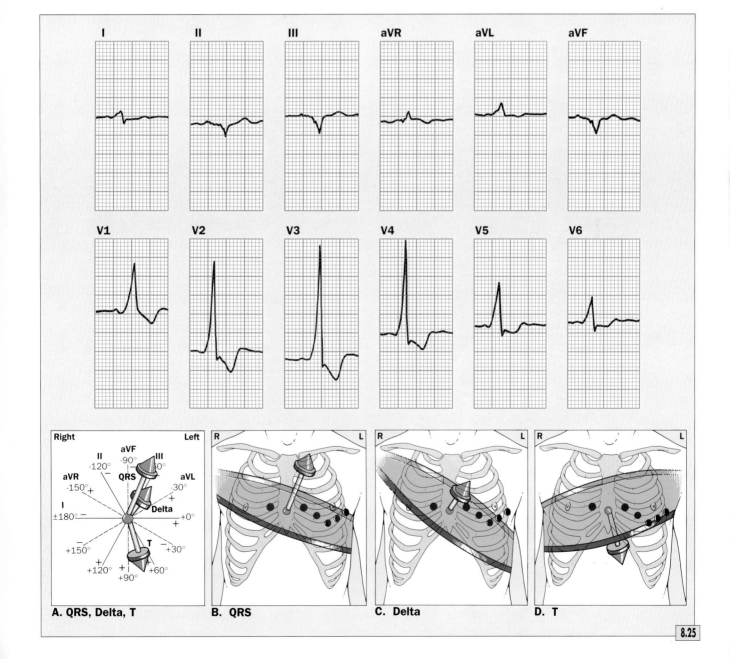

A. QRS, Delta, T   B. QRS   C. Delta   D. T

8.25

FIGURE 8.26

This electrocardiogram, showing pre-excitation of the ventricles, was recorded from a 23-year-old man. The rhythm is normal and the heart rate is 80 complexes per minute. The duration of the PR interval is 0.10 second, that of the QRS complex is 0.12 second and that of the QT interval is 0.32 second.

P waves: The P waves are normal. The PR interval is very short (0.10 second).

QRS complex: The mean QRS vector is directed at about +17° and an uncertain number of degrees (probably about 30°) anteriorly. The initial portion of the QRS complex is slurred; this is the delta wave. A mean vector representing this wave is directed 0° to the left and to an uncertain number of degrees anteriorly.

T waves: The mean T vector is directed at +40° and an uncertain number of degrees (probably about 50°) anteriorly.

A. The frontal plane projections of the mean QRS vector, a vector representing the delta wave, and the mean T vector. **B.** The frontal plane projection of the mean QRS vector. **C.** The spatial orientation of a mean vector representing the delta wave. **D.** The spatial orientation of the mean T vector.

Summary: The short PR interval, delta wave, and abnormally wide QRS complexes signify the presence of pre-excitation of the ventricles. The discussion in the legend of Figure 8.25 also applies here.

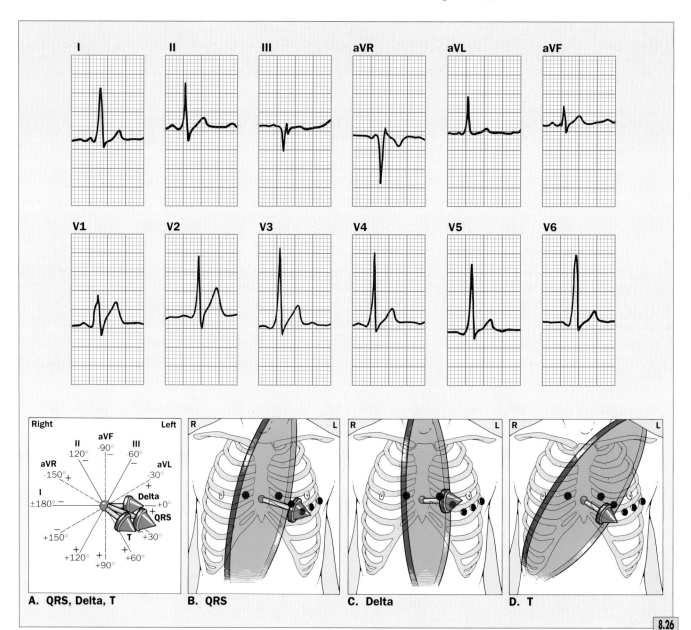

A. QRS, Delta, T   B. QRS   C. Delta   D. T

8.26

FIGURE 8.27

This electrocardiogram, showing a short PR interval with a normal QRS complex, was recorded from a 13-year-old girl. The rhythm is most likely normal and the heart rate is 62 complexes per minute. The duration of the PR interval is 0.10 second. The duration of the QRS complex is 0.07 second and the duration of the QT interval is 0.36 second.

P waves: The mean P vector is directed 0° to the left, and P waves are barely seen in the precordial leads. The PR interval is very short, and there is a possibility that these findings are due to an ectopic focus in the atrium.

QRS complex: The duration of the QRS complex is 0.07 second. No delta wave is present. The mean QRS vector is directed +70° inferiorly and 20° posteriorly.

T waves: The mean T vector is directed +30° inferiorly and about 20° posteriorly. This is normal for an adolescent.

A. The frontal plane projections of the mean P, mean QRS, and mean T vectors. **B.** The spatial orientation of the mean QRS vector. **C.** The spatial orientation of the mean T vector.

Summary: This electrocardiogram illus-trates a short PR interval with normal QRS complexes. The rhythm may represent an atrial ectopic beat but this cannot be stated with certainty. Patients with extremely short PR intervals and normal QRS complexes represent a group with pre-excitation of the ventricles. They are prone to episodes of supraventricular tachycardia. When the electrocardiographic abnormalities and the arrhythmias are present, these patients are said to have the Lown-Ganong-Levine syndrome. (This electrocardiogram is reproduced by the courtesy of Dr. John R. Morgan of Chattanooga, Tennessee.)

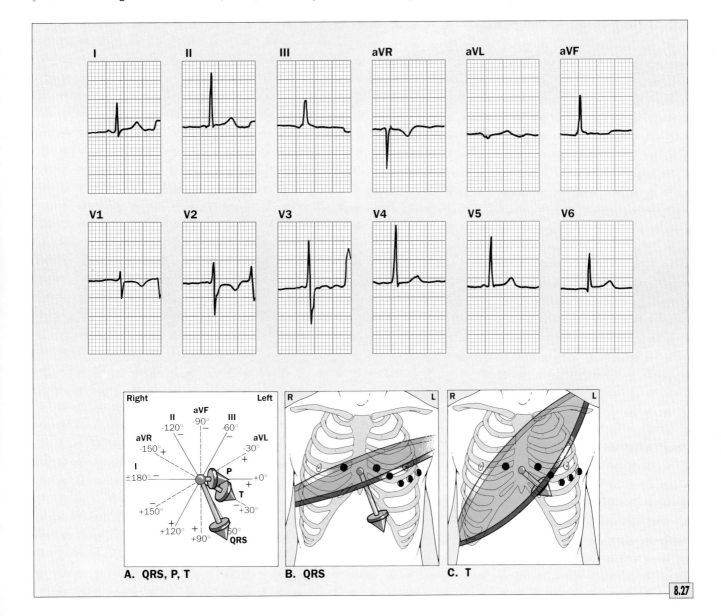

A. QRS, P, T   B. QRS   C. T

8.27

REFERENCES

1. Brechenmacher C: Atrio-His bundle tracts. *Br Heart J* 1975;37:853-855.

FIGURE CREDITS

Figure 8.3 From Estes EH: Electrocardiography and Vectorcardiography in Hurst JW, Logue RB (eds): *The Heart,* Ed 1. New York, McGraw–Hill, 1966, p 136.

Figure 8.10 From Hurst JW, Woodson GC Jr: *Atlas of Spatial Vector Electrocardiography.* New York, Blakiston, 1952, p 177.

Figure 8.15 From Graybiel A, White PD, Wheeler L, Williams C: *Electrocardiography in Practice.* Philadelphia, W.B. Saunders, 1952, p 154.

Figure 8.18 From Chung EK: *Cardiac Arrhythmias: Self-Assessment.* Baltimore, Williams & Wilkins, 1977, p 257.

Figure 8.19 From Hurst JW, Woodson GC Jr: *Atlas of Spatial Vector Electrocardiography.* New York, Blakiston, 1952, p 161.

Figure 8.20 From Marriot HJL: *Practical Electrocardiography* Ed 4. Baltimore, Williams & Wilkins, 1968, p 75.

Figure 8.21 From Hurst JW, Woodson CG Jr: *Atlas of Spatial Vector Electrocardiography.* New York, Blakiston, 1952, p 165.

Figure 8.22 From Clements SD, Hurst JW: Diagnostic value of electrocardiographic abnormalities observed in subjects accidentally exposed to cold. *Am J Cardiol* 1972; 29:729.

Figure 8.24 From Ferrer MI: *Electrocardiographic Notebook* Ed 4. New York, Futura, 1973.

SECONDARY AND PRIMARY VENTRICULAR HYPERTROPHY

Secondary ventricular hypertrophy develops in response to another condition such as hypertension, cardiac valve disease, or congenital heart disease. In contrast, *primary ventricular hypertrophy* occurs in the absence of the etiologies listed above; it is due to disease of the heart muscle itself. The disease may be isolated to the myocardium or may be part of a generalized disease.

SECONDARY VENTRICULAR HYPERTROPHY

SECONDARY LEFT VENTRICULAR HYPERTROPHY

There are no electrocardiographic criteria that permit the identification of left ventricular hypertrophy in all adults who have this condition, nor are there criteria that exclude it in all adults who do not have it. This is because normal adults exhibit left ventricular dominance, and the normal range of the direction and amplitude of the mean QRS vector overlaps the abnormal range. The electrocardiographic abnormalities associated with left ventricular hypertrophy vary according to whether the hypertrophy is due to systolic or diastolic pressure overload of the left ventricle. Eventually, at a later stage of the condition, diastolic pressure overload produces electrocardiographic signs similar to those of systolic pressure overload. The concept of systolic or diastolic pressure overload appears to be more applicable to children and young adults than to older adults. The explanation for this is partly related to the duration of the conditions responsible for the electrocardiographic abnormalities (see Chapter 6).

SYSTOLIC PRESSURE OVERLOAD OF THE LEFT VENTRICLE: The electrocardiographic abnormalities indicating left ventricular hypertrophy associated with systolic pressure overload are different from those associated with diastolic pressure overload. This is more evident when the diastolic pressure overload is mild or has existed for only a short time. Patients with moderately severe diastolic pressure overload that has been present for a number of years will often develop the electrocardiographic signs described for systolic pressure overload of the left ventricle.

The electrocardiographic characteristics related to systolic pressure overload of the left ventricle are listed in Table 9.1, and those that must be differentiated from systolic pressure overload are listed in Table 9.2. Electrocardiographic examples of this condition are shown in Figures 9.1 through 9.5.

Systolic pressure overload of the left ventricle may be caused by: aortic valve stenosis due to congenital bicuspid valve abnormalities, rheumatic fever, or calcific disease of the elderly; supravalvular aortic stenosis; systemic hypertension; longstanding, moderately severe diastolic pressure overload due to mitral or aortic regurgitation of any cause, dilated cardiomyopathy, or atherosclerotic coronary heart disease, which only rarely causes left ventricular hypertrophy.

DIASTOLIC PRESSURE OVERLOAD OF THE LEFT VENTRICLE: The electrocardiogram in diastolic pressure overload of the left ventricle varies according to the magnitude and duration of the condition causing it. When the diastolic pressure overload is mild to moderate or has been present for only a short time, the electrocardiogram is more likely to reveal the features of diastolic pressure overload; when the pressure overload is severe or has been present for a long time, the electrocardiogram reveals evidence of systolic pressure overload (see Table 9.1).

The electrocardiographic characteristics related to diastolic pressure overload of the left ventricle are listed in Table 9.3, and the electrocardiographic abnormalities that must be differentiated from these are listed in Table 9.4. Examples of the condition are shown in Figures 9.6 through 9.8.

Diastolic pressure overload of the left ventricle may be caused by: aortic valve regurgitation due to rheumatic heart disease; myxomatous degeneration of the aortic valve; endocarditis of the aortic valve; trauma; congenital bicuspid aortic valve; aorto-annular dysplasia; mitral valve regurgitation due to ruptured cords to the mitral valve secondary to myxomatous degeneration, endocarditis, or trauma; a ruptured papillary muscle secondary to myocardial infarction or trauma; papillary muscle dysfunction due to myocardial infarction; or congenital heart disease with patent ductus arteriosus or a ventricular septal defect.

SECONDARY RIGHT VENTRICULAR HYPERTROPHY

There are no electrocardiographic criteria that permit the identification of right ventricular hypertrophy in all neonates and infants. This is because normal neonates and infants exhibit right ventricular dominance, and the normal and abnormal ranges of mean QRS vector direction and amplitude overlap.

There is a difference between the electrocardiographic signs of right ventricular hypertrophy when due to congenital versus acquired heart disease. The child with right ventricular hypertrophy due to pulmonary valve stenosis never loses the "normal" right ventricular dominance that was present at birth. Accordingly, the mean QRS vector is directed to the right and anteriorly, and never shifts to the left and posteriorly as it does when the normal subject grows older. On the other hand, right ventricular hypertrophy due to an acquired disease such as mitral stenosis, must gradually overcome the electrocardiographic features of normal left ventricular dominance. Accordingly, the mean QRS vector of the adult with acquired right ventricular hypertrophy is directed inferiorly at about +80° and posteriorly. As time passes the direction of the mean QRS vector tends to shift rightward and may eventually become anterior. When a rightwardly, anteriorly directed mean QRS vector suggests right ventricular hypertrophy in an adult with an acquired disease, the clinician can deduce that the condition is rather far advanced, and that pulmonary hypertension is present. A right atrial abnormality may become evident when this develops.

Note: As stated in several places in this book, the model presented here is a clinically useful approximation of the real situation within the heart. At times, the explanation moves beyond the known evidence. When this occurs, every effort has been made to extend the facts in a logical manner.

The electrocardiographic signs of right ventricular hypertrophy are different when the condition is due to systolic as opposed to diastolic pressure overload of the right ventricle. These differences are more likely to be apparent in the child than in the adult, because the child has not lived sufficiently long to develop the advanced electrocardiographic changes observed in older patients. When moderately severe diastolic pressure overload of the right ventricle has been present for a long time, it produces the electrocardiographic abnormalities of systolic pressure overload (see Chapter 5).

SYSTOLIC PRESSURE OVERLOAD OF THE RIGHT VENTRICLE: The electrocardiographic characteristics related to right ventricular systolic pressure overload are listed in Table 9.5. Electrocardiographic abnormalities that must be differentiated from those due to systolic pressure overload of the right ventricle are listed in Table 9.6. Examples are shown in Figures 9.9 and 9.10.

Systolic pressure overload of the right ventricle may be caused by congenital heart disease such as pulmonary valve stenosis, the tetralogy of Fallot, and rare causes of right ventricular hypertension or acquired heart disease such as mitral stenosis, primary pulmonary hypertension, repeated pulmonary emboli, or the gradual development of Eisenmenger physiology due to an interventricular septal defect, patent ductus arteriosus, or interatrial septal defect. The electrocardiograms of patients with Eisenmenger physiology due to patent ductus arteriosus or an interventricular septal defect may initially show diastolic pressure overload of the *left* ventricle, while those of patients with an interatrial septal defect may initially show diastolic pressure overload of the *right* ventricle. As pulmonary hypertension develops, the electrocardiogram shows systolic pressure overload of the right ventricle. Chronic obstructive lung disease and emphysema may also produce right ventricular hypertrophy.

The S1, S2, S3 type of conduction defect, with large terminal QRS forces, may be associated with acquired causes of right ventricular hypertrophy such as mitral stenosis, chronic obstructive lung disease, or pulmonary emphysema.

DIASTOLIC PRESSURE OVERLOAD OF THE RIGHT VENTRICLE: The electrocardiographic characteristics of right ventricular hypertrophy related to diastolic pressure overload of the right ventricle are listed in Table 9.7, and the electrocardiographic abnormalities that must be differentiated from them are listed in Table 9.8. An electrocardiographic example of the condition is shown in Figure 9.11.

This condition may be caused by: a secundum type of atrial septal defect; the anomalous entrance of some of the pulmonary veins into the right atrium; absence of the pulmonary valve; or pulmonary regurgitation due to endocarditis. Theoretically, isolated tricuspid regurgitation due to endocarditis or carcinoid involvement of the tricuspid valve can cause it as well.

COMBINED SECONDARY LEFT AND RIGHT VENTRICULAR HYPERTROPHY

The electrocardiographic characteristics of combined secondary left and right ventricular hypertrophy are listed in Table 9.9. An example of combined left and right ventricular hypertrophy is given in Figure 7.5. The electrocardiographic abnormalities that must be differentiated from those due to combined left and right ventricular hypertrophy are listed in Table 9.10.

The cardiac abnormalities responsible for combined left and right ventricular hypertrophy are: aortic valve disease plus mitral stenosis due to rheumatic heart disease; aortic or mitral valve disease with heart failure and pulmonary hypertension; and dilated cardiomyopathy with heart failure and pulmonary hypertension.

PRIMARY VENTRICULAR HYPERTROPHY (CARDIOMYOPATHY)

The electrocardiographic abnormalities of dilated cardiomyopathy include: an abnormal heart rhythm; left and right atrial abnormalities; left ventricular or combined ventricular hypertrophy; left or right bundle branch block; left bundle branch and left anterior-superior division block; primary T wave abnormalities; and abnormal Q waves suggesting myocardial infarction. These abnormalities are discussed in Chapters 6, 7, 8, and 11.

Restrictive cardiomyopathy may exhibit electrocardiographic abnormalities similar to those found for dilated cardiomyopathy. The electrocardiographic abnormalities associated with *hypertrophic cardiomyopathy* are sufficiently different from those of dilated cardiomyopathy and restrictive cardiomyopathy to deserve additional discussion; they are listed in Table 9.11.

Many patients with hypertrophic cardiomyopathy exhibit electrocardiograms that show left ventricular hypertrophy plus some rather unique abnormalities of the QRS complex, ST segments, and T waves, all of which may not be observed early in the course of the disease. As a rule, however, when other clinical clues are present, the electrocardiogram is usually abnormal. Right ventricular hypertrophy may occur in the absence of left ventricular hypertrophy, but this is rare. Examples of primary left ventricular hypertrophy due to hypertrophic cardiomyopathy are shown in Figures 9.12 through 9.16. Electrocardiographic abnormalities that must be differentiated from those due to primary ventricular hypertrophy are listed in Table 9.12.

Some cases of primary ventricular hypertrophy are genetically determined, and rare cases are related to acromegaly. The condition is relatively common, often overlooked in the elderly, and in most cases, of unknown cause. Magnetic resonance images of hypertrophic cardiomyopathy are shown in 9.17.

TABLE 9.1 ELECTROCARDIOGRAPHIC CHARACTERISTICS OF SECONDARY LEFT VENTRICULAR HYPERTROPHY DUE TO SYSTOLIC PRESSURE OVERLOAD OF THE LEFT VENTRICLE

- A left atrial abnormality may be present (see Table 7.2).

- The QRS duration in adults is usually 0.10 second or less, but may be 0.11 second. It may be less than this in children.

- The mean QRS vector is usually directed from -30° to +30°, but may be directed vertically, especially in children. It is always directed posteriorly.

- The mean initial 0.01- and 0.02-second QRS vectors should be anterior to the subsequent QRS forces. The mean initial 0.04-second QRS vector should be directed to the left of a vertically-directed mean QRS vector. It may be directed to either side of an intermediate mean QRS vector, but must be inferior to a horizontal or leftward mean QRS vector. It is anterior to the mean QRS vector, but may be rotated leftward and posteriorly to such a degree that there may be no Q waves or only small Q waves in leads I, V5, and V6, and absent or small R waves in leads V1 and V2.

- The QRS amplitude is increased (see Table 5.3). The total 12-lead QRS amplitude is usually greater than 185 mm.

- The QRS amplitude may be abnormally large, and the intrinsicoid deflection of the QRS complex, measured in leads V5 or V6, may be greater than 0.04 second.

- The mean T vector gradually rotates to a position opposite the mean QRS vector. Initially, the QRS-T angle may be normal. Later it may be 70°, then 90°, and still later, 180°. The direction of the mean T wave vector gradually shifts increasingly to the right of a large horizontal mean QRS vector, and becomes increasingly anterior to a large vertical mean QRS vector. The mean T vector is always anterior to the mean QRS vector. (The T wave is never inverted in leads V1, V2, and V3.)

- The mean ST segment vector tends to be parallel with the mean T vector.

- The U wave may become prominent in the precordial leads.

TABLE 9.2 ELECTROCARDIOGRAPHIC ABNORMALITIES THAT MUST BE DIFFERENTIATED FROM THOSE DUE TO SYSTOLIC PRESSURE OVERLOAD OF THE LEFT VENTRICLE

- The greatest problem is to distinguish the normal electrocardiogram from the one showing only an increase in QRS voltage secondary to left ventricular hypertrophy due to systolic pressure overload of the left ventricle (see Table 5.3).

- The normal total 12-lead QRS amplitude is usually less than 185 mm (see Fig. 5.8; the reader is also referred to Table 5.3 for the criteria established by Romhilt and Estes). Consider the possibility of left ventricular hypertrophy when the amplitude of the QRS complexes is at the upper end of the normal range. The predictability of left ventricular hypertrophy increases with an increase in amplitude of the QRS complexes.

- Although the mean QRS vector is almost always directed from +80° to -30° in the frontal plane, and from 40° to 80° posteriorly, the predictive value of the mean QRS vector direction is not as high as that of the QRS amplitude in determining the presence of left ventricular hypertrophy. However, left ventricular hypertrophy is more likely to be present when the mean QRS vector is directed from +30° to -30°, than from +30° to +80°.

- When systolic pressure overload is the cause of left ventricular hypertrophy, and the mean QRS vector is horizontal, the mean T vector shifts rightward and anteriorly. When the mean QRS vector is vertical, it shifts anteriorly and superiorly. Some of the T wave abnormalities that are often interpreted as "nonspecific T wave changes" are early electrocardiographic signs of left ventricular hypertrophy. Such changes may be suspected when there is an apparent cause for left ventricular hypertrophy.

- Left anterior-superior division block may simulate left ventricular hypertrophy. In such cases, the duration of the QRS complex is

0.10 second, whereas in patients with left ventricular hypertrophy, it is often less than 0.10 second. The mean QRS vector is directed beyond -30° to the left when left anterior-superior division block is present. Left ventricular hypertrophy alone does not produce a mean QRS vector that is directed more than -30° to the left.

- Left bundle branch block may simulate left ventricular hypertrophy in that the mean QRS vector is large and the mean ST and T vectors are opposite the mean QRS vector. When there is left bundle branch block, however, the QRS duration is 0.12 second or more. In left ventricular hypertrophy, it is usually less than 0.10 second. Q waves are usually present in leads 1 and V6, and a small R wave is usually present in lead V1 when there is left ventricular hypertrophy; these waves are absent when there is left bundle branch block.

- Left ventricular conduction delay may simulate left ventricular hypertrophy. In this condition, the QRS duration is about 0.10 second, the mean QRS vector is directed less than -30° to the left, there are no Q waves in leads I and V6, and no R wave in lead V1. The QRS complex resembles that of left bundle branch block, but the duration is less than 0.12 second. Left ventricular hypertrophy is often present, but the electrocardiographic abnormalities are those of left ventricular conduction delay.

- The calibration of the electrocardiograph machine may be improper. Overstandardization causes all complexes to appear large, and this may lead to the misinterpretation of left ventricular hypertrophy.

FIGURE 9.1

Left ventricular hypertrophy due to systolic pressure overload of the left ventricle. This electrocardiogram was recorded from a 42-year-old woman with severe aortic valve stenosis and mild aortic regurgitation. The peak instantaneous gradient across the aortic valve, determined by the echo Doppler technique, was 100 mm Hg, and the mean gradient was 64 mm Hg. There was echocardiographic evidence of concentric left ventricular hypertrophy, and the left ventricular wall motion was normal.

The PR interval is 0.13 second. The duration of the QRS complex is 0.08 second, and the QT interval is 0.36 second.

A. The frontal plane projections of the mean QRS and mean T wave vectors.
B. The spatial orientation of the mean QRS vector. Its direction is normal, but the total 12-lead amplitude is greater than 230 mm, whereas the upper limit of normal is 185 mm. **C.** The spatial orientation of the mean T vector. It is directed slightly anterior to the mean QRS vector, and the QRS-T angle is normal.

Summary: The only abnormality in this electrocardiogram is the increased amplitude of the normally directed mean QRS vector; the direction and amplitude indicate left ventricular hypertrophy. The normal ST segment and T wave vectors favor early systolic pressure overload of the left ventricle. In this case, the left ventricular hypertrophy is caused by moderately severe aortic stenosis.

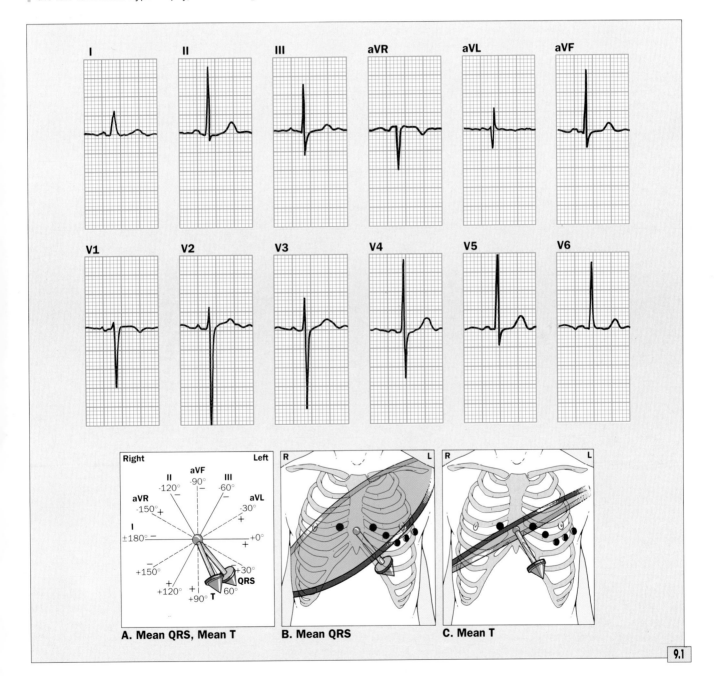

A. Mean QRS, Mean T   B. Mean QRS   C. Mean T

9.1

FIGURE 9.2

Left ventricular hypertrophy due to systolic pressure overload of the left ventricle. This electrocardiogram and vectorcardiogram were recorded from a 32-year-old man with severe hypertensive cardiovascular disease.

The PR interval is 0.20 second. The QRS duration is 0.08 second, and the QT interval is 0.32 second.

QRS complex: The duration of the QRS complex is 0.08 second, and the mean QRS vector is directed at +20° in the frontal plane; compare this with the direction of the QRS loop as viewed in the frontal plane (F) of the vectorcardiogram. The 12-lead amplitude of the QRS complex is greater than 188 mm. Note that the mean QRS vector is directed about 45° posteriorly; the transitional pathway for the QRS courses between the electrode positions for leads V3 and V4. Compare this with the direction of the QRS loop shown in the transverse (T) and sagittal (S) planes.

ST-T segment: The frontal plane projections of the mean T vector and mean ST segment vector are small. The former is directed to +30° because it is perpendicular to lead axis III. It is also directed 80° to 90° anteriorly. The mean ST vector is perpendicular to lead axis III, but opposite the T vector because it is negative in leads I and II. The mean ST vector is directed -150° in the frontal plane and about 80° anteriorly. Because both the T and ST vectors are directed anteriorly and barely visible in the frontal plane, one can conclude that they are almost parallel with each other, directed about 125° away from an abnormally large mean QRS vector. The short QT interval suggests a digitalis effect.

Summary: This electrocardiogram is characteristic of left ventricular hypertrophy due to systolic pressure overload. The small R wave in leads V1 and V2 must not be interpreted as being due to myocardial infarction because this commonly occurs as a result of systolic pressure overload of the left ventricle. (Reproduced with permission from the publisher and author; see Figure Credits. The orientation of the vectorcardiogram in the transverse plane has been changed from that of the original publication, with the permission of Dr. Estes, so that it now conforms to the orientation of the magnetic resonance images presented in this book.)

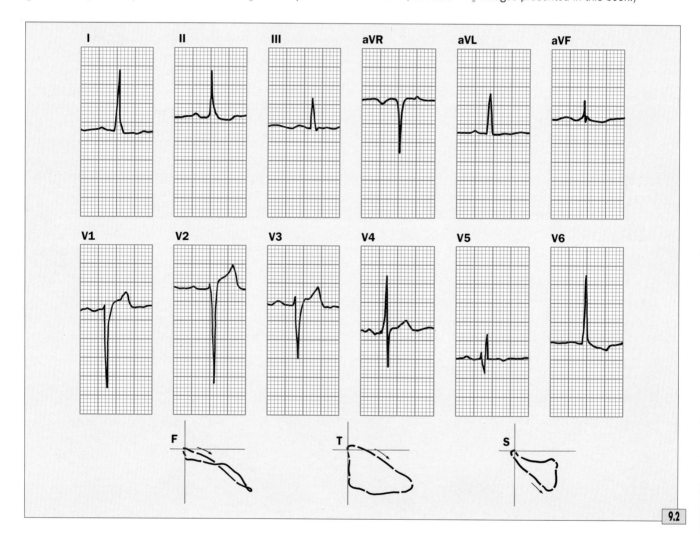

9.2

FIGURE 9.3

Left ventricular hypertrophy due to systolic pressure overload of the left ventricle. This electrocardiogram was recorded from an 85-year-old woman with severe calcific aortic valve stenosis. Murmurs of aortic stenosis and regurgitation were present. Cardiac catheterization, performed because of angina-like chest pain and heart failure, revealed a systolic blood pressure of 145 mm Hg and a diastolic pressure of 50 mm Hg. The left ventricular systolic pressure was 260 mm Hg. Slight aortic regurgitation was present.

The PR interval is 0.17 second. The duration of the QRS complex is 0.095 second, and the QT interval is 0.36 second.

QRS complex: The intrinsicoid deflection is slightly more than 0.04 second. The mean QRS vector is directed to about +28°, and the 12-lead QRS amplitude is more than 281 mm. The mean QRS vector is directed about 30° posteriorly.

T wave: The mean T vector is directed inferiorly at about +58°, and anteriorly at 80°.

ST segment: The mean ST vector is directed superiorly at about -148°, and anteriorly at 30°.

A. The frontal plane projections of the mean QRS, T, and ST vectors. **B.** The spatial orientation of the mean QRS vector. **C.** The spatial orientation of the mean T vector. **D.** The spatial orientation of the mean ST vector.

Summary: The abnormalities in this electrocardiogram indicate left ventricular hypertrophy due to systolic pressure overload of the left ventricle. The predictive value of the abnormalities is 100 percent. In this case the abnormalities were caused by severe calcific aortic valve stenosis.

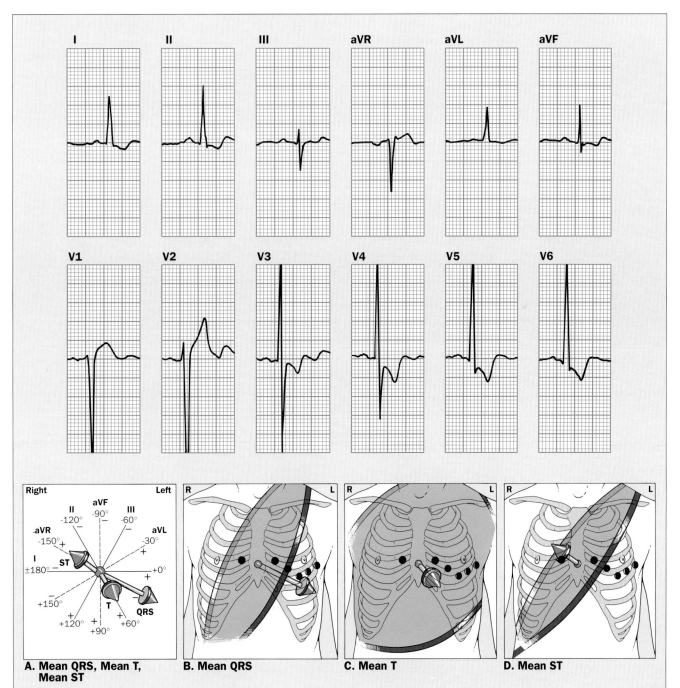

A. Mean QRS, Mean T, Mean ST

B. Mean QRS

C. Mean T

D. Mean ST

F I G U R E   9 . 4

Left ventricular hypertrophy due to systolic pressure overload of the left ventricle. The systolic pressure overload in this case was due to very advanced, long-standing diastolic pressure overload of the left ventricle. The patient was a 67-year-old woman with extremely severe mitral regurgitation due to myxomatous degeneration of the mitral valve. Cardiac catheterization revealed normal coronary arteries, a huge left atrium, left ventricular enlargement, and pulmonary hypertension.

The PR interval is 0.20 second, the duration of the QRS complex is 0.08 second, and the QT interval is 0.40 second.

P waves: The duration of the P wave in lead II is 0.12 second, and its amplitude is 0.15 mm. The mean P vector is directed at +65°. The mean P1 vector is direc-

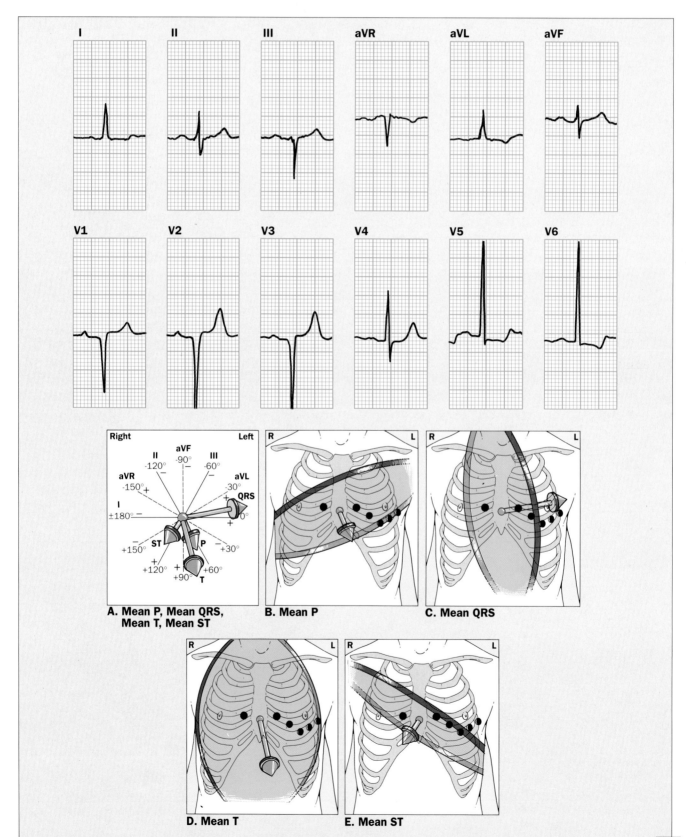

A. Mean P, Mean QRS, Mean T, Mean ST

B. Mean P

C. Mean QRS

D. Mean T

E. Mean ST

(Figure 9.4 continued.)
ted anteriorly (note the tall P1 in lead V1), and the P wave suggests a right atrial abnormality. This undoubtedly occurred because of pulmonary hypertension resulting from severe mitral regurgitation. Although there was angiographic evidence of an enlarged left atrium, the abnormal P waves are due to a *right* atrial abnormality. Remember, abnormal P waves are often due to atrial conduction defects rather than atrial enlargements.

QRS complex: The initial mean 0.04-second QRS vector is directed to the left and posteriorly. Accordingly, no R waves are recorded in leads V1, V2, and V3. There are no Q waves in leads I and V6. The intrinsicoid deflection of the QRS complex is greater than 0.04 second, and the direction of the mean QRS vector is -10° in the frontal plane and 45° posteriorly. The 12-lead QRS amplitude is greater than 176 mm.

T waves: The frontal plane direction of the mean T vector is +75°; it is directed about 80° anteriorly.

ST segment: The frontal plane direction of the mean ST segment vector is +125°.

A. The frontal plane projections of the mean P, QRS, T, and ST vectors. **B.** The spatial orientation of the mean P vector. Note that it is directed vertically and anteriorly, indicating a right atrial abnormality. **C.** The spatial orientation of the

mean QRS vector. Note that it is directed about 45° posteriorly. **D.** The spatial orientation of the mean T vector. Note that it is directed inferiorly and more than 80° anteriorly. The QRS-T angle is about 125°. **E.** The spatial orientation of the mean ST vector.

Summary: The abnormalities in this electrocardiogram are characteristic of systolic pressure overload of the left ventricle. It is an example of the systolic pressure overload that eventually occurs when there is longstanding, progressive diastolic pressure overload of the left ventricle. A left ventricular conduction defect may be causing the absence of R waves in leads V1, V2 and V3, though this could be misinterpreted as being due to myocardial infarction. The P wave abnormality indicates a right atrial abnormality secondary to pulmonary hypertension, and this is likely, even though the left atrium was found to be enlarged on angiography.

FIGURE 9.5

Left ventricular hypertrophy due to systolic pressure overload of the left ventricle. The hypertrophy is due to a late stage of diastolic pressure overload. The patient was a 24-year-old man with severe aortic regurgitation and mild aortic stenosis due to rheumatic heart disease.

The PR interval is 0.16 second. The QRS duration is 0.08 second, and the QT interval is 0.36 second.

P waves: The P wave is abnormal. Its duration in lead II is 0.12 second, and its amplitude is 2 mm. The terminal P2 in lead V1 is -0.06 mm-sec, indicating a left atrial abnormality.

QRS complex: The duration of the QRS complex is 0.08 second, and the intrinsicoid deflection is 0.042 second. The direction of the mean QRS vector is +60° in the frontal plane and about 45° posteriorly. Compare this with the orientation of the frontal plane (F), transverse plane (T), and sagittal plane (S) QRS loop. The 12-lead amplitude of the QRS complex is about 220 mm.

T waves: The mean T vector is directed at +80° in the frontal plane and 80° anteriorly. The QRS-T angle is 120°.

ST segment: The mean ST vector is directed anteriorly. It is difficult to identify in the frontal plane; it seems to be directed toward the right shoulder (it is isoelectric in lead aVL).

Summary: The presence of a left atrial abnormality, an abnormal intrinsicoid deflection of the QRS complex, an abnormally large amplitude of the QRS complexes, abnormal ST-T vectors, and an abnormal QRS-T angle indicates left ventricular hypertrophy.

(Figure 9.5 continued on page 9.10.)

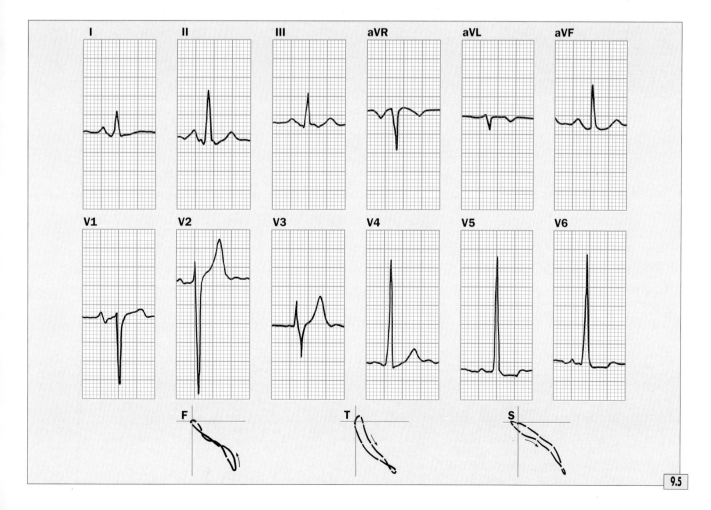

(Figure 9.5 continued.)

The predictive value of these abnormalities approaches 100 percent. This electrocardiogram, as well as that in Figure 9.4, illustrates the point that severe, longstanding, and progressive diastolic pressure overload will eventually produce an abnormal electrocardiogram characteristic of systolic pressure overload. (Reproduced with permission from the publisher and author; see Figure Credits. The orientation of the vectorcardiogram in the transverse plane has been changed from that in the original publication, with the permission of Dr. Estes, so that it conforms to the orientation of the magnetic resonance images used in this book.)

FIGURE 9.6

Left ventricular hypertrophy due to diastolic pressure overload of the left ventricle.

The patient was a 24-year-old man with aortic regurgitation due to a congenital bicuspid aortic valve. An echocardiogram and Doppler study revealed aortic regurgitation. The left ventricular diastolic diameter was 60 mm.

The PR interval is 0.16 second; the direction of the mean T vector indicates a lower atrial rhythm. The duration of the QRS complex is 0.10 second, and the QT interval is 0.36 second.

P waves: The mean P vector is directed at -40°. This indicates a lower atrial rhythm. The P wave in lead III shown in this illustration appears to be positive; it was negative in the other deflection of the original recording.

QRS complex: The intrinsicoid deflection of the QRS complex is slightly greater than 0.04 second, and the direction of the mean QRS vector is +75°. The 12-lead QRS amplitude is greater than

233 mm. The QRS complex is definitely negative in leads V1, V2, V3, and V4. Accordingly, the mean QRS vector is directed about 60° posteriorly. The transitional pathway courses between leads V4 and V5. As diagrammed, the deflections at V5 and V6 would be almost transitional, but in reality they are positive. It is highly likely that the electrodes were placed a little higher than they should have been, or that the transitional pathway took a slightly different course than is depicted in the diagram.

T waves: The mean T vector is large and is directed at +65°; it is parallel with the frontal plane.

ST segment: The mean ST vector is directed at +80° and relatively parallel with the mean T vector.

A. The frontal plane projections of the mean P, QRS, T, and ST vectors. **B.** The spatial orientation of the mean P vector.

TABLE 9.3 ELECTROCARDIOGRAPHIC CHARACTERISTICS OF SECONDARY LEFT VENTRICULAR HYPERTROPHY DUE TO DIASTOLIC PRESSURE OVERLOAD OF THE LEFT VENTRICLE

- A left atrial abnormality may be present (see Table 7.2).

- The QRS duration in adults is usually 0.10 second or less, but may be 0.11 second. It may be less than 0.10 second in children.

- The mean QRS vector may be directed from +80° to -30°, but always posteriorly. The mean QRS vector tends to be further to the left than in systolic pressure overload, but this finding is not sufficient to distinguish systolic from diastolic pressure overload.

- The QRS amplitude is increased (see Table 5.3), and the total 12-lead QRS amplitude is often greater than 185 mm (see Fig. 5.8).

- The initial QRS forces become larger than normal but may retain their normal direction. The Q waves become more prominent in leads I, V5, and V6, and the R waves become more prominent in leads V1 and V2.

- The direction of the mean T vector and the QRS-T angle may remain normal.

- The T waves may become larger.

- The mean ST vector is parallel with the mean T vector.

- The U waves may be prominent.

- Late in the natural history of this condition, the electrocardiographic abnormalities become similar to those due to systolic pressure overload of the left ventricle (see Table 9.1).

TABLE 9.4 ELECTROCARDIOGRAPHIC ABNORMALITIES THAT MUST BE DIFFERENTIATED FROM THOSE DUE TO DIASTOLIC PRESSURE OVERLOAD OF THE LEFT VENTRICLE

- The greatest problem is to separate the normal electrocardiogram from that showing only an increased QRS amplitude secondary to left ventricular hypertrophy due to diastolic pressure overload (see Table 5.3). The normal total 12-lead QRS amplitude can be as much as 185 mm (see Fig. 5.8). This problem is especially worrisome during the stage of diastolic pressure overload in which the mean ST-T vectors are large and relatively parallel with the mean QRS vector. Normal early repolarization can produce the same ST-T changes. The predictability of left ventricular hypertrophy increases as the QRS amplitude increases.

- Electrocardiographically, left bundle branch block does not resemble diastolic overload of the left ventricle; in left bundle branch block, the mean ST and T vectors are opposite the mean QRS vector, and the QRS duration is 0.12 second or greater. In addition, the Q waves are absent in leads I and V6, and no R wave is present in lead V1. These waves are prominent when there is left ventricular hypertrophy due to diastolic pressure overload.

- Left ventricular conduction delay may simulate diastolic pressure overload in that the QRS duration may be about 0.10 second, and the amplitude of the QRS complex may be large. In diastolic pressure overload, the Q waves are prominent in leads I and V6, and the R waves are prominent in lead V1. These deflections are absent in left ventricular conduction delay. Left ventricular hypertrophy may, however, be associated with left ventricular conduction delay.

- In left anterior-superior division block, the mean QRS vector is directed more than -30° to the left; left ventricular hypertrophy alone will not cause this degree of leftward shifting.

- The calibration of the electrocardiograph machine may be over-standardized, leading to misinterpretation of the size of the QRS complexes.

(Figure 9.6 continued.)
It is abnormal because of the patient's lower atrial rhythm. **C.** The spatial orientation of the mean QRS vector.
D. The spatial orientation of the large mean T vector. The mean QRS-T angle is about 60°. **E.** The spatial orientation of the mean ST vector. Note that this vector is relatively parallel with the mean T vector.

Summary: These abnormalities indicate a lower atrial rhythm. The 12 lead QRS amplitude is increased, with a predictive value of 100 percent for left ventricular hypertrophy. The mean vectors representing the ST segments and T waves are characteristic of diastolic pressure overload of the left ventricle.

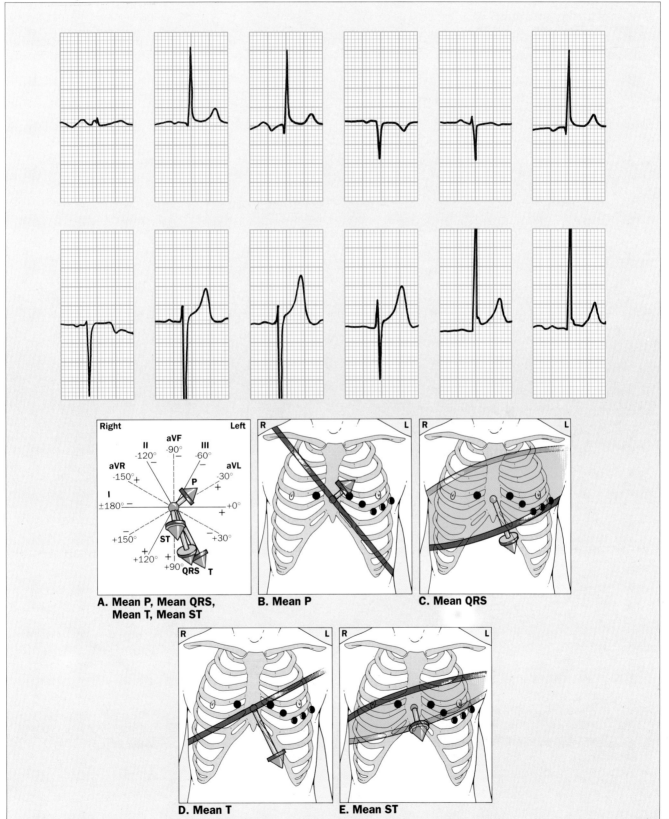

A. Mean P, Mean QRS, Mean T, Mean ST

B. Mean P

C. Mean QRS

D. Mean T

E. Mean ST

9.6

FIGURE 9.7

Left ventricular hypertrophy due to diastolic pressure overload of the left ventricle. This electrocardiogram was recorded from a seven-year-old child with a ventricular septal defect of moderate size.

The PR interval is 0.13 second, the duration of the QRS complex is 0.08 second, and the QT interval is 0.32 second.

QRS complexes: The mean QRS vector is directed at + 70° in the frontal plane and about 60-70° posteriorly. The 12-lead QRS amplitude is about 184 mm.

T waves: The mean T wave vector is directed at +60°; it is directed 20° posteriorly.

ST segment: The mean ST vector is directed at 60°, and parallel with the frontal plane.

A. The frontal plane projections of the mean QRS, T, and ST vectors. **B.** The spatial orientation of the mean QRS vector. The transitional pathway courses between leads V4 and V5; leads V5 and V6 record positive deflections. A small change in the electrode positions of leads V5 and V6 could change the deflections from positive to negative. **C.** The spatial orientation of the mean T vector. This vector can be directed posteriorly in a normal seven-year-old child. **D.** The spatial orientation of the mean ST vector.

Summary: This electrocardiogram could be normal for a seven-year-old child. The 12-lead QRS amplitude is at the upper limits of normal, but this type of measurement has not been studied in normal children of this age. This case illustrates the thought process to take when observing a tracing of this sort: the electrocardiogram is either normal or consistent with diastolic pressure overload of the left ventricle. When a patent ductus arteriosus or ventricular septal defect is detected on the physical examination, the electrocardiogram is considered to be consistent with such an abnormality. (Reproduced with permission from the publisher and author; see Figure Credits.)

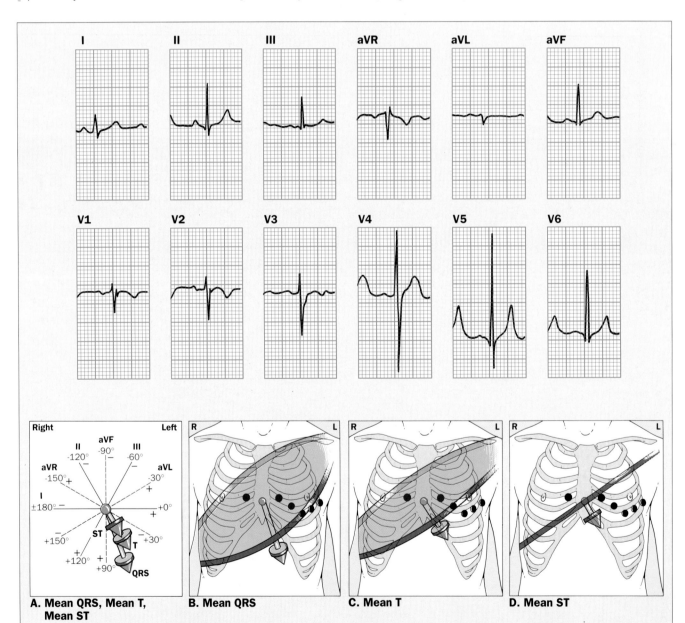

A. Mean QRS, Mean T, Mean ST

B. Mean QRS

C. Mean T

D. Mean ST

FIGURE 9.8

Left ventricular hypertrophy due to diastolic pressure overload of the left ventricle. This electrocardiogram and vectorcardiogram were recorded from a 22-year-old man with rheumatic heart disease and aortic regurgitation.

The PR interval is 0.18 second. The duration of the QRS complex is 0.10 second, and the QT interval is 0.40 second.

QRS complexes: The mean QRS vector is directed at +70° in the frontal plane and at about 45° posteriorly. The 12-lead QRS amplitude is 288 mm. Note that a prominent R wave is present in lead V1 and that Q waves are present in leads V5 and V6.

T waves: The mean T vector is directed at -15° in the frontal plane. It is flush with the frontal plane when viewed in space.

ST segment: The ST segment is isoelectric in the frontal plane and is directed anteriorly.

Summary: The direction and amplitude of the mean QRS vector indicate left ventricular hypertrophy. The predictive value of these findings for this abnormality approaches 100 percent. The early QRS forces and ST and T vectors are consistent with diastolic pressure overload of the left ventricle. In this case, the overload was due to aortic regurgitation. (Reproduced with permission from the publisher and author; see Figure Credits. The orientation of the vectorcardiogram in the transverse plane has been changed from the original, with the permission of Dr. Estes, so that it conforms to the orientation of the magnetic resonance images presented in this book.)

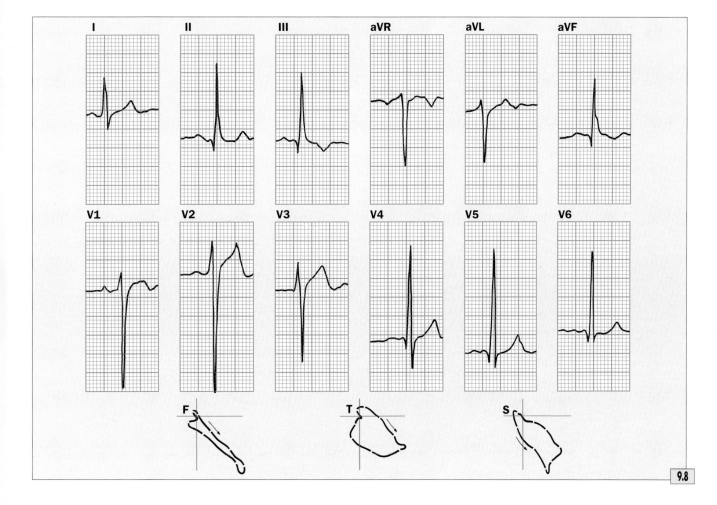

9.8

TABLE 9.5 ELECTROCARDIOGRAPHIC CHARACTERISTICS OF SECONDARY RIGHT VENTRICULAR HYPERTROPHY DUE TO SYSTOLIC PRESSURE OVERLOAD OF THE RIGHT VENTRICLE

- A right atrial abnormality may be present.

- A left atrial abnormality may be present when the right ventricular hypertrophy is due to mitral stenosis.

- Biatrial abnormality may be present in patients with mitral stenosis or cardiomyopathy with pulmonary hypertension.

- The QRS duration is usually 0.08 to 0.10 second in adults. It may be less in children.

- The initial QRS forces may be directed in such a way that a large initial R wave is written in lead V1. A Q wave, followed by a prominent R wave, may be seen in lead V1 in some patients. This, and other variations of the initial portion of the QRS complex in lead V1 are caused by remodeling of the septum due to right ventricular hypertension. The remodeled septum produces electrical forces that are directed to the right, superiorly, and posteriorly.

- When the systolic pressure overload is due to congenital heart disease, the mean QRS vector is usually directed more than +90° to the right and anteriorly, and the middle QRS forces are increased in size. When systolic pressure overload due to acquired heart disease develops in adults, the mean QRS vector may initially be directed vertically and posteriorly. It may be directed vertically no more than +80°, and may gradually rotate further to the right and anteriorly.

- The mean T vector is directed away from the mean QRS vector. The QRS-T angle may be 180°. This is common in congenital heart disease such as pulmonary valve stenosis. It develops late in the course of right ventricular hypertrophy due to acquired heart disease.

- The mean ST segment vector tends to be parallel with the mean T vector.

- The S1, S2, S3 type of conduction disturbance may be a normal variant, but when the terminal QRS forces are large, it is proper to consider the possibility of right ventricular hypertrophy.

TABLE 9.6 ELECTROCARDIOGRAPHIC ABNORMALITIES THAT MUST BE DIFFERENTIATED FROM THOSE DUE TO SYSTOLIC PRESSURE OVERLOAD OF THE RIGHT VENTRICLE

- Lateral myocardial infarction may produce a mean QRS vector directed more than +90° to the right, and posterior-inferior myocardial infarction or true posterior myocardial infarction may cause an anterior rotation of the initial QRS forces that produces a prominent initial R wave in lead V1. Other electrocardiographic signs of infarction are usually present to assist in distinguishing such electrocardiograms from those showing right ventricular hypertrophy.

- Right bundle branch block produces a mean QRS vector that is directed to the right and anteriorly, but the QRS duration is 0.11 to 0.12 second. The middle forces may be larger than normal, suggesting, but not proving the presence of right ventricular hypertrophy.

- Right ventricular conduction delay may produce a mean QRS vector that is directed to the right and anteriorly. The QRS duration is usually 0.08 to 0.10 second. The initial QRS forces may be normal. Right ventricular hypertrophy may be recognized when the middle QRS forces are larger than normal. The problem here is that it is difficult to determine whether or not the middle QRS forces are abnormally large.

- Left posterior-inferior division block may produce a mean QRS vector that is directed about +120° to the right and posteriorly. It is not possible to identify this abnormality without a series of electrocardiograms in which the mean QRS vector is seen to shift abruptly from its normal direction to the new, abnormal direction.

- Some patients with the electrocardiographic signs of pre-excitation of the ventricles (associated with the Wolff-Parkinson-White syndrome) exhibit tall R waves in lead V1. The other features of pre-excitation are evident, however, and serve to distinguish this abnormality from right ventricular hypertrophy.

- The electrocardiogram associated with pulmonary emphysema may suggest that of right ventricular hypertrophy (see Figure 13.1), but the QRS voltage is usually diminished in these patients.

- The electrocardiogram of acute pulmonary embolism may also mimic the electrocardiogram of right ventricular hypertrophy (see Figures 13.2-13.4); however, its transient nature serves to eliminate the presence of right ventricular hypertrophy.

- The normal child may exhibit a mean QRS vector that is directed to the right and anteriorly. There is a tall R wave in lead V1. In young children, it is difficult to distinguish the normal electrocardiogram from the one indicating right ventricular hypertrophy (see Chapters 5 and 6).

FIGURE 9.9

Systolic pressure overload of the right ventricle. This electrocardiogram was recorded from a seven-year-old child with an interventricular septal defect and Eisenmenger's syndrome. The standardization is normal in leads I, II, III, aVR, aVL, aVF, and V4R; one half normal in lead V1; and one quarter normal in leads V2, V4, V5, and V6. The PR interval is 0.16 second. The duration of the QRS complex is 0.09 second, and the QT interval is 0.36 second.

P waves: The P waves are extremely large in the precordial leads (recall that the deflections seen in lead V1 are half-standardized, and those in leads V2, V4, V5, and V6 are one quarter standardized). The mean P vector (Pm) is directed inferiorly at about +30° and slightly posteriorly. The P waves probably represent left and right atrial abnormalities.

QRS complex: The mean QRS vector is directed at about +160° in the frontal plane and about 60° anteriorly. The middle QRS forces are huge.

T waves: The mean T vector is directed -25° to the left and about 70° posteriorly.

A. The frontal plane projections of the mean P (Pm), QRS, and T vectors. **B.** The spatial orientation of the mean QRS vector. Note the course of the transitional pathway. **C.** The spatial orientation of the mean T vector. Note the course of the transitional pathway.

Summary: The P waves are clearly abnormal. Right and left atrial abnormalities are probably present. The mean QRS vector is huge, directed to the right and anteriorly, while the mean T vector has an opposite direction. This electrocardiogram is characteristic of systolic pressure overload of the right ventricle. In this case, it was due to Eisenmenger's syndrome secondary to an interventricular septal defect. (Reproduced with permission from the publisher and author; see Figure Credits.)

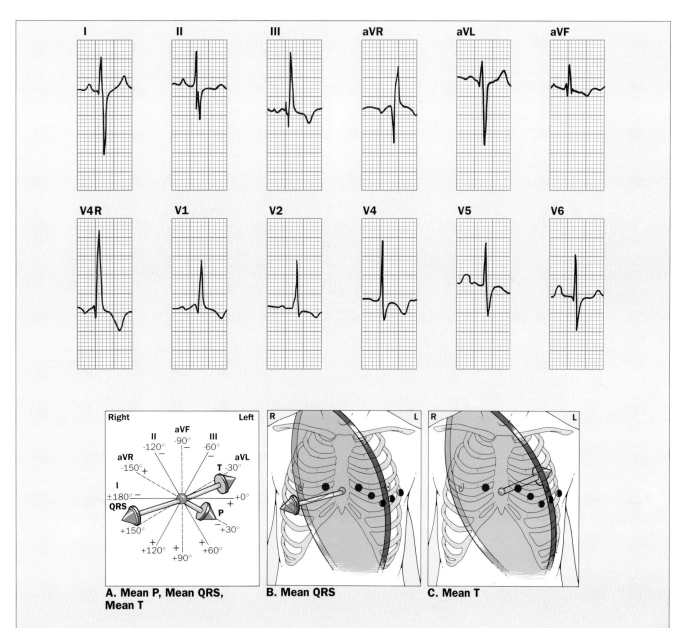

A. Mean P, Mean QRS, Mean T

B. Mean QRS

C. Mean T

FIGURE 9.10

Right ventricular hypertrophy due to systolic pressure overload of the right ventricle. This electrocardiogram and vectorcardiogram were recorded from a 39-year-old man with an atrial septal defect and pulmonary hypertension.

The PR interval is 0.16 second. The duration of the QRS complex is 0.09 second, and the QT interval is 0.36 second.

P waves: The mean P vector (Pm) is directed at +60° in and flush with the frontal plane.

QRS complex: The mean QRS vector is directed at +110° in, and parallel with,

the frontal plane, suggesting right ventricular hypertrophy.

T waves: The mean T vector is directed at about -90° in the frontal plane and slightly posteriorly. Note that the T vector need not be directed very far posteriorly for all of the precordial T waves to be negative, and the T wave in V6 to be isoelectric.

Summary: This electrocardiogram is characteristic of right ventricular hypertrophy due to systolic pressure overload of the right ventricle. In this case, the electrocardiographic abnormalities were caused by an atrial septal defect with pulmonary hypertension (Eisenmenger's

physiology). (Reproduced with permission from the publisher and author; see Figure Credits. The orientation of the vectorcardiogram in the transverse plane has been changed from that in the original publication, with the permission of Dr. Estes, so that it conforms to magnetic resonance images presented in this book.)

FIGURE 9.11

Right ventricular conduction defect associated with diastolic pressure overload of the right ventricle. This electrocardiogram was recorded from a

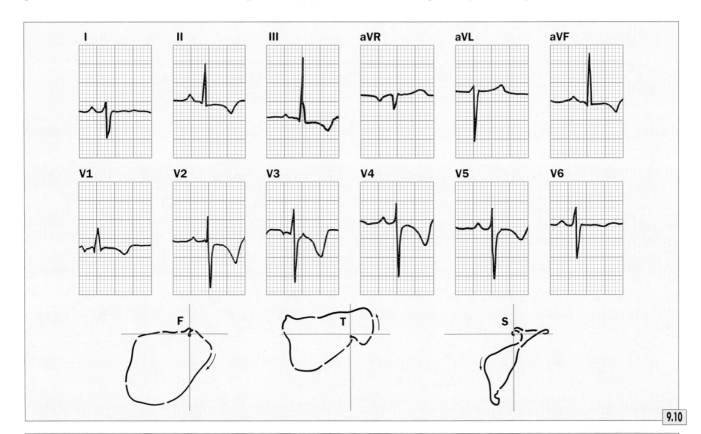

9.10

TABLE 9.7 ELECTROCARDIOGRAPHIC CHARACTERITICS OF SECONDARY RIGHT VENTRICULAR HYPERTROPHY DUE TO DIASTOLIC PRESSURE OVERLOAD OF THE RIGHT VENTRICLE

- A right atrial abnormality may be present (see Table 7.1).

- The electrocardiographic abnormalities of diastolic overload of the right ventricle are those of right ventricular conduction delay.

- The QRS duration is 0.08 to 0.10 second.

- The initial QRS forces may be directed normally but may be larger than normal. The terminal QRS forces are directed to the right and anteriorly, signifying a right ventricular conduction delay.

- Right ventricular hypertrophy is more likely to be present when the middle QRS forces are directed to the right and anteriorly. The earlier in the cycle the QRS forces shift to the right and anteriorly, and the larger they are, the more likely the finding will be related to right ventricular hypertrophy.

- The mean QRS vector is usually directed more than +110° to the right.

- The mean T wave vector may be normally directed but tends to be directed away from the mean QRS vector.

- The ST segment vector is parallel with the mean T vector.

- Right bundle branch block may develop when the QRS duration becomes 0.11 to 0.12 second. Right ventricular hypertrophy is more likely in patients with right bundle branch block when the middle QRS forces are large and point to the right and anteriorly. Regrettably, this is not a reliable sign of right ventricular hypertrophy.

(Figure 9.11 continued.)
49-year-old woman with an atrial septal defect. (The left-to-right shunt ratio was 5:1.) The tracing shows a right ventricular conduction defect that is often associated with right ventricular hypertrophy secondary to diastolic pressure overload of the right ventricle.

The PR interval is 0.12 second. The duration of the QRS complex is 0.08 second, and the QT interval is 0.36 second.

P waves: The P waves are normal in this electrocardiogram.

QRS complex: The mean QRS vector is directed inferiorly at about +70°, and parallel with the frontal plane. The terminal 0.04-second QRS vector is directed to the right and anteriorly, pointing toward the right ventricle.

T waves: The mean T vector is directed to the left at 0° and about 60° posteriorly. It is directed away from the right ventricle.

A. The frontal plane projections of the mean QRS, mean terminal 0.04-second QRS, and mean T vectors. **B.** The spatial orientation of the mean QRS vector. Note the course of the transitional pathway on the chest. **C.** The spatial orientation of the mean terminal 0.04-second QRS vector. Note the course of the transitional pathway on the chest. **D.** The spatial orientation of the mean T vector. Note the course of the transitional pathway on the chest.

Summary: The mean terminal 0.04-second QRS vector points toward the right ventricle, and the mean T vector is directed away from the right ventricle. The last portion of the heart to undergo depolarization is the right ventricle. This electrocardiographic abnormality often accompanies right ventricular diastolic pressure overload. There are few causes of this condition, and in this case, it appears that the

(Figure 9.11 continued on page 9.18.)

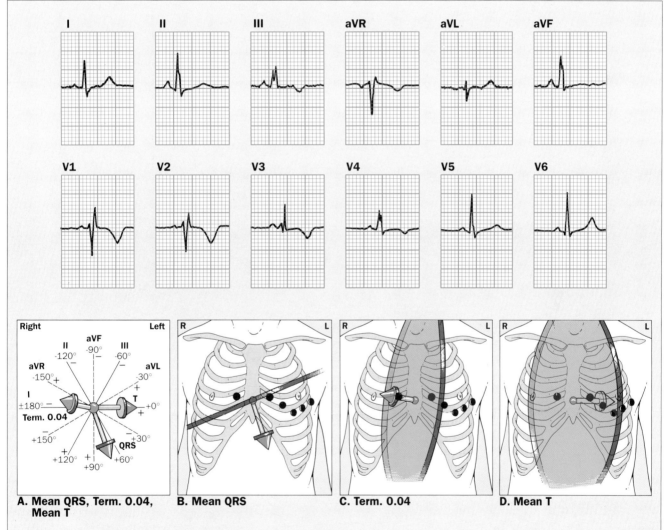

A. Mean QRS, Term. 0.04, Mean T   B. Mean QRS   C. Term. 0.04   D. Mean T

9.11

TABLE 9.8 ELECTROCARDIOGRAPHIC ABNORMALITIES THAT MUST BE DIFFERENTIATED FROM THOSE DUE TO DIASTOLIC PRESSURE OVERLOAD OF THE RIGHT VENTRICLE

- It is not always possible to distinguish the right ventricular conduction delay associated with diastolic pressure overload, such as occurs with a secundum atrial septal defect, from that which is a variant of normal.

- Right ventricular hypertrophy is more likely to be present when the middle QRS forces are large and directed to the right and anteriorly.

- Terminal QRS forces that are small, directed to the right, and flush with the frontal plane or slightly anterior may be a normal variant.

(Figure 9.11 continued.)
right ventricular conduction defect actu- ally dominates the electrical field and masks the abnormalities that might be caused by right ventricular diastolic pressure overload. This creates the fol- lowing relationship: a right ventricular conduction defect may be caused by

diastolic pressure overload of the right ventricle, which in turn may correlate with the presence of right ventricular hypertrophy.

F I G U R E   9 . 1 2
Idiopathic hypertrophic subaortic stenosis. This electrocardiogram was

recorded from a 28-year-old man who has primary cardiomyopathy, as do two other members of his family. The mag- netic resonance images of his heart, made when he was 31-years-old, are shown in Figure 9.17.
The PR interval is 0.17 second. The duration of the QRS complex is 0.08

TABLE 9.9 ELECTROCARDIOGRAPHIC CHARACTERISTICS OF COMBINED SECONDARY LEFT AND RIGHT VENTRICULAR HYPERTROPHY

- Right and left atrial abnormalities may be present (see Tables 7.1 and 7.2).
- The QRS duration is less than 0.12 second.
- The mean QRS vector may be large, and may be directed inferiorly and slightly posteriorly, or horizontally and more anteriorly than normal.

- The QRS duration may be 0.12 second, but when this occurs, conduction defects are often present, and the electrocardio- graphic abnormalities are not solely due to ventricular hypertrophy.
- The mean T and mean ST vectors are usually directed opposite the mean QRS vector.

TABLE 9.10 ELECTROCARDIOGRAPHIC ABNORMALITIES THAT MUST BE DIFFERENTIATED FROM THOSE OF COMBINED SECONDARY RIGHT AND LEFT VENTRICULAR HYPERTROPHY

- The direction and magnitude of the mean QRS vector are used to determine the presence of combined left and right ventricular hypertrophy.
- It is not always possible to separate the normal electrocardio- gram, or that of left ventricular hypertrophy, from that of com- bined right and left secondary ventricular hypertrophy.

- When accompanied by right and left atrial abnormalities, the abnormally large mean QRS vector that is directed inferiorly and slightly posteriorly, or horizontally and slightly anteriorly, indicates right and left ventricular hypertrophy with a predictive value of more than 75 percent.

TABLE 9.11 ELECTROCARDIOGRAPHIC CHARACTERISTICS OF PRIMARY LEFT VENTRICULAR HYPERTROPHY (HYPERTROPHIC CARDIOMYOPATHY)

- A left atrial abnormality may be present (see Figure 7.2).
- The electrocardiographic abnormalities of systolic pressure overload of the left ventricle may be present.
- The following abnormalities occur in hypertrophic cardiomyopa- thy but not in left ventricular hypertrophy due to other causes:
- The PR interval may be short, and the initial portion of the QRS complex may have the characteristics of pre-excitation of the ventricles, suggesting the Wolff-Parkinson-White syndrome. In addition, the QRS magnitude is usually abnormally large.
- The mean initial 0.04-second QRS vector may have the charac- teristics of myocardial infarction. Inferior, anterior, and lateral infarction may be simulated.

- The ST-T waves may be bizarre. The mean T vector may be directed away from the mean QRS vector to varying degrees, and the QRS-T angle may be as wide as 90° to 180°. The mean ST segment vector may be relatively parallel with the mean QRS vector and may simulate that of epicardial injury accompanying myocardial infarction. The abnormality remains constant when due to hypertrophic cardiomyopathy, and usually disappears or becomes smaller when due to myocardial infarction.
- Bizarre T wave abnormalities may occur. The mean T vector may be large and directed far to the right and anteriorly. This produces extremely large and inverted T waves in leads I, II, III, V4, V5, and V6, and is more likely to occur when there is apical hypertrophic cardiomyopathy.

(Figure 9.12 continued.)
second, and the QT interval is 0.36 second.

P waves: The mean P vector (Pm) is directed at +30° in the frontal plane and slightly posteriorly. The duration of the P wave in lead II is 0.08 second, and its amplitude is 2.5 mm. The duration-amplitude product for last half of the P wave (P2) in V1 is 0.04 mm-sec. These measurements suggest a left atrial abnormality and hint at a right atrial abnormality.

QRS complex: The mean QRS vector is directed inferiorly at about +60° and posteriorly at about 60°. The total 12-lead QRS amplitude is 166 mm.

T wave: The direction of the mean T vector is -45° in the frontal plane; it is directed markedly anteriorly.

A. The frontal plane projections of the mean P, QRS, and T vectors. **B.** The spatial orientation of the mean P vector. The mean vector representing P2 is abnormal, indicating a left atrial abnormality The tall, narrow P waves in lead II suggest a right atrial abnormality.
C. The spatial orientation of the mean QRS vector. Note the course of the transitional pathway on the chest.
D. The spatial orientation of the mean T vector. Note that there is no transitional complex recorded in the precordial leads. Additional leads from the

right side of the chest would be needed to identify the transitional pathway. It is definite, however, that the mean T vector is directed moderately anteriorly, because the T wave in V1 is larger than the T wave in V6.

Summary: The 12-lead QRS amplitude in this case is not sufficient to identify left ventricular hypertrophy. The QRS amplitude in V2 is about 28 mm, and P2 is abnormal, signifying a left atrial abnormality. The clinical features in this patient, including the magnetic resonance image and cardiac catheterization, indicate severe idiopathic hypertrophic subaortic stenosis.

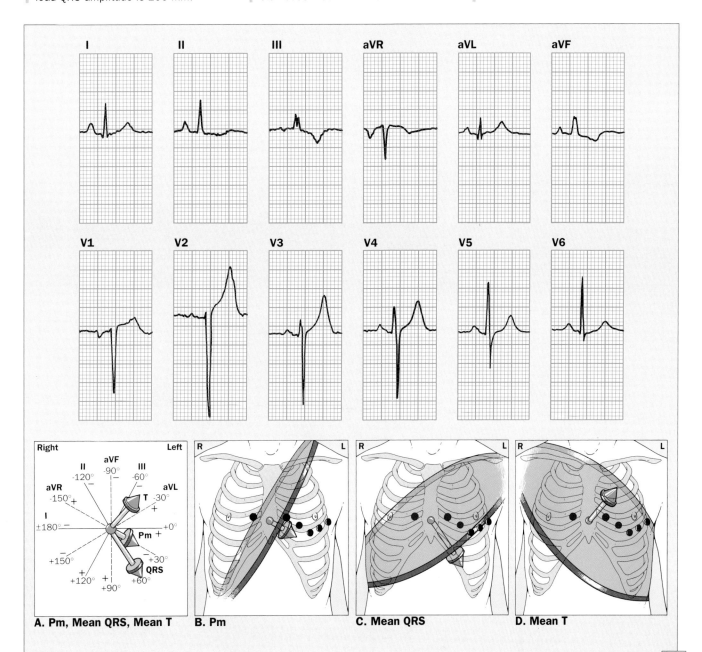

A. Pm, Mean QRS, Mean T   **B. Pm**   **C. Mean QRS**   **D. Mean T**

9.12

FIGURE 9.13

Primary hypertrophic cardiomyopathy. This electrocardiogram was recorded from a 43-year-old man, and is characteristic of hypertrophic subaortic stenosis.

The PR interval is 0.17 second. The duration of the QRS complex is 0.08 second; the QT interval is 0.44 second.

P waves: The P wave duration in lead II is about 0.12 second, and its amplitude is 1.5 mm. The mean P vector (Pm) is directed at +30° in the frontal plane, and about 30° posteriorly. P2 is abnormal; it is directed about 40° posteriorly, with a duration-amplitude product of about -0.04 mm-sec in lead V1. This signifies a left atrial abnormality.

QRS complex: The QRS complex is directed about -45° to the left, and about 60° posteriorly. The total 12-lead QRS amplitude is 131 mm. The mean initial 0.04-second QRS vector is directed to the right at +180°, flush with the frontal plane. This produces Q waves that simulate massive anterolateral myocardial infarction in leads V3, V4, V5 and V6.

T waves: The mean T vector is directed at +10° in, and parallel with, the frontal plane. **A.** The frontal plane projections of the mean P, mean QRS, mean initial 0.04-second QRS, mean T, and mean ST vectors. Note the courses of the transitional pathways on the chests

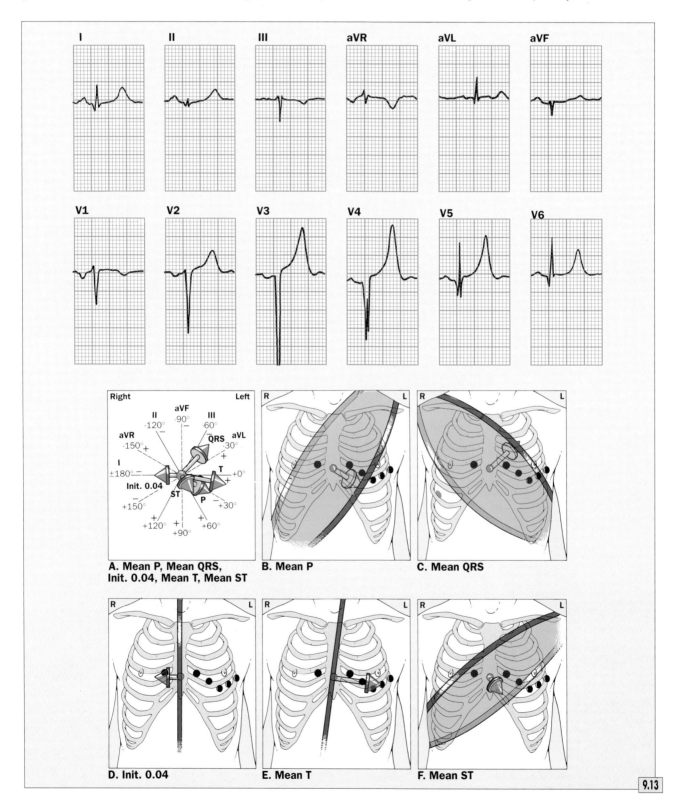

A. Mean P, Mean QRS, Init. 0.04, Mean T, Mean ST

B. Mean P

C. Mean QRS

D. Init. 0.04

E. Mean T

F. Mean ST

(Figure 9.13 continued.)
depicted in parts B-F. **B.** The spatial orientation of the mean P vector. It is abnormally directed posteriorly. **C.** The spatial orientation of the mean QRS vector; it is also abnormally directed posteriorly. **D.** The spatial orientation of the mean initial 0.04-second QRS vector. It is abnormal and could be mistaken for an abnormality due

to myocardial infarction. **E.** The spatial orientation of the mean T vector. Note the course of the transitional pathway on the chest. **F.** The spatial orientation of the ST segment vector.

Summary: There is evidence of a left atrial abnormality. An abnormally-directed mean QRS vector and an abnormal mean initial 0.04-second QRS vector suggest

anterolateral infarction. These abnormalities are among the many that may be seen in patients with hypertrophic cardiomyopathy.

FIGURE 9.14
Hypertrophic cardiomyopathy and subaortic stenosis. This electrocardiogram was recorded from a 49-year-old man.
(Figure 9.14 continued on page 9.22.)

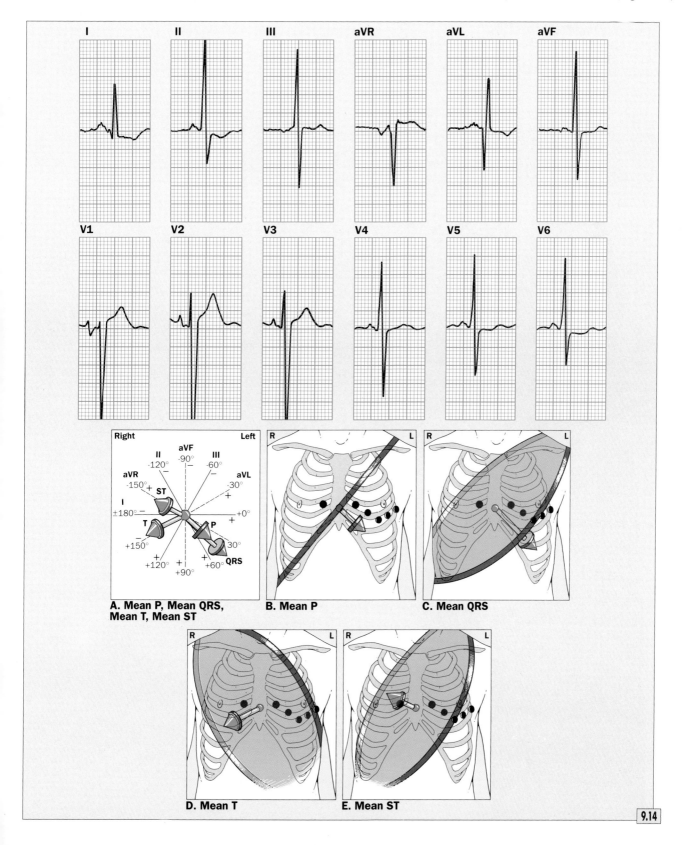

A. Mean P, Mean QRS, Mean T, Mean ST

B. Mean P

C. Mean QRS

D. Mean T

E. Mean ST

(Figure 9.14 continued.)

The PR interval is 0.13 second. The duration of the QRS complex is 0.11 second, and the QT interval is 0.40 second.

P waves: The duration of the P wave in lead I is 0.11 second; its amplitude is 2.5 mm. The duration-amplitude product of P2 in lead V1 is -0.05 mm-sec, indicating a left atrial abnormality.

QRS complex: The mean QRS vector is directed inferiorly at about +45°, and posteriorly at about 60°. The mean terminal 0.04-second QRS vector is directed far to the left and posteriorly, signifying a left ventricular conduction defect. The middle QRS forces indicate left ventricular hypertrophy, and the terminal forces indicate a left ventricular conduction defect. The total QRS amplitude is greater than 360 mm.

T waves: The mean T vector is directed at about +150° in the frontal plane, and about 85° anteriorly. The QRS-T angle is about 150°.

ST segment: The mean ST segment vector is relatively parallel with the mean T vector.

A. The frontal plane projections of the mean P, QRS, T, and ST vectors. In the following representations, note the courses of the transitional pathways on the chests. **B.** The spatial orientation of the mean P vector. **C.** The spatial orientation of the mean QRS vector. **D.** The spatial orientation of the mean T vector. It is abnormally directed away from the mean QRS vector. **E.** The spatial orientation of the mean ST vector. It is relatively parallel with the mean T vector.

Summary: Evidence of a left atrial abnormality, a large QRS amplitude, the presence of a left ventricular conduction defect, and abnormal ST and T vectors may be observed in patients with hypertrophic cardiomyopathy.

FIGURE 9.15

Apical hypertrophic cardiomyopathy. This electrocardiogram was recorded from a 28-year-old man. The PR interval is 0.14 sec-ond. The duration of the QRS complex is 0.09 second, and the QT interval is 0.32 second.

P waves: The duration of the P wave in lead II is 0.08 second; its amplitude is 2.25 mm. The mean P vector (Pm) is directed inferiorly and slightly anteriorly. It is not definitely abnormal.

QRS complex: The mean QRS vector is directed superiorly at about -105°, and posteriorly, to an unknown degree. The mean initial 0.04-second QRS vector is directed to the left at about -45°, parallel with the frontal plane or directed slightly posteriorly. The mean terminal 0.04-second QRS vector is directed far to the right and posteriorly. The 12-lead QRS amplitude is about 282 mm, indicating left ventricular hypertrophy.

T waves: The mean T vector is directed inferiorly at about +40°, and anteriorly to an unknown degree.

A. The frontal plane projections of the mean QRS, mean initial 0.04-second QRS,

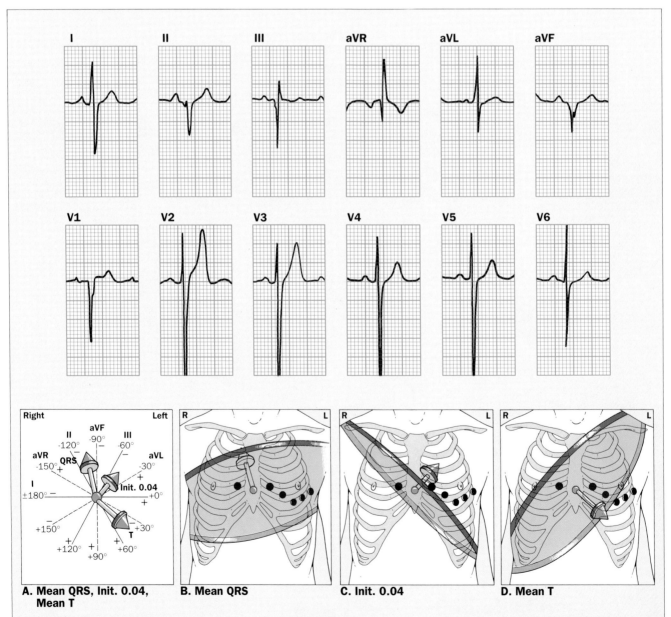

A. Mean QRS, Init. 0.04, Mean T   **B. Mean QRS**   **C. Init. 0.04**   **D. Mean T**

(Figure 9.15 continued.)
and mean T vectors. **B.** The spatial orientation of the mean QRS vector. **C.** The spatial orientation of the mean initial 0.04-second QRS vector. This vector simulates the abnormality of inferior infarction. **D.** The spatial orientation of the mean T vector. It is directed anteriorly to an unknown degree.

Summary: The increase in QRS amplitude indicates left ventricular hypertrophy. The direction of the mean initial 0.04-second QRS vector is abnormal; it simulates inferior myocardial infarction. The abnormality of the mean terminal 0.04-second QRS vector indicates a type of conduction abnormality that may be in the left or right ventricle. All of these abnormalities may occur with hypertrophic cardiomyopathy.

FIGURE 9.16
Apical hypertrophic cardiomyopathy. This electrocardiogram was recorded from an 81-year-old woman.

(Figure 9.16 continued on page 9.24.)

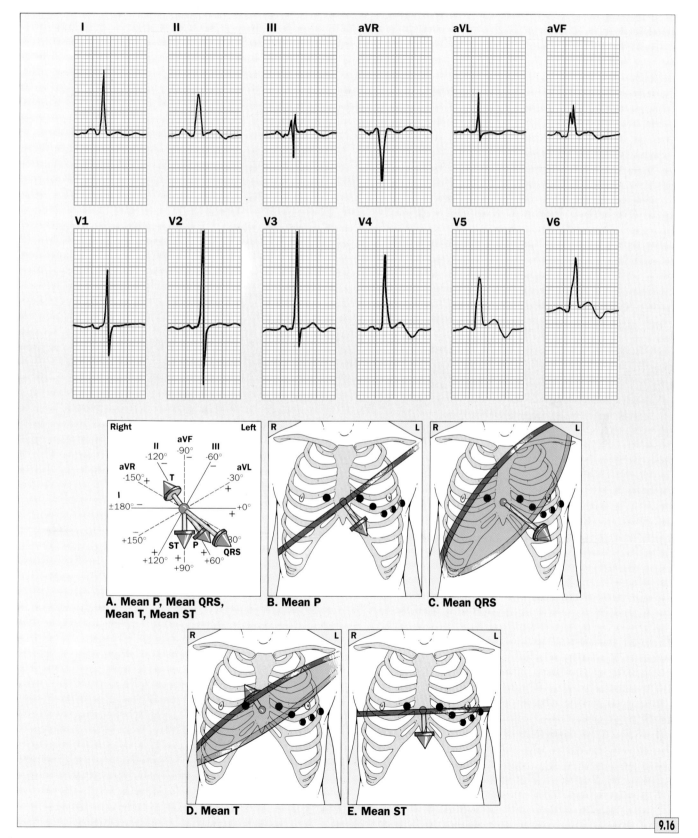

A. Mean P, Mean QRS, Mean T, Mean ST

B. Mean P

C. Mean QRS

D. Mean T

E. Mean ST

(Figure 9.16 continued.)

The PR interval is 0.16 second. The duration of the QRS complex is 0.09 second, and the QT interval is 0.36 second.

P waves: The duration of the P wave in lead II is 0.12 second; its amplitude is 2 mm. The terminal P wave (P2) is abnormal in V1; its duration-amplitude product measures -0.04 mm-sec. This indicates a left atrial abnormality.

QRS complex: The mean QRS vector is directed inferiorly at about +40°, and anteriorly to an undetermined degree; probably about +30-40°. This unusual direction probably signifies combined left and right ventricular hypertrophy.

T wave: The mean T vector is directed at about -122° in the frontal plane, and slightly posteriorly.

ST segment: The mean ST vector is directed inferiorly at +90° and parallel with the frontal plane.

A. The frontal plane projections of the mean P, QRS, ST, and T vectors. **B.** The spatial orientation of the mean P vector. The mean P2 vector, although not plotted, is abnormal, and indicates a left atrial abnormality. **C.** The spatial orientation of the mean QRS vector. **D.** The spatial orientation of the mean T vector. It is abnormally directed opposite the mean QRS vector. The T wave abnormality did not change over many years. Note the course of the transitional pathway on the chest. **E.** The spatial orientation of the large ST vector. The ST segment

---

TABLE 9.12 ELECTROCARDIOGRAPHIC ABNORMALITIES THAT MUST BE DIFFERENTIATED FROM THOSE DUE TO PRIMARY VENTRICULAR HYPERTROPHY

- The electrocardiogram of primary ventricular hypertrophy usually shows left ventricular hypertrophy, but may show right or combined ventricular hypertrophy as well; it may not be possible to distinguish the electrocardiogram of secondary hypertrophy due to systolic pressure overload from that of primary ventricular hypertrophy.

- The electrocardiogram of myocardial infarction may simulate that of primary ventricular hypertrophy. The following distinctions apply:

- When due to myocardial infarction, the abnormal initial QRS forces, ST segment, and T wave abnormalities usually evolve through a set of stages, but these features rarely change when they are due to primary hypertrophy.

- Electrocardiographic signs of left ventricular hypertrophy (i.e., an increase in QRS amplitude) rarely occur with myocardial infarction unless there is associated systemic hypertension, aortic valve disease, or mitral regurgitation. Signs of left ventricular hypertrophy are often present when the pseudoinfarction pattern is due to hypertrophic cardiomyopathy.

- There are many causes for an abnormal mean T vector: left ventricular ischemia, left ventricular hypertrophy, pericarditis, or subarachnoid hemorrhage, among others. When due to apical hypertrophy, the large mean T vector is directed to the right and anteriorly.

- The electrocardiographic abnormalities associated with the Wolff-Parkinson-White syndrome may occur with primary ventricular hypertrophy. It is not possible to distinguish the signs of isolated bypass tracts from those associated with primary hypertrophy. When signs of a bypass tract are identified, one must search for the clues to primary ventricular hypertrophy, atrial septal defect, Ebstein's anomaly, or another source of this condition.

- The ST segment abnormality of idiopathic hypertrophy is persistent, unlike that of pericarditis or epicardial injury of infarction, which evolves toward normal (although it may persist if a ventricular aneurysm develops).

(Figure 9.16 continued.)
abnormality did not change over a period of many years. Note the course of the transitional pathway on the chest.

Summary: Evidence of left atrial abnormality, probable signs of both right and left ventricular hypertrophy, and a bizarre ST-T wave abnormality may be found in patients with hypertrophic cardiomyopathy. A different electrocardiogram of this

patient, when she was 77 years of age, was published on page 5.14 of the *Atlas of the Heart* (New York: Gower Medical Publishing, 1988).

FIGURE 9.17

Hypertrophic cardiomyopathy. These magnetic resonance images were made from the patient whose electrocardiogram is shown in Figure 9.12. He had experienced

two episodes of syncope. The transverse sections were made during (**A**) end-diastole, (**B**) mid-diastole, and (**C**) end systole. An image in the coronal plane (**D**) was also made during mid-systole. Left ventricular hypertrophy is evident, and systolic anterior motion of the mitral valve is seen in all of the systolic images. (Reproduced with permission from the publisher and author; see Figure Credits.)

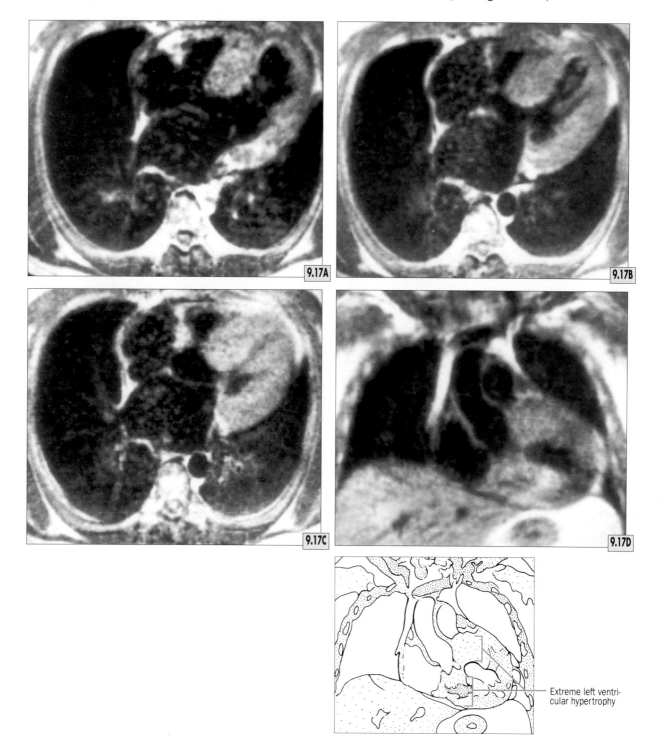

Extreme left ventricular hypertrophy

FIGURE CREDITS

Figure 9.2 From Estes EH: Routine diagnostic procedures: electrocardiography and vectorcardiography, in Hurst JW, Logue RB (eds): *The Heart*, Ed 1. New York: Blakiston, 1966, p 137.

Figure 9.5 From Estes EH: Routine diagnostic procedures: electrocardiography and vectorcardiography, in Hurst JW, Logue RB (eds): *The Heart*, Ed 1. New York: Blakiston, 1966, p 138.

Figure 9.7 From Hurst JW, Nugent EW, Anderson RH, Wilcox BR: Congenital heart disease, in Hurst JW (ed): *Atlas of the Heart*. New York: McGraw-Hill and Gower, 1988, p 3.6. (The electrocardiogram was originally supplied by the Electrocardiographic Laboratory of Henrietta Egleston Hospital for Children, Atlanta, Georgia.)

Figure 9.8 From Estes EH: Routine diagnostic procedures: electrocardiography and vectorcardiography, in Hurst JW, Logue RB (eds): *The Heart*, Ed 1. New York: Blakiston, 1966, p.139.

Figure 9.9 From Hurst JW, Nugent EW, Anderson RH, Wilcox BR: Congenital heart disease, in Hurst JW (ed): *Atlas of the Heart*. New York: McGraw-Hill and Gower, 1988, p 3.6.(Redrawn courtesy of the Electrocardiography Laboratory, Henrietta Egleston Hospital for Children, Atlanta, Georgia.)

Figure 9.10 From Estes EH: Routine diagnostic procedures: electrocardiography and vectorcardiography, in Hurst JW, Logue RB (eds): *The Heart*, Ed 1. New York: Blakiston, 1966, p 141.

Figure 9.17 From Hurst JW, Wenger NK, Goodwin JF, Becker AE, Wilcox BR: Cardiomyopathy, in Hurst JW (ed): *Atlas of the Heart*. New York: McGraw-Hill and Gower, 1988, p 5.16. (Courtesy of Roderic I. Pettigrew, PhD, MD, Atlanta, Georgia.)

CHAPTER TEN

PERICARDIAL DISEASE

The electrocardiogram may be abnormal in patients with acute pericarditis because the disease process involves the epicardium of the atria and ventricles. A pericardial effusion may blanket the propagation of electrical activity, resulting in a decrease in voltage of the QRS-T complexes and electrical alternans. Constrictive pericarditis may also produce a decrease in the QRS-T voltages because the thick pericardium alters the propagation of electrical activity. Atrial arrhythmias may accompany both acute and constrictive pericarditis.

The mechanisms responsible for the electrocardiographic abnormalities related to pericardial disease are discussed below.

ACUTE PERICARDITIS

The electrocardiographic characteristics of acute pericarditis are listed in Table 10.1. The electrocardiographic abnormalities that must be differentiated from those due to acute pericarditis are listed in Table 10.2. Examples of electrocardiograms associated with this disease are shown in Figures 10.1 and 10.2.

The electrocardiogram cannot assist in the establishment of the etiology of acute pericarditis. The condition may be idiopathic, in which case it is probably of viral origin,or it may be caused by myocardial infarction, collagen disease, neoplastic disease, bacterial infection uremia or trauma. Acute pericarditis can also be a consequence of myocardial infarction (Dressler's syndrome), or cardiac surgery.

PERICARDIAL EFFUSION

The electrocardiographic characteristics of pericardial effusion are listed in Table 10.3. The electrocardiographic abnormalities that must be differentiated from those due to pericardial effusion are listed in Table 10.4. An example electrocardiogram shown in Figure 10.3.

The electrocardiogram cannot assist in establishing the etiology of pericardial effusion. Pericardial fluid may be caused by idiopathic pericarditis, viral pericarditis, collagen disease, bac-

terial infection, neoplastic disease, myxedema, uremia, Dressler's syndrome, following cardiac surgery, trauma, or congestive heart failure.

CONSTRICTIVE PERICARDITIS

The electrocardiographic characteristics associated with constrictive pericarditis are listed in Table 10.5. Electrocardiographic abnormalities that must be differentiated from those due to constrictive pericarditis are listed in Table 10.6. An example of an electrocardiogram recorded from a patient with this condition is shown in Figure 10.4.

Constrictive pericarditis may be caused by or follow idiopathic or viral pericarditis, bacterial pericarditis, radiation treatment for neoplastic disease of the breast or mediastinum, cardiac surgery, collagen disease including rheumatoid arthritis, or trauma.

TABLE 10.1
ELECTROCARDIOGRAPHIC ABNORMALITIES
OF ACUTE PERICARDITIS

- Can occur without electrocardiographic abnormalities.

- Atrial arrhythmias may be present.

- Epicardial injury of the atria produces displacement of the PR segment. The mean PR segment vector is directed opposite the cardiac apex and relatively opposite the mean ST vector.

- The QRS complex remains normal unless the voltage is diminished by pericardial fluid (see Table 10.3).

- The mean ST vector is directed toward the centroid of generalized epicardial injury. It is directed toward the cardiac apex and is usually relatively parallel with, but slightly anterior to the mean QRS vector.

- As the mean ST segment vector diminishes in size, an abnormal T vector develops.

- The mean T vector tends to run opposite its normal direction; it is usually directed opposite the mean ST vector. It is directed away from the centroid of epicardial ischemia.

- The electrocardiogram may eventually return to normal, or low-amplitude T waves may persist. An abnormally wide QRS-T angle may persist.

TABLE 10.2
ELECTROCARDIOGRAPHIC ABNORMALITIES
THAT MUST BE DIFFERENTIATED FROM THOSE
DUE TO ACUTE PERICARDITIS

The mean PR segment vector of acute pericarditis must be differentiated from the vector due to the Ta wave. This is not always possible, but the PR segment displacement of pericarditis generally does not persist, while the Ta wave does.

Early repolarization may occur in a small percentage of normal subjects. The following points apply:

- The mean ST vector of a normal subject is directed relatively parallel with the mean T vector, and is usually located within 45° of the mean QRS vector.

- The mean T vector in normal subjects is larger than average and is directed normally, dragging the ST vector with it. The mean T vector of acute pericarditis is normal or small.

- The ST-T abnormality of pericarditis evolves in a predictable way; that of the normal subject is static.

The electrocardiographic abnormalities of acute pericarditis must be differentiated from those produced by myocardial infarction. The following points apply:

- Extremely large ST segment abnormalities of localized epicardial injury with large T waves due to localized epicardial ischemia are more common in myocardial infarction than in pericarditis. With pericarditis, the smaller abnormal ST segment vector of generalized epicardial injury tends to decrease prior to the development of the abnormal mean T vector of generalized epicardial ischemia.

- The ST vector produced by myocardial infarction is directed toward a localized segment of the left ventricular wall; the mean ST segment vector of pericarditis is directed toward the cardiac apex.

- Acute myocardial infarction may be the etiology of pericarditis; both conditions may occur simultaneously.

- Abnormal initial QRS forces (abnormal Q waves) may indicate infarction; but all infarcts do not produce abnormal Q waves.

- An apical infarction may not produce abnormal QRS forces (abnormal Q waves), because there is no myocardium opposite it, and the mean ST vector may be directed toward the cardiac apex. This particular infarction may simulate pericarditis. One needs other clinical data to distinguish the two conditions.

FIGURE 10.1

This electrocardiogram was recorded from a patient with acute pericarditis. **A.** Frontal plane projections of the mean PR, mean QRS, mean ST, and mean T vectors. **B.** The spatial orientation of the mean PR segment vector. **C.** The spatial orientation of the mean QRS vector. **D.** The spatial orientation of the mean ST vector. **E.** The spatial orientation of the mean T vector.

Summary: Note that the PR segment vector is directed opposite the mean ST segment vector, which is directed toward the centroid of generalized epicardial injury. The mean QRS vector is directed to the left and posteriorly because left anterior-superior division block is present; the QRS duration is 0.10 second and the mean QRS vector is directed -45° to the left. The centroid of the epicardial injury is in the region of the cardiac apex which is located slightly anteriorly. (Reproduced with permission from the publisher and author; see Figure Credits.)

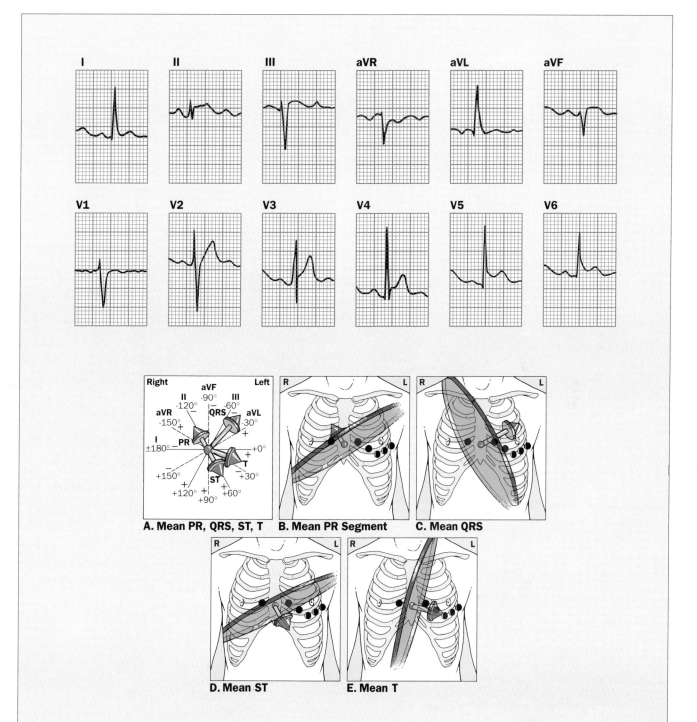

A. Mean PR, QRS, ST, T   B. Mean PR Segment   C. Mean QRS

D. Mean ST   E. Mean T

F I G U R E   1 0 . 2
This electrocardiogram was recorded from a 37-year-old patient with clinical evidence of acute pericarditis. **A.** The frontal plane projections of the mean PR segment, mean QRS, mean ST, and mean T vectors. **B.** Spatial orientation of the mean PR segment vector. **C.** Spatial orientation of the mean QRS vector. **D.** Spatial orientation of the mean ST vector. **E.** Spatial orientation of the mean T vector.

Summary: This electrocardiogram illustrates a later phase of pericarditis than that shown in Figure 10.1. Note that the mean ST segment vector is directed at +60° and posteriorly, while the mean T vector is relatively opposite the mean ST vector. There are no QRS abnormalities. (Reproduced with permission from the publisher and author; see Figure Credits.)

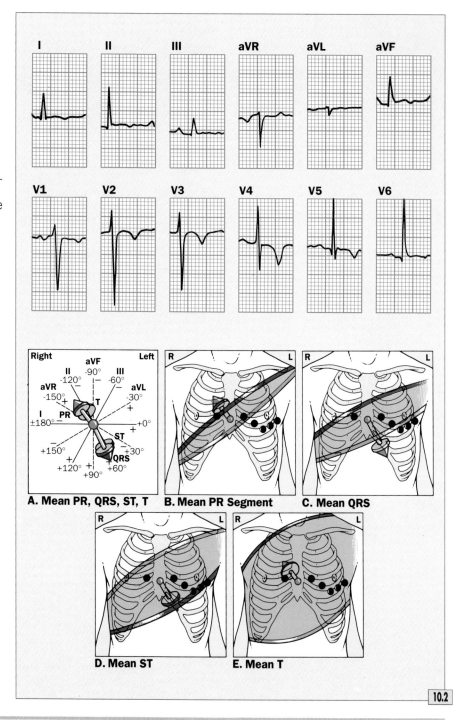

TABLE 10.3 ELECTROCARDIOGRAPHIC ABNORMALITIES OF PERICARDIAL EFFUSION

- The electrocardiogram may be normal.

- The amplitudes of the QRS complex and T wave may be less than normal. The amplitude of the QRS complex may be as low as 3 mm, but is usually 5 to 7 mm. The total 12-lead QRS amplitude may be 80 mm or less.

- The electrocardiographic signs of acute pericarditis may also be present.

- Abnormalities of the initial QRS forces do not occur.

- Electrical alternans may be present.

FIGURE 10.3

This electrocardiogram was recorded from a patient with pericardial effusion. It illustrates low voltage of the QRS complexes and T waves, and electrical alternans. This particular patient also had cardiac tamponade. **A.** The amplitude of the QRS complex is 6–7 mm (measured in leads V1 and V2). The total 12-lead QRS amplitude is 65 mm; the lower limit of normal is about 80 mm. The first QRS complex shown in each lead is larger than the second, indicating electrical alternans. The frontal plane projection of each of the complexes is shown in this illustration. **B.** The spatial orientation of the mean QRS vector representing the first QRS complex shown in each lead. **C.** The spatial orientation of the mean QRS vector representing the second QRS complex shown in each lead.

Summary: The presence of QRS complexes of low voltage plus electrical alternans, is almost pathognomonic of pericardial effusion. (Reproduced with permission from the publisher and author; see Figure Credits.)

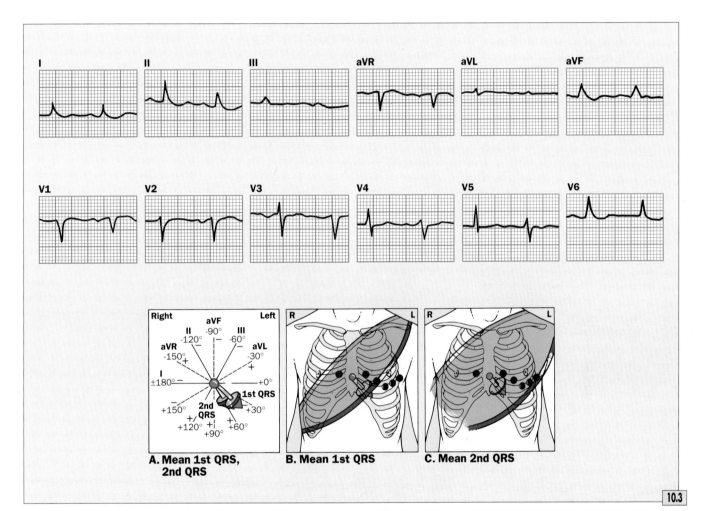

A. Mean 1st QRS, 2nd QRS **B. Mean 1st QRS** **C. Mean 2nd QRS**

10.3

TABLE 10.4 ELECTROCARDIOGRAPHIC ABNORMALITIES THAT MUST BE DIFFERENTIATED FROM THOSE DUE TO PERICARDIAL FLUID

Low amplitude of the QRS complexes and T waves may be caused by:

- Hypothyroidism, which may produce low voltage of the QRS complexes and T waves. In such cases, bradycardia is often present. Some patients with myxedema who have low voltage actually have pericardial effusion and others do not.

- Cardiomyopathy, especially due to amyloid infiltration, which may cause low voltage in the electrocardiogram. Initial QRS abnormalities, bundle branch block, and primary T wave abnormalites may be present.

- The electrocardiographic abnormalities of constrictive pericarditis listed in Table 10.5.

- Emphysema, which may cause low voltage of the QRS complexes and T waves. In such patients, other abnormalities are usually present.

- Improper standardization of the electrocardiographic tracing.

- Electrical alternans in a patient who exhibits low voltage in the electrocardiogram indicates pericardial effusion rather than myocardial disease. However, the clinician must remember that both diseases can occur in the same patient. Electrical alternans may also occur with atrial tachycardia.

FIGURE 10.4
This electrocardiogram was recorded from a 39-year-old woman in 1950. She had evidence of constrictive pericarditis 20 years earlier, at which time a large area of pericardium was removed, as well as a band constricting the inferior vena cava. **A.** Frontal plane projections of the mean QRS and T vectors. Note that the QRS vector is directed vertically. The mean T vector is abnormal in that it is opposite the mean QRS vector. The amplitude of the QRS complex is low in all leads except V2 and V3. The total 12- lead QRS amplitude is 116 mm. **B.** The spatial orientation of the mean QRS vector. **C.** The spatial orientation of the mean T vector.

Summary: Although this patient underwent surgery for constrictive pericarditis 20 years before the electrocardiogram was recorded, she undoubtedly had residual areas of thick pericardium and epicardial scarring, even though constrictive physiology was not present. (Reproduced with permission from the publisher and author; see Figure Credits.)

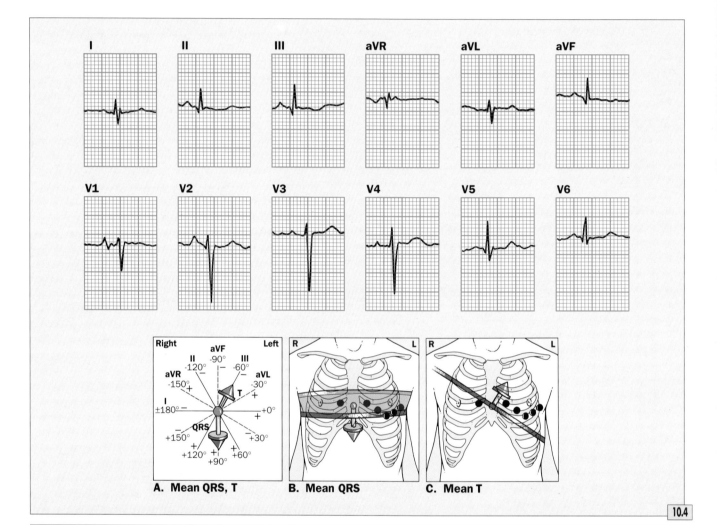

A. Mean QRS, T   B. Mean QRS   C. Mean T

10.4

TABLE 10.5 ELECTROCARDIOGRAPHIC ABNORMALITIES OF CONSTRICTIVE PERICARDITIS

- Atrial arrhythmias may be present.
- The amplitude of the QRS complexes and T waves may be diminished.
- The QRS complex may be abnormal in addition to exhibiting low voltage.

- The mean QRS vector is usually directed normally but may shift to the right.
- Abnormal initial QRS forces and bundle branch block may occasionally occur due to calcification of the deeper portion of the myocardium.

TABLE 10.6 ELECTROCARDIOGRAPHIC ABNORMALITIES THAT MUST BE DIFFERENTIATED FROM THOSE DUE TO CONSTRICTIVE PERICARDITIS

- The electrocardiographic abnormalities associated with pericardial fluid may simulate those due to constrictive pericarditis. Other clinical data may be needed to distinguish between the two.

- Constrictive pericarditis cannot always be electrocardiographically differentiated from dilated cardiomyopathy, restrictive cardiomyopathy due to amyloid infiltration, neoplastic invasion of the heart, sarcoidosis, and other diseases. Other clinical data may be needed to distinguish these diseases.

FIGURE CREDITS

Figure 10.1 Redrawn from Shabetai R: *The Pericardium*. New York, Grune & Stratton, 1981, p 359.

Figure 10.2 From Hurst JW, Woodson GC Jr: *Atlas of Spatial Vector Electrocardiography*. New York, Blakiston Company, 1952, p 199.

Figure 10.3 From Surawicz B, Lasseter KC: Electrocardiogram in pericarditis. *Am J Cardiol* 26:472, 1970.

Figure 10.4 From Graybiel A, White PD, Wheeler L, Williams C: *Electrocardiography in Practice*. Philadelphia, W. B. Saunders Company, 1952, p 195.

Myocardial Ischemia, Injury and Infarction

MYOCARDIAL ISCHEMIA, MYOCARDIAL INJURY AND MYOCARDIAL INFARCTION

A mismatch of coronary artery blood flow and myocardial oxygen requirements produces myocardial damage. This is usually discussed in terms of a myocardial oxygen supply which is inadequate to meet myocardial oxygen demands. Two mechanisms are responsible for this condition: coronary artery blood flow may be impeded by chronically narrowed coronary arteries, with a mismatch occurring when there is an increased myocardial requirement for oxygen; or when the already narrowed coronary arteries become more acutely narrowed by coronary artery thrombosis, coronary spasm, or both. The disease most commonly responsible for the mismatch is coronary atherosclerosis, but many other causes are listed later in this chapter.

The electrocardiographic consequences of the mismatch are ischemia, injury, and a myocardial dead zone. In the context of the mismatch, T wave abnormalities indicate myocardial ischemia, ST segment abnormalities indicate myocardial injury, and Q wave abnormalities indicate a myocardial dead zone. The electrophysiological mechanisms responsible for these abnormalities are discussed in chapter 6 and throughout this chapter.

The electrocardiographic abnormalities produced by the mismatch are determined by the intensity of the myocardial hypoxia, the duration and the locations of the hypoxia in the myocardium, as well as the coexistence of other heart disease. Electrocardiographic abnormalities secondary to myocardial hypoxia are almost always due to damage to the left ventricle, although the right ventricle and atria may also be damaged.

Severe myocardial ischemia, including infarction, may not produce electrocardiographic abnormalities. This fact must be emphasized repeatedly. The antithesis to this is that many other disease processes may produce electrocardiographic abnormalities suggesting myocardial ischemia, injury, or dead zone. Under these circumstances, the electrocardiographic abnormalities are referred to as *pseudoinfarctions*. The conditions causing pseudoinfarctions will be discussed later; they must be remembered to prevent the possibility of a grave diagnostic error.

T WAVE ABNORMALITIES (ISCHEMIA)

The T wave abnormalities related to hypoxia may be located predominantly in the endocardial or epicardial area. Endocardial ischemia tends to be generalized, whereas epicardial ischemia tends to be localized to specific areas of the ventricular myocardium. Myocardial ischemia usually occurs in the left ventricle, including the septum, but it may also occur in the right ventricle. A T wave abnormality may be the only sign of infarction, and such infarctions are referred to as T wave infarctions (see later discussion).

ST SEGMENT ABNORMALITIES (INJURY)

The ST segment abnormalities related to hypoxia may be located predominantly in the endocardial or epicardial area. Endocardial injury tends to be generalized, and epicardial injury tends to be localized to specific areas of the ventricular myocardium. Like myocardial infarction, myocardial injury usually occurs in the left ventricle, including the septum, but it may also occur in the right ventricle.

Q WAVE INFARCTION (DEAD ZONE)

Myocardial damage may be sufficiently severe to cause the death of myocytes, which removes electrical forces from certain areas of the heart[1]. When this occurs, the electrical forces generated by the diametrically opposite side of the heart will dominate the electrical field. This may create abnormal Q waves in the electrocardiogram. Such abnormalities usually occur in the left ventricle, but may also occasionally involve the right ventricle. The myocardial damage responsible for the Q wave abnormality is located predominately in the endocardial area, and diminishes in magnitude as it approaches the epicardium. It is sometimes referred to as a *transmural infarction*. It seems proper, however, to discontinue the use of the term "transmural infarction" because abnormal Q waves may occur with an infarct that is not transmural [1]; the electrocardiogram is more accurately referred to as showing a Q *wave infarction*. Areas of injured and ischemic tissue surround the dead zone; they are usually located predominantly in the epicardial areas of the myocardium.

Abnormal Q waves due to myocardial infarction are shown in Figure 6.7, along with the ST and T wave abnormalities. Whereas a mean initial 0.04-second QRS vector is used to represent the infarcted area, it must be emphasized that a Q wave may be abnormal even when its duration is less than 0.04 second. In such cases, the identification of an abnormality depends on determination of the relationship of the initial QRS forces to the subsequent QRS forces.

NON-Q WAVE INFARCTION

The term "subendocardial infarction" has fallen into disrepute. For many years, I have asked hundreds of individuals to describe their criteria for subendocardial infarction. The criteria varied greatly from one individual to another. I discovered that the criteria being used were "made up," and seemed to be "hand-me-downs of misinformation." Many of the persons who used the term had no notion of the pathophysiological mechanism involved in the process they described.

In the past, those using the term "subendocardial infarction" usually applied it to an electrocardiogram that showed the development of ST and T wave abnormalities without the development of abnormal Q waves. Although this approaches the truth, it misses the mark in that there are several reasons why abnormal Q waves may not appear in the electrocardiograms of many patients with myocardial infarction (Table 11.1). Note that a transmural infarction may be present, yet the electrocardiogram may not reveal abnormal Q waves. Consequently, it is more accurate to refer to such an infarction as a *non-Q wave* infarction than to presume that the infarction is located in the subendocardial area.

There is one circumstance in which it seems proper to use the term "subendocardial infarction": when subendocardial injury persists for hours, it is often the first stage of a generalized subendocardial infarction. This type of infarct, one could argue, should be referrered to as a "generalized endocardial infarction." The pathophysiology is often different from that of a spontaneous infarction associated with epicardial injury. Persistent subendocardial injury may occur when a patient with significant coronary atherosclerosis develops hypotension. It is especially likely in a patient with coronary atherosclerosis complicated by left ventricular hypertrophy and elevated left ventricular diastolic pressure, as may occur

---

Note: As stated in several places in this book, the model presented here is a clinically useful approximation of the real situation within the heart. At times, the explanation moves beyond the known evidence. When this occurs, every effort has been made to extend the facts in a logical manner.

with severe aortic valve stenosis. Accordingly, patients with significant coronary atherosclerosis and aortic stenosis, hypertension, aortic regurgitation, or even cardiomyopathy are at greater risk for generalized subendocardial injury and subendocardial infarction. Recognized by an abnormal and persistent ST segment vector directed away from the centroid of the left ventricle, subendocardial injury may last for several hours, during which time a generalized endocardial infarction may develop. This, however, often gives way to the usual electrocardiographic signs of non-Q wave infarction.

ELECTROCARDIOGRAPHIC ABNORMALITIES DUE TO MYOCARDIAL ISCHEMIA, INJURY, AND MYOCARDIAL DEAD ZONE

The electrocardiographic characteristics of myocardial ischemia, injury, and abnormal Q waves of myocardial dead zone are listed in Table 11.2. Examples are shown in Figures 11.1 through 11.18.

The etiologic considerations related to myocardial ischemia, myocardial injury, and development of a myocardial dead zone are: atherosclerotic coronary heart disease; atherosclerotic coronary heart disease plus coronary artery spasm; coronary spasm without coronary atherosclerosis;coronary embolism; coronary thrombosis without evidence of other disease; dissection of the coronary artery; coronary arteritis; Kawasaki's disease; trauma of the heart muscle or coronary artery; involvement of the coronary arteries with amyloid; and congenital anomalies of the coronary arteries.

SPECIAL CONSIDERATIONS

CORONARY ARTERY SPASM (PRINZMETAL'S ANGINA OR VARIANT ANGINA)

The electrocardiographic abnormalities associated with coronary artery spasm were first identified by Frank Wilson and Franklin Johnston in 1941(2), and the clinical syndrome associated with it was described by Prinzmetal and associates in 1959(3). Most patients with coronary spasm also have obstructive coronary atherosclerosis, although a few do not. The patient with chest discomfort due to coronary artery spasm exhibits transient electrocardiographic abnormalities that simulate those of an acute myocardial infarction. The mean ST vector is directed toward the area of epicardial injury. The mean T vector may be directed away from the area of epicardial ischemia, but the ST segment abnormality usually dominates the tracing. There may be abnormal but transient Q wave abnormalities, with the initial mean 0.04-second QRS vector being directed away from the transiently "dead" or "stunned" myocytes. Atrioventricular block and other arrhythmias may be present. These abnormalities occur with the usual infarction, but, when caused by transient coronary artery spasm, they disappear as chest discomfort subsides. The only other time this disappearance occurs is when thrombolytic therapy is successful in patients in whom thrombosis is superimposed on high-grade obstructive coronary atherosclerosis. In such cases, the electrocardiographic abnormalities and chest discomfort often subside as the clot is lysed. The electrocardiogram of a patient with coronary artery spasm is shown in Figure 11.19.

EXERCISE ELECTROCARDIOGRAPHY

There are many different protocols available for exercise electrocardiography. While I have used the Bruce protocol almost exclusively, I recognize that other techniques are equally good. An abnormal electrocardiographic response to exercise is said to be present when an arrhythmia, an abnormal ST segment displacement, or a T wave abnormality occurs. The ST segment displacement is more likely to indicate myocardial hypoxia than are the other abnormalities, and this displacement is usually due to generalized subendocardial injury. Accordingly, the mean ST segment is directed approximately opposite the mean QRS vector. An ST segment displacement of 1 mm that continues horizontally for more than 0.08 second, or slopes downward, is more likely due to myocardial injury than is an ST segment displacement characterized by a displaced J point, but which rapidly ascends in an up-sloping manner. The predictive value of a positive electrocardiographic response, indicating injury due to myocardial ischemia, is about 80 percent in adult males and 50 percent in females under 45 years of age. The predictive value varies according to the amount of ST segment displacement during the test, and the duration of displacement after completion of the exercise.

The lead system used for exercise electrocardiography does not permit determination of the spatial characteristics of the electrical forces responsible for the mean ST segment vector. Therefore, the details of this particular abnormality are not discussed here. Suffice it to say that ST segment displacement due to exercise can be caused by transient subendocardial injury; but as stated earlier, false positive tests also occur, especially in young women. While the causes of these false positive tests are usually unknown, they are likely to occur in hypokalemic patients or those receiving digitalis. Patients with ST segment displacement due to left ventricular hypertrophy, left bundle branch block, or ventricular pre-excitation may be exercised to determine if there is exercise-induced angina, but it is not possible to accurately interpret the electrocardiographic response.

PSEUDOINFARCTION

Several conditions produce electrocardiographic abnormalities that must be differentiated from those due to myocardial infarction. Such abnormalities are called *pseudoinfarctions*. The electrocardiographic abnormalities associated with pseudoinfarction are listed in Table 11.3 and the causes of pseudoinfarction are listed in Table 11.4. Electrocardiograms illustrating pseudoinfarction are shown in Figures 11.20 through 11.23

ELECTROCARDIOGRAPHIC CORRELATES

Many patients with extensive coronary atherosclerosis have normal resting electrocardiograms, and as I have already stressed, there are multiple reasons why myocardial infarction may not be reflected in the electrocardiogram.

It is not possible to accurately predict the ejection fraction of the left ventricle, or to predict abnormalities in the contractility of segments of the left ventricular wall, by studying the electrocardiogram. For example, a large initial QRS abnormality may be associated with normal contractility of the left ventricular wall, and poor contractility of the ventricular wall may be associated with normal QRS complexes in the electrocardiogram. One clinical point that should be emphasized is that congestive heart failure is usually associated with an abnormal electrocardiogram. The opposite is not true: an abnormal electrocardiogram need not be associated with congestive heart failure.

The ability to predict the particular coronary artery that is obstructed and, therefore, responsible for an infarction, is fraught with difficulty. Before the advent of coronary arteriography, an effort was made to correlate the electrocardiographic abnormalities of myocardial infarction with autopsy data. It was then discovered that the location of an infarct determined by electrocardiography did not correlate perfectly with the abnormalities found at autopsy. One reason for this is that on the autopsy table, the orientation of the anatomic parts of the heart is not the same as within the thorax of a living patient. Recent studies using coronary arteriography have yielded more insight into this problem and, as indicated by the following discussion, the ability to predict the artery responsible for an infarct has improved, though it still remains relatively crude.

The prediction of the culprit artery is more accurate when one uses the mean ST vector of an acute infarction, and less accurate when one uses the Q waves of an old infarction. Clearly, such a prediction does not indicate the severity of the disease in other vessels. It should also be emphasized that the prediction does not eliminate the need to estimate the risk of other coronary events through other techniques such as coronary arteriography, radionuclide testing, or exercise electrocardiography.

The relationships between the electrocardiographic abnormalities of infarction and the culprit coronary arteries are discussed below:

• When the mean ST vector associated with a myocardial infarction is directed to the right, inferiorly, and anteriorly, the cause is often an obstruction of the *proximal portion of the right coronary artery.* The initial 0.04-second QRS vector may be directed leftward, superiorly, and posteriorly in such patients. When this occurs, the *inferior portions of the left and right ventricles* are likely to be involved by the infarction.

• Whenever the mean ST vector is directed inferiorly and parallel with the frontal plane, an obstruction in the *middle portion of the right coronary artery* is likely. The initial mean 0.04-second QRS vector may be directed to the left, superiorly, and parallel with the frontal plane. These abnormalities signify an *inferior myocardial infarction.*

• A mean ST vector that is directed inferiorly and slightly posteriorly may signify an obstruction of either the *distal portion of the right coronary artery or the distal portion of the left circumflex coronary artery.* The initial mean 0.04-second QRS vector may be directed to the left, superiorly, and slightly anteriorly. These abnormalities signify an *inferior-posterior myocardial infarction.*

• Whenever the mean ST vector is directed only slightly inferiorly but markedly posteriorly, it is likely that the obstruction is located in the *proximal portion of the left circumflex coronary artery.* The initial mean 0.04-second QRS vector is usually directed to the left, superiorly, and anteriorly in such patients; this produces a prominent R wave in lead V1. These abnormalities signify a *true posterior myocardial infarction.*

• There is an interesting exception to the usual assumption that an inferior infarction is due to obstruction of the right coronary or circumflex coronary arteries. A small percentage of inferior infarctions are due to obstruction of the proximal left anterior descending coronary artery(4). This artery, in such cases, "wraps around the apex." Isoembolism may be the cause.

• Whenever the mean ST segment vector is directed slightly to the left and markedly anteriorly, it is likely that the obstruction is located in the *proximal portion of the left anterior descending coronary artery.* The mean initial 0.04-second QRS vector is often posterior to the subsequent QRS forces. These abnormalities signify an *anteroseptal myocardial infarction.*

• A mean ST vector directed to the left and slightly anteriorly indicates that the obstruction is most likely located in the *proximal portion of the left anterior descending artery, with possible compromise of the diagonal branches.* The mean initial 0.04-second QRS vector is directed to the right, and may be directed slightly posteriorly or parallel with the frontal plane. These electrocardiographic abnormalities signify an *anterolateral myocardial infarction.*

COMMENTS REGARDING THE DIAGRAMS SHOWN IN THIS CHAPTER

The reader will note that in some of the diagrams in this chapter, the actual electrocardiographic deflections do not match those that would be predicted by studying the spatial orientation of the vectors that have been drawn to represent them. For example, the T waves may be positive in leads V5 and V6 but the direction of the vector representing the T waves may be oriented so that negative T waves would be recorded in leads V5 and V6 (see Fig. 11.14). Whereas similar problems occur in several illustrations throughout the book, the diagrams shown in this chapter can serve as examples of a problem that deserves reemphasis (see discussion following the table of contents).

The *frontal plane direction* of a mean vector can usually be determined without difficulty. This is true because the extremity lead electrodes are almost electrically equidistant from the heart, and the distance varies very little from one person to another. Consequently, a rigid display system changes little from one subject to another, and the hexaxial reference system is used to display the frontal plane projection of the vectors.

The *anterior and posterior directions* of a vector are determined by studying the deflections in the precordial leads. There are several problems associated with this method, and an accurate, rigid display system cannot be created.

The problems are as follows:

• The precordial electrodes are nearer to the heart than the extremity leads, and they are influenced by their nearness to the center of the electrical field. Accordingly, one cannot assume that the largest deflection is written by an electrical force that is parallel to a given lead axis. However, one can assume that the electrical force that produces the smallest deflection is *relatively* perpendicular to the lead axis in which it appears.

• Whereas the locations of the precordial electrode sites are determined by strict anatomic guidelines, these may vary from person to person. For example, the precordial electrodes located at V2, V3 and V4 are positioned almost vertically, one above the other, in tall individuals. The same electrode positions are located almost side by side in broad chested individuals. In preparing the book, I was forced to use a replica of the chest that represents only one chest shape and size; I could not make a diagram that accurately reproduced the shape of the chest for each person from whom an electrocardiogram was recorded. This leads to occasional situations in which the actual deflections seen in the electrocardiogram are different from those that would be predicted from the vector diagrams.

• It is difficult for some individuals to visualize electrical forces in three-dimensional space. Accordingly, in an effort to assist the reader to accomplish this goal, I suggested that the artist use several techniques which would convert a two-dimensional, flat-surface image into a three-dimentional image. The artistic rendition of the zero potential plane, the transitional pathway, the rim of the arrowhead, and the base of the arrowhead are helpful in this regard. Again, in the interest of creating three-dimensional diagrams, I have depicted electrode positions V5, and V6 as though they were located a little higher on the lateral chest wall than the V4 electrode (V6 appears a little higher on the chest wall than V5, and V5 is located a little higher on the chest wall than V4). Actually, the position of electrodes V4, V5 and V6 should be in the same transverse plane. *This deviation from the true positions was permitted in order to depict the thorax as three-dimensional structure, but it may, at times, make it difficult to diagram the spatial orientation of the vectors.*

Owing to the aforementioned reasons, it is impossible for one to always determine, and then to display on a rigid replica of the chest, the exact number of degrees to which vector is anteriorly or posteriorly directed in the frontal plane. It is usually possible, in such cases, to identify several precordial electrode deflections in which there is no argument about polarity, and these deflections should be used to determine the anterior or posterior direction of the vector. Often, when the deflections in the other precordial leads do not match what was predicted, it is because these other electrodes record electrical impulses from near the transitional pathway for the vector.

Whenever there is an apparent "lack of a fit" between the actual and the predicted deflections of an electrocadiogram, I have indicated such in the legend, and I refer the reader to this section and to the discussion following the table of contents for an appropriate explanation.

TABLE 11.1 REASONS FOR NON-Q-WAVE INFARCTION

- The "dead zone" in the myocardium may not be sufficiently large to produce an abnormal Q wave. This may occur even if the infarction is transmural.
- The "dead zone" may be located in the "mid area" of the left ventricular wall, and abnormal Q waves may not be produced.
- The "dead zone" may be located at the cardiac apex; there is no left ventricular muscle located diametrically opposite the apex (the left atrioventricular valve area is opposite the apex). Consequently, no abnormal Q waves can be generated.

- The "dead zone" may involve the papillary muscle or the basilar portion of the left ventricle and, for this reason, may not produce abnormal Q waves.
- A previous infarct located diametrically opposite the new infarct may eliminate the condition required for production of a new abnormal Q wave, since there will be no normal myocardium opposite the new infarct.
- A left ventricular conduction defect such as left bundle branch block may prevent the development of abnormal Q waves.
- Abnormal Q waves may shrink in size as time passes.

TABLE 11.2 ELECTROCARDIOGRAPHIC CHARACTERISTICS OF MYOCARDIAL ISCHEMIA, MYOCARDIAL INJURY, AND ABNORMAL Q WAVES

T Wave Abnormalities:

- The mean T vector of subendocardial ischemia is directed normally but is abnormally large.
- The mean T vector of epicardial ischemia is directed away from the area of damage. The angle between the mean QRS vector and mean T vector may be greater than 60°.
- The mean T vector is abnormal when it is located to the right of a vertical mean QRS vector even when the QRS-T angle is normal.
- The mean T vector is abnormal when it is directed to the left of, and superior to a horizontal mean QRS vector, even when the QRS-T angle is normal.
- The mean T vector is abnormal in adults when it is posterior to the mean QRS vector, even when the QRS-T angle is normal.

ST Segment Abnormalities:

- The mean ST vector of prolonged subendocardial injury is directed opposite the mean QRS vector. No Q waves may be present; this is *rarely* due to subendocardial infarction. This abnormality may be followed by abnormal Q waves, giving way to the electrocardiographic abnormalities of epicardial injury and ischemia.
- The mean ST vector is directed toward the area of localized epicardial injury. This vector points toward an area of the left ventricle, and occasionally, toward an area of right ventricular infarction associated with inferior infarction.

Abnormal Q waves:

- Abnormal Q waves, represented as an abnormality of the mean initial 0.04-second QRS vector, may occur with infarction. The mean initial 0.04-second QRS vector is directed away from the infarcted area of the left ventricle. The mean initial 0.04-second QRS vector is usually located more than 60° away from the mean QRS vector. Exceptions to this are mean initial 0.04-second QRS vectors due to infarction which are located to the right of a vertical mean QRS vector, superior to a horizontal mean QRS vector, or posterior to the mean QRS vector, even when the angle between the mean QRS vector and mean initial 0.04-second QRS vector is less than 60°. Electrocardiograms with abnormal Q waves due to infarction are referred to as showing *"Q wave infarctions"* rather than transmural infarctions.
- Visualization of the QRS loop is useful. An infarct should be considered when the first portion of a vertical QRS loop is inscribed in a counterclock-wise direction; when the first portion of a horizontal QRS loop is inscribed in a clockwise direction; and when the mean initial QRS forces are posterior to the subsequent QRS forces. These features of infarction assist in identification of abnormal Q waves of less than 0.04 second duration.
- The term *"non-Q wave infarction"* has replaced the ill-defined term "subendocardial infarction." The ST segment and T wave vectors indicate myocardial infarction especially when the diagnosis is supported by other clinical data, such as characteristic chest discomfort and an increased concentration of the MB isoenzyme of serum creatine kinase (CK).

FIGURE 11.1

This electrocardiogram was recorded from a 55-year-old patient with an acute inferolateral and posterior myocardial infarction. The heart rate is 72 complexes per minute, with a lower atrial rhythm. The duration of the QRS complex is 0.09 second and the duration of the QT interval is 0.36 second.

P waves: The mean P vector is directed superiorly; this signifies that atrial excitation originates in the lower portion of the atrium rather than in the sinus node.

QRS complex: The mean QRS vector is directed about -35° to the left. It is parallel with the frontal plane, whereas normally, it would be directed more posteriorly. The mean initial 0.04-second QRS vector is directed about -85° to the left. This is abnormal since the vector should be inferior to a horizontally-directed mean QRS vector. The mean initial 0.04-second QRS vector has an abnormal anterior direction, producing tall R waves in leads V1 and V2. It is directed away from the inferolateral and posterior portion of the left ventricle.

ST segment: The mean ST segment vector is huge. It is directed toward the epicardial injury located in the inferior, slightly posterior, and lateral portion of the left ventricle.

T waves: The mean T vector is enormous. It may represent generalized endocardial ischemia in that it is direct-

ed toward the centroid of the left ventricle. The mean T vector, during this hyperacute phase, has not yet become directed away from the epicardial area of the inferior, posterior, and lateral portion of the left ventricle.

A. The frontal plane projections of the mean P, mean initial 0.04-second QRS, mean QRS, mean ST, and mean T vectors. **B.** The spatial orientation of the mean P vector. It indicates a lower atrial rhythm because it is directed superiorly. The P waves are barely visible in the precordial leads; this makes it difficult to determine the degree of anterior or posterior deflection of the mean P vector. It is likely that all of the precordial electrode positions are near the transitional pathway for the mean P vector. **C.** The spatial orientation of the mean QRS vector. Note the course of the transitional pathway in the precordial leads. **D.** The spatial orientation of the mean initial 0.04-second QRS vector. It is abnormally directed anteriorly, superiorly, and away from the inferolateral and posterior portion of the left ventricle. It is the major cause of abnormal left axis deviation of the mean QRS vector. Leads V4, V5 and V6 are near the transitional pathway for the mean initial 0.04-second vector. Accordingly, the predicted deflections related to the mean initial 0.04-second vector do not fit the actual deflections shown in leads V4, V5,

and V6 (see previous discussions of discrepancies between predicted and actual deflections). **E.** The spatial orientation of the mean ST vector. Note the course of the transitional pathway in the precordial leads. The mean ST vector is directed toward epicardial injury in the inferolateral and posterior portions of the left ventricle. **F.** The spatial orientation of the mean T vector. Note that the transitional pathway cannot be identified in the precordial leads, making it impossible to identify how far anteriorly the vector is directed. The T wave is about the same size in V1 as in V6, suggesting that the mean T vector is directed about 30° to 45° anteriorly. The hyperacute mean T vector is probably due to endocardial ischemia. At a later stage of myocardial infarction, it would be directed away from epicardial ischemia in the inferolateral and posterior region of the left ventricle.

Summary: This electrocardiogram shows abnormalities of the mean initial 0.04-second QRS vector, the mean ST vector, and the mean T vector that are characteristic of an early stage of inferolateral and posterior myocardial infarction. The direction of the mean ST vector suggests, but does not prove that obstruction of the circumflex coronary artery is the culprit. (Reproduced with permission from the publisher and author; see Figure Credits.)

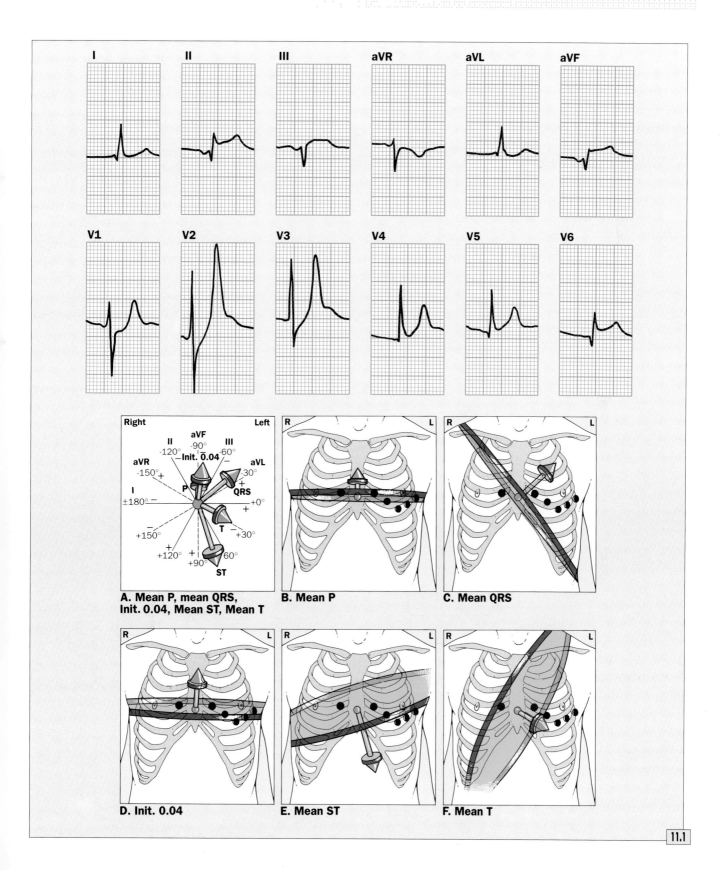

A. Mean P, mean QRS, Init. 0.04, Mean ST, Mean T

B. Mean P

C. Mean QRS

D. Init. 0.04

E. Mean ST

F. Mean T

11.1

FIGURE 11.2

This electrocardiogram, showing inferior myocardial infarction, was recorded from a 52-year-old man with chest pain. He gave a history of previous myocardial infarction. Coronary arteriography revealed 61 percent occlusion of the left anterior descending artery beyond its first branch, 41 percent occlusion of the first diagonal branch, and 16 percent occlusion of the left circumflex coronary artery.

The rhythm is normal, and the heart rate is 75 complexes per minute. The PR interval is 0.16 second. The duration of the QRS complex is 0.08 second, and the duration of the QT interval is 0.36 second.

P waves: The P waves are normal.

QRS complex: The mean QRS vector is directed about -18° to the left, and parallel with the frontal plane; normally, it should be directed slightly posteriorly. The mean initial 0.04-second QRS vector is abnormal; it is directed about -55° to the left, away from the inferior portion of the left ventricle. It is parallel with the frontal plane. Normally, it should be inferior to a horizontally-directed mean QRS vector.

T waves: The mean T vector is large, and directed away from an area of epicardial ischemia located in the inferior portion of the left ventricle. It shows an abnormal shift to the left of the horizontal mean QRS vector. Normally, the mean T vector would also be inferior to a horizontally directed mean QRS vector.

A. The frontal plane projections of the mean QRS, mean initial 0.04-second QRS, and mean T vectors. **B.** The spatial orientation of the mean QRS vector. Note the course of the transitional pathway in the precordial leads. The mean QRS vector is more anteriorly directed than it is normally. **C.** The spatial orientation of the mean initial 0.04-second QRS vector. Note the course of the transitional pathway in the precordial leads. The mean initial 0.04-second QRS vector is directed away from a dead zone in an inferior portion of the left ventricle.

D. The spatial orientation of the mean T vector. Note that the transitional pathway cannot be identified in the precordial leads. The T wave in lead V1 is much smaller than in lead V6. Accordingly, the mean T vector is directed about 20 to 30° anteriorly.

Summary: The mean initial 0.04-second QRS vector is directed away from a dead zone in the inferior portion of the left ventricle. The mean T vector points away from the area of epicardial ischemia in the inferior portion of the left ventricle. Coronary arteriography revealed a

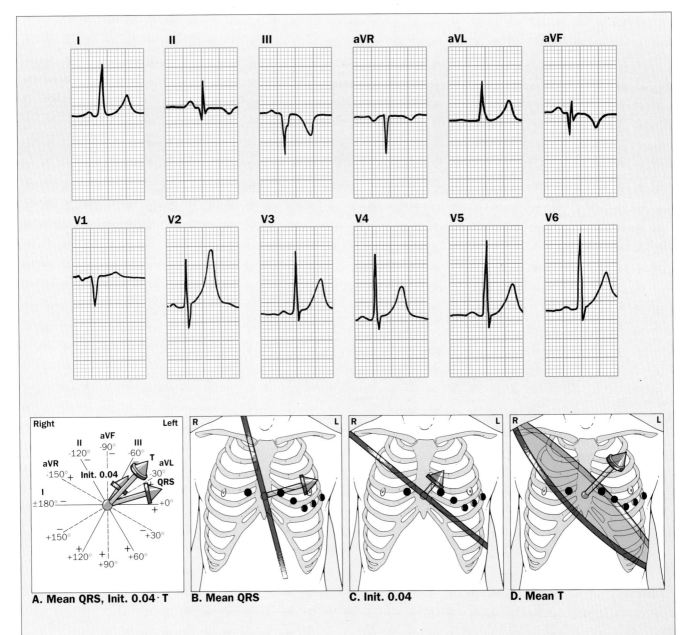

A. Mean QRS, Init. 0.04·T   B. Mean QRS   C. Init. 0.04   D. Mean T

(Figure 11.2 continued.)
significant obstruction in the left anterior descending coronary artery after its first branch. This type of infarction is usually caused by obstruction of the right coronary arteries. On rare occasions, as in this patient, it can be caused by obstruction of a "wraparound" left anterior descending artery (4).

FIGURE 11.3

This electrocardiogram was recorded from a 59-year-old woman with an acute inferoposterior myocardial infarction. She had previously undergone coronary bypass surgery, and underwent coronary arteriography following unstable angina pectoris. This revealed that the vein grafts to the left anterior descending and right coronary arteries were closed. The circumflex coronary artery was totally obstructed, and the left anterior descending coronary artery was 60 percent occluded. There were three sequential obstructions in the right coronary artery, the most severe being a 90 percent occlusion. The patient was given tissue plasminogen activator (tPA), which resulted in a marked decrease in the size of the ST segment vector. Intravenous nitroglycerin and heparin were administered, and coronary bypass surgery was performed the following day.

The heart rate is 48 complexes per minute; sinus bradycardia is present. The PR interval is 0.18 second. The duration of the QRS complex is 0.12 second, and the duration of the QT interval is 0.40 second.

P waves: The P waves are normal.
QRS complex: The duration of the QRS complex is 0.12 second. The mean QRS vector is directed about +118° inferiorly, and about 45° anteriorly. The mean terminal 0.04-second QRS vector is directed to the right and slightly anteriorly; this signifies right bundle branch block.

ST segment: The mean vector representing the ST segment is directed +120° inferiorly and slightly posteriorly. When there is uncomplicated right bundle branch block, the mean T and ST vectors should be directed to the left and posteriorly, opposite the mean QRS vector. In this case of complicated right bundle branch block, the mean ST segment vector is directed inferiorly and posteriorly, toward an area of epicardial myocardial injury in the inferior and posterior portion of the left ventricle.

T waves: The mean T vector is directed about +90° inferiorly, and markedly posteriorly. This probably represents early endocardial ischemia of the inferoposterior portion of the left ventricle. It is likely that this vector will, at a later time, be directed away from an area of inferior and posterior epicardial ischemia.

A. The frontal plane projections of the mean QRS, mean ST vector, and mean T vectors. **B.** The spatial orientation of the mean QRS vector. The features are characteristic of right bundle branch block. **C.** The spatial orientation of the mean ST vector. **D.** The spatial orientation of the mean T vector.

Summary: The abnormalities in this electrocardiogram can be used to illustrate several points. They indicate the way in which the ST segment and early T wave abnormalities of inferoposterior infarction can be identified in the presence of right bundle branch block. The mean vectors representing the ST and T abnormalities of uncomplicated right bundle branch block should be directed opposite the mean QRS vector of right bundle branch block. Such is not the

(Figure 11.3 continued on page 11.10.)

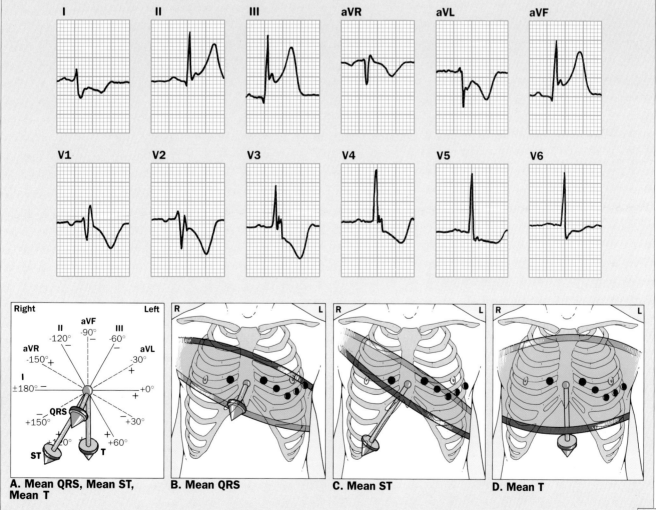

A. Mean QRS, Mean ST, Mean T **B. Mean QRS** **C. Mean ST** **D. Mean T**

(Figure 11.3 continued.)
case in this patient with complicated right bundle branch block. The mean ST and T vectors are abnormal as the result of an inferior-posterior infarction. The ST segment abnormality almost disappeared following the use of tPA, indicating the lysis of a clot.

F I G U R E   1 1 . 4

This electrocardiogram was recorded from a 58-year-old man with an inferolateral myocardial infarction and stable angina pectoris. He had a history of two previous myocardial infarctions requiring bypass surgery in 1980. He had class 2 to 3 stable angina pectoris (Canadian Cardiovascular Society Classification). A coronary arteriogram made in June, 1983, showed 100 percent occlusion of the left anterior descending artery, distal to the first septal perforator. The first diagonal branch and the circumflex coronary arteries were 100 percent occluded. The bypass grafts were patent. The ejection fraction was 58 percent. The distal right coronary artery was normal. The

apex and inferior apical areas of the myocardium were noncontractile, and the inferior basal area showed a moderate decrease in contractility.

The rhythm is normal and the heart rate is 107 complexes per minute. The PR interval is 0.16 second. The duration of the QRS complex is 0.10 second, and that of the QT interval is 0.32 second.

P waves: The P waves are normal.

QRS complexes: The QRS complexes are abnormal. The mean QRS vector is directed at -100° superiorly, and about 60° posteriorly. The mean initial 0.04-second QRS vector is directed at -85° superiorly and about 30° anteriorly, away from an inferoposterior dead zone (see later discussion).

T waves: The T waves are abnormal. The mean T vector is directed about +5° in the frontal plane, and 85° to 90° anteriorly. It is directed away from an area of epicardial ischemia located in the posterior portion of the left ventricle.

A. The frontal plane projections of the mean QRS, mean initial 0.04-second QRS, and mean T vectors. **B.** The spatial

orientation of the mean QRS vector. Note that the QRS complexes are all negative in the precordial leads. The QRS complex in lead V1 is more negative than it is in lead V6; accordingly, the mean QRS vector is directed at least 60° posteriorly.

C. The spatial orientation of the mean initial 0.04-second QRS vector. It is directed superiorly and anteriorly, away from the inferoposterior and lateral portions of the left ventricle. The transitional pathway for the mean initial 0.04-second vector is located near electrode positions V5 and V6. Accordingly, the diagram, which is constructed using a rigid format, does not match the actual deflections of the mean initial 0.04-second vector as reflected in leads V5 and V6 (see previous discussions). **D.** The spatial orientation of the mean T vector. It is directed anteriorly at 85° to 90°, so that the T wave is isoelectric in lead V6, and upright in all other precordial leads; it is directed away from an area of epicardial injury in the posterior portion of the left ventricle.

Summary: This electrocardiogram illustrates the presence of an inferior-

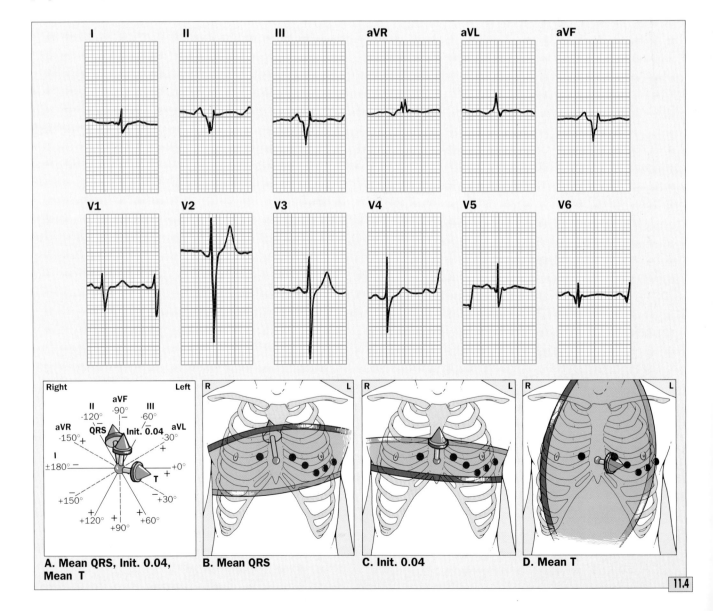

A. Mean QRS, Init. 0.04, Mean T   **B. Mean QRS**   **C. Init. 0.04**   **D. Mean T**

(Figure 11.4 continued.)
posterior dead zone and a posterior area of epicardial ischemia. These abnormalities could be due to two separate infarcts or a single infarct that is located in the proper area of the left ventricle.

FIGURE 11.5

This electrocardiogram, showing inferolateral infarction, was taken from a 78-year-old man with a history of myocardial infarction and angina pectoris occurring at rest.

The rhythm is normal, and the heart rate is 75 complexes per minute. A coronary arteriogram revealed 60 percent occlusion of the third marginal branch of the left circumflex coronary artery.

The PR interval is 0.13 second. The duration of the QRS complex is 0.08 second, and the duration of the QT interval is 0.40 second.

P waves: The P waves are normal.

QRS complex: The mean QRS vector is directed -50° to the left and about 45° posteriorly. The mean initial 0.04-second QRS vector is directed -40° to the left, and parallel with the frontal plane. It is directed away from the inferior portion of the left ventricle. The marked left axis deviation is due to the inferior infarction.

ST segment: The mean ST vector is directed toward an inferior area of epicardial injury.

T waves: The mean T vector is directed away from an inferior-posterior area of epicardial ischemia.

A. The frontal plane projections of the mean QRS, mean initial 0.04-second QRS, mean ST, and mean T vectors. **B**. The spatial orientation of the mean QRS vector. Note the course of the transitional

(Figure 11.5 continued on page 11.12.)

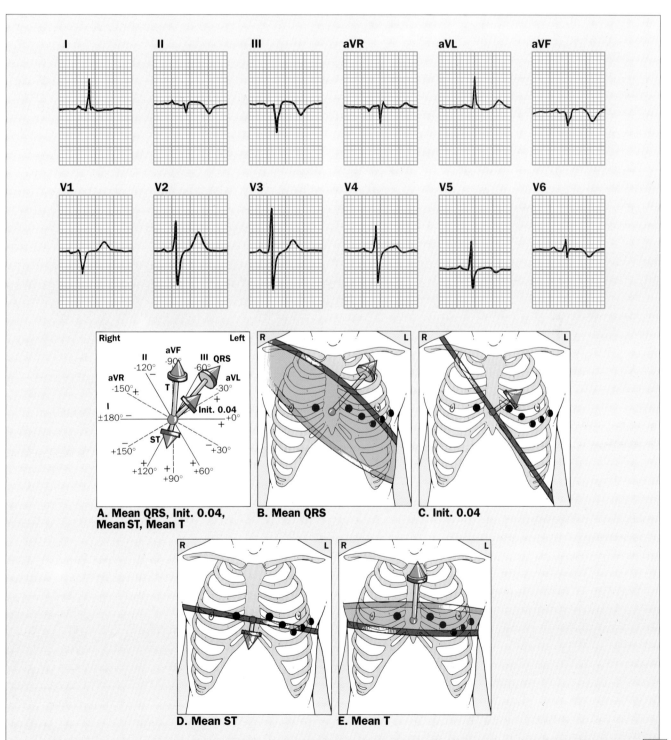

A. Mean QRS, Init. 0.04, Mean ST, Mean T

B. Mean QRS

C. Init. 0.04

D. Mean ST

E. Mean T

(Figure 11.5 continued.)
pathway in the precordial leads. **C**. The spatial orientation of the mean initial 0.04-second QRS vector. It points away from an inferior area of the left ventricle. Note the course of the transitional pathway in the precordial leads. **D**. The spatial orientation of the mean ST vector. All precordial electrode positions are located near the transitional pathway for the mean ST vector **E**. The spatial orientation of the mean T vector. Note the course of the transitional pathway in the precordial leads. The V4, V5, and V6 electrode positions are located near the transitional pathway for the mean T vector. Because of this, the diagram, based on a rigid format, does not match the deflections. Note that the T waves are inverted in leads V5 and V6, whereas the diagram suggests that they would be upright (see discussion of discrepancies between actual and predicted deflections earlier in this chapter).

Summary: The mean initial 0.04-second QRS vector is directed away from an inferior left ventricular dead zone, and the mean ST segment vector points toward the same area. The mean T vector points away from an inferoposterior area of left ventricular epicardial ischemia. Note that the culprit artery was the third marginal branch of the circumflex coronary artery.

FIGURE 11.6

This electrocardiogram was recorded from an 89-year-old man with an inferior myocardial infarction. He had class 2 to 3 angina pectoris (Canadian Cardiovascular Society Classification), a history of three infarctions, and systemic hypertension. He was receiving digoxin for heart failure. Coronary bypass surgery had been performed in 1976, and arteriography performed at that time revealed 90 percent obstruction of the left main coronary artery, 80 percent obstruction of the left anterior descending coronary artery, 80 percent obstruction of the circumflex coronary artery, and 100 percent obstruction of the right coronary artery. The inferior portion of the left ventricle was akinetic.

The rhythm is normal and the heart rate is 68 complexes per minute. The PR interval is 0.16 second. The duration of the QRS complex is 0.09 second, and that of the QT interval is 0.39 second.

P waves: The mean P vector is directed +85° inferiorly, and slightly posteriorly. The second halves of the P waves in leads V1 and V2 suggest a left atrial abnormality. The P waves are not definitely abnormal.

U waves: The U waves are large in leads V2 and V3.

QRS complexes: The QRS complexes are abnormal. The mean QRS vector is directed about +8° in the frontal plane, and about 30° posteriorly. The total 12-lead QRS amplitude is greater than 124 mm, and the QRS amplitude in lead V5 is greater than 25 mm. The mean initial 0.04-second QRS vector is directed -70° to the left, about 10° posteriorly, and abnormally to the left of a horizontal mean QRS vector. This is due to a dead zone in the inferior portion of the left ventricle.

ST segment: The mean ST (early T) vector is directed +150° to the right and parallel with the frontal plane. This is probably due to the digitalis medication.

T waves: The mean late T vector is directed +85° inferiorly, and 85° anteriorly.

A. The frontal plane projections of the mean QRS, mean initial 0.04-second QRS, mean ST (early T), and mean late T vectors. **B**. The spatial orientation of the mean QRS vector. Note the course of the transitional pathway in the precordial leads. **C**. The spatial orientation of the mean initial 0.04-second QRS vector. The electrode positions for leads V2, V3, and V4 are all near the transitional pathway for the mean 0.04-second vector. **D**. The spatial orientation of the mean ST (early T) segment vector. **E**. The spatial orientation of the mean late T vector. The abnormal anterior direction is not due to digitalis because the vector is directed about 115° anterior to the mean QRS vector. This wide QRS-T angle is due either to left ventricular hypertrophy or left ventricular ischemia.

Summary: This electrocardiogram exhibits evidence of an inferior dead zone, posterior ischemia, and a digitalis effect.

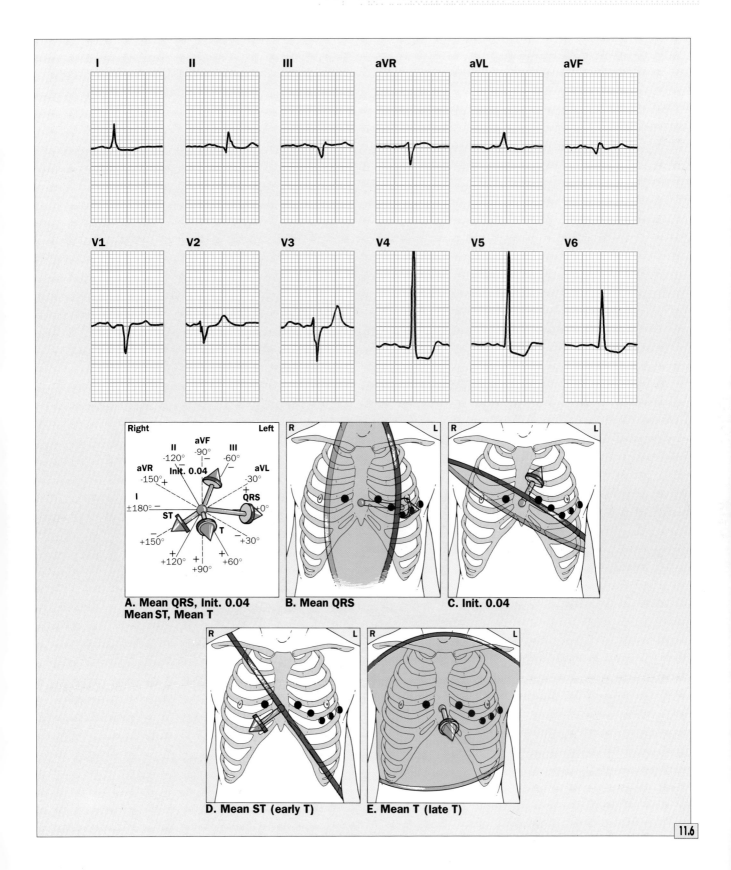

A. Mean QRS, Init. 0.04
Mean ST, Mean T

B. Mean QRS

C. Init. 0.04

D. Mean ST (early T)

E. Mean T (late T)

FIGURE 11.7

This electrocardiogram was recorded in the intensive care unit from a 59-year-old man who had just undergone coronary bypass surgery. The previous electrocardiogram showed inferior infarction. The coronary arteriogram showed 100 percent occlusion of the left anterior descending coronary artery after its first branch, 79 percent occlusion of the first diagonal branch, 59 percent occlusion of the mid and 57 percent occlusion of the distal portion of the circumflex coronary artery, and 95 percent occlusion of the distal portion of the right coronary artery. The ejection fraction was 40 percent, and there was anterobasal and anterior mild hypokinesis, apical, septal and postero-lateral moderate hypokinesis, and inferoapical inferior akinesis. The conduction abnormality shown in this electrocardiogram was not present prior to coronary bypass surgery; it was observed for only a few hours after surgery.

The rhythm is normal and the heart rate is 90 complexes per minute. The PR interval is 0.16 second. The duration of

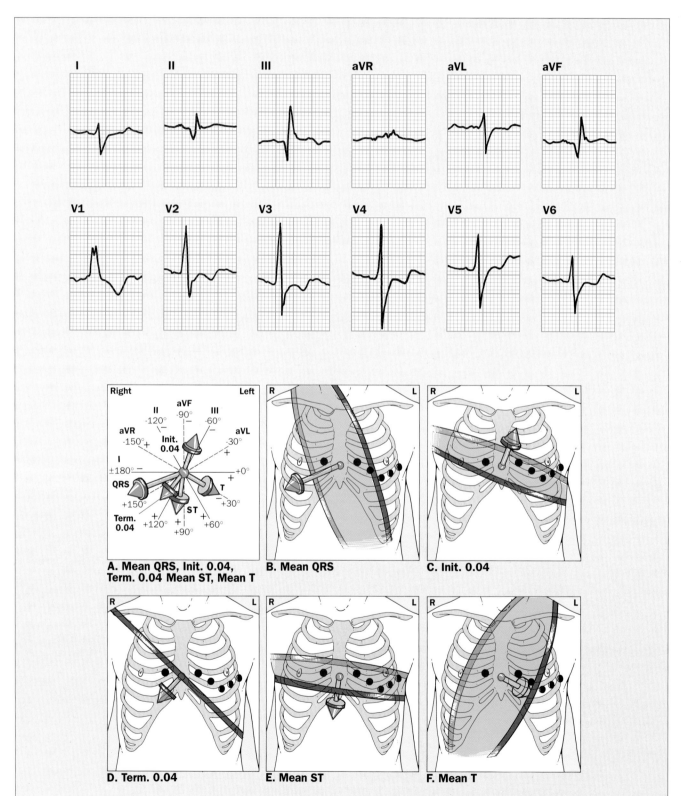

A. Mean QRS, Init. 0.04, Term. 0.04 Mean ST, Mean T

B. Mean QRS

C. Init. 0.04

D. Term. 0.04

E. Mean ST

F. Mean T

(Figure 11.7 continued.)
the QRS complex is 0.14 second and the QT interval is 0.44 second.

P waves: The P waves are normal.

QRS complexes: The QRS duration is 0.14 second. The mean QRS vector is directed +160° to the right and about +35° anteriorly, signifying complicated right bundle branch block. The mean initial 0.04-second QRS vector is abnormal; it is directed -70° superiorly and anteriorly. The anterior direction of the vector could be caused by a true posterior infarction or right ventricular hypertrophy. In this patient, the anterior direction of the vector was transient; it persisted for only a few hours, ruling out right ventricular hypertrophy. The leftward deviation of the vector is due to inferior infarction because it was present throughout the period of observation. However, its anterior direction changed, suggesting a posterior area of "stunned" myocardium. The orientation of the mean terminal 0.04-second QRS vector was also transient. It is directed +135° to the right and parallel with the frontal plane, suggesting left pos-

terior-inferior division block and right bundle branch block.

ST segment: The mean ST vector is directed +100° inferiorly and slightly posteriorly, in the direction of the epicardial injury in the inferior portion of the left ventricle.

T waves: The mean T vector is directed +30° in the frontal plane, and about 35° posteriorly, away from an area of anterior left ventricular epicardial ischemia.

A. The frontal plane projections of the mean QRS, mean initial 0.04-second QRS, mean terminal 0.04-second QRS, mean ST, and mean T vectors. **B.** The spatial orientation of the mean QRS vector. **C.** The spatial orientation of the mean initial 0.04-second QRS vector. **D.** The spatial orientation of the mean terminal 0.04-second QRS vector. It is directed so far to the right that right bundle branch block alone does not account for it. **E.** The spatial orientation of the mean ST vector. **F.** The spatial orientation of the mean T vector.

Summary: This unusual electrocardiogram reveals signs of inferoposterior

infarction. The leftward and slightly anterior direction of the mean initial 0.04-second QRS vector is due to an inferoposterior dead zone. Its anterior direction may be due to an area of temporarily "stunned" posterior myocardium.

The mean terminal 0.04-second QRS vector is abnormal, owing to transient right bundle branch block; it is directed so far to the right and anteriorly that additional, transient posterior-inferior division block should be considered. The mean T vector indicates anterior epicardial ischemia. The cause of the transient conduction disturbance in this patient is related to ischemia or hypothermia which may have occurred during bypass surgery. There may be many different explanations for these transient electrocardiographic abnormalities, but those given here seem plausible in this patient.

FIGURE 11.8
This electrocardiogram was recorded from a 59-year-old hypertensive man with angina pectoris and a history of
(Figure 11.8 continued on page 11.16.)

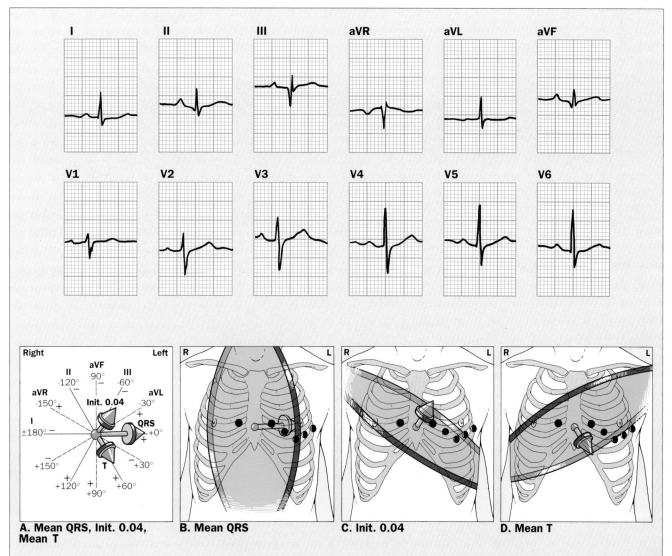

A. Mean QRS, Init. 0.04, Mean T   **B. Mean QRS**   **C. Init. 0.04**   **D. Mean T**

11.8

(Figure 11.8 continued.)
inferior myocardial infarction. The coronary arteriogram revealed 100 percent occlusion of the left anterior descending coronary artery beyond its first branch, 100 percent occlusion of the distal portion of the left circumflex coronary artery, and 100 percent occlusion of the third marginal branch of the circumflex coronary artery.

The rhythm is normal and the heart rate is 78 complexes per minute. The PR interval is 0.20 second. The duration of the QRS complex is 0.08 second and the duration of the QT interval is 0.36 second.

P waves: The P waves are normal.

QRS complex: The mean QRS vector is directed at 0° in the frontal plane and about 50° to 60° posteriorly. The mean initial 0.04-second QRS vector is directed about -50° to the left and to an undetermined degree anteriorly. The mean initial 0.04-second QRS vector is abnormal for two reasons: it is superior to a horizontally directed mean QRS vector, and the spatial angle between the initial 0.04-second QRS vector and the mean QRS vector is greater than 60°. This vector is directed away from a dead zone located in the inferior and slightly posterior portion of the left ventricle.

T waves: The mean T vector is directed at +60°, and at least 45° anteriorly (the T wave amplitude in leads V1 and V6 is about equal). The QRS-T angle is abnormal because it is greater than 90°.

A. The frontal plane projections of the mean QRS, mean 0.04-second QRS, and mean T vectors. **B.** The spatial orientation of the mean QRS vector. Note the course of the transitional pathway in the precordial leads. **C.** The spatial orientation of the mean initial 0.04-second QRS vector. Note the difficulty in identifying the transitional pathway in the precordial leads. One can assume, however, that the vector has a moderately anterior orientation. **D.** The spatial orientation of the mean T vector. Note the difficulty in identifying

the transitional pathway in the precordial leads. One can assume that the mean T vector is directed about 45° anteriorly, because the size of the T waves is about equal in leads V1 and V6.

Summary: This interesting electrocardiogram is included to make a single point: the clinician should not assume that the QRS-T angle abnormality is due to inferior infarction. Even though the direction of the mean initial 0.04-second QRS vector indicates an infero-posterior infarction, the QRS-T angle indicates another abnormality; it does not conform to the changes expected with such an infarct. The QRS-T angle is abnormal owing to either an early stage of left ventricular systolic pressure overload due to hypertension, or posterior-superior epicardial ischemia of obstructive coronary disease.

FIGURE 11.9

This electrocardiogram, showing a tall R wave in lead V1 secondary to a true posterior infarction, was recorded from a 75-year-old man. The patient had unstable angina pectoris for two months. A coronary arteriogram made on June 9, 1988, revealed 79 percent obstruction of the left anterior descending coronary artery beyond the first septal perforator. The first diagonal branch was 52 percent obstructed, and the proximal right coronary artery was 66 percent obstructed. The circumflex coronary artery was normal, and the third marginal branch and left posterior descending coronary arteries were absent. The ejection fraction was 65 to 70 percent. Coronary bypass surgery was performed on June 13, 1988.

The heart rhythm is normal and the heart rate is 75 complexes per minute. The PR interval is 0.17 second. The duration of the QRS complex is 0.07 second and the duration of the QT interval is 0.38 second.

P waves: The P waves are normal.

QRS complex: The mean QRS vector is directed about +65° to the right, and

10° anteriorly; this is abnormal. The mean initial 0.04-second QRS vector is directed about +45° to the right and about 40° anteriorly. It is impossible to determine how far anteriorly it is directed, because the initial forces are positive in all of the precordial leads. The fact that the R wave in lead V1 is almost as large as that in lead V6 indicates that the initial 0.04-second QRS vector is directed moderately anteriorly. This is due to a dead zone located in the true posterior portion of the left ventricle. Right ventricular hypertrophy could cause this, but the frontal plane orientations of the mean QRS and initial 0.04-second QRS vectors rule against such a view.

T waves: The T waves are normal. The mean T vector is directed +30° in, and parallel with, the frontal plane.

A. The frontal plane projections of the mean QRS, mean initial 0.04-second QRS, and mean T vectors. **B.** The spatial orientation of the mean QRS vector. **C.** The spatial orientation of the mean initial 0.04-second QRS vector. **D.** The spatial orientation of the mean T vector.

Summary: This electrocardiogram illustrates three points: first, hasty inspection of the tracing could lead the observer to conclude that it was normal, whereas the patient actually had severe coronary disease. Second, the tracing also illustrates how a true posterior infarction can produce tall R waves in leads V1 and V2 because the initial 0.04-second QRS vector is directed anteriorly to an abnormal degree. There are no abnormal Q waves in the tracing; they would be found in a recording made from the patient's back. This figure also illustrates that the location of an infarction does not always signify which coronary artery has the greatest chronic obstruction. In this patient, the greatest obstruction was in the left anterior descending coronary artery, which was not responsible for the electrocardiographic abnormalities.

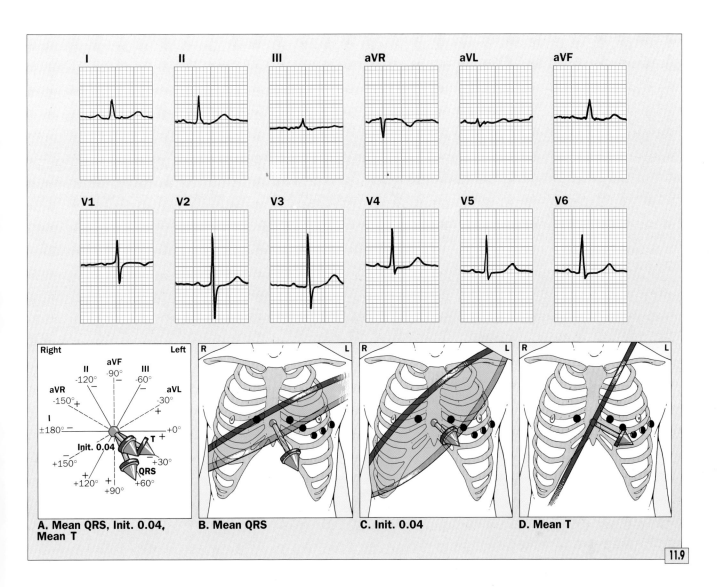

A. Mean QRS, Init. 0.04, Mean T

B. Mean QRS

C. Init. 0.04

D. Mean T

11.9

FIGURE 11.10 (I AND II)

These electrocardiograms, showing the development of a right ventricular infarction, were recorded from a 51-year-old man. He had an anterior infarction in August, 1988. A coronary arteriogram made at that time revealed total obstruction of the first diagonal coronary artery and the left anterior descending coronary artery after the first septal perforator. The patient had coronary bypass surgery the same month. He developed a recurrent ventricular tachycardia that could not be controlled with drugs, including amiodarone. Electrophysiologic testing with endocardial mapping and possible endocardial surgical resection was planned. It seemed wise to take a coronary arteriogram prior to these procedures in order to determine whether myocardial ischemia might be responsible for the patient's arrhythmia.

The arteriogram was made on November

29, 1988. Unfortunately, the procedure precipitated severe dissection of the right coronary artery, which became completely occluded. The patient was transferred to Emory University Hospital where percutaneous transluminal coronary angioplasty was unsuccessful; the proximal portion of the right coronary artery became completely obstructed. These events made it possible to study the evolution of a right ventricular myocardial infarction occurring in the presence of a former anteroseptal myocardial infarction. The patient responded to the specific treatment for right ventricular infarction.

I. This electrocardiogram was recorded at 7:24 pm on November 29, 1988, after coronary arteriography, at which time a severe dissection of the right coronary artery occurred. It shows the previous anteroseptal infarction due to total occlusion of the left anterior descending artery.

The rhythm is normal; there are 72 complexes per minute. The duration of the PR interval is 0.17 second. The duration of the QRS complex is 0.09 second and that of the QT interval is 0.37 second.

P waves: The P waves are normal.

QRS complex: The mean QRS vector is directed at 0° in the frontal plane. It is directed at about 20° to 30° posteriorly, and the mean initial 0.04-second vector is directed about 20° posteriorly—a little more than it should be for this particular mean QRS vector.

T waves: The mean T vector is directed at 0° in the frontal plane, and 80° posteriorly, away from an area of anterior epicardial ischemia.

A. The frontal plane projections of the mean QRS, mean initial 0.04-second QRS, mean ST segment, and mean T vectors. **B-D.** The spatial orientations of the mean QRS, mean initial 0.04-second QRS, and mean T vectors, respectively.

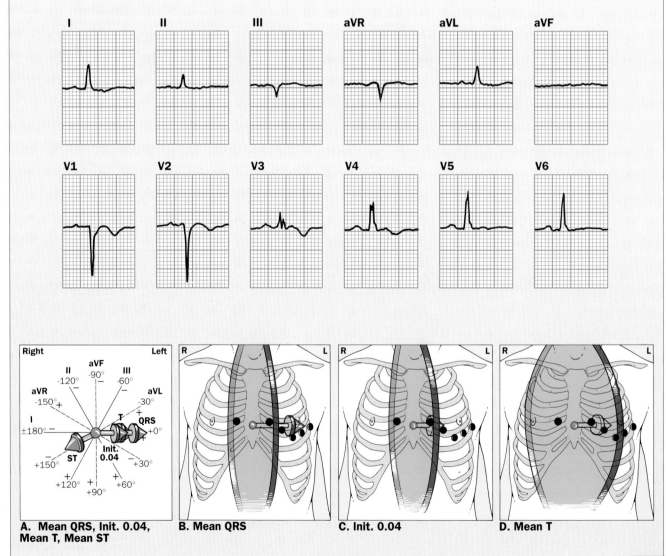

A. Mean QRS, Init. 0.04, Mean T, Mean ST   B. Mean QRS   C. Init. 0.04   D. Mean T

(Figure 11.10 continued.)

II. This electrocardiogram was recorded at 11:46 pm, after an attempted angioplasty to open the totally occluded right coronary artery. A more proximal portion of this vessel became completely obstructed, at which time the electrocardiogram showed evidence of right ventricular infarction.

The rhythm is normal. There are 80 complexes per minute. The duration of the PR interval is 0.20 second. The duration of the QRS complex is 0.10 second, and the duration of the QT interval is 0.36 second.

P waves: The P waves are normal, although the mean P vector is a little more posteriorly directed than in the tracing shown in Figure 11.10(I).

QRS complex: The mean QRS vector is directed +45° inferiorly, and 15° posteriorly. The mean initial 0.04-second QRS vector is directed a little more to the left than it was in Figure 11.10(I); this may be due to a new inferior dead zone.

ST segment: The mean ST vector is huge. It is directed about +130° to the right, and 40° to 60° anteriorly. This is characteristic of epicardial injury associated with inferior and right ventricular infarction.

T waves: The mean T vector shows a markedly posterior direction. It is difficult to identify the frontal plane projection of the mean T vector, but the T waves are definitely inverted in leads V1 through V5. The vector is directed away from an area of anterior epicardial ischemia.

(Figure 11.10 continued on page 11.20.)

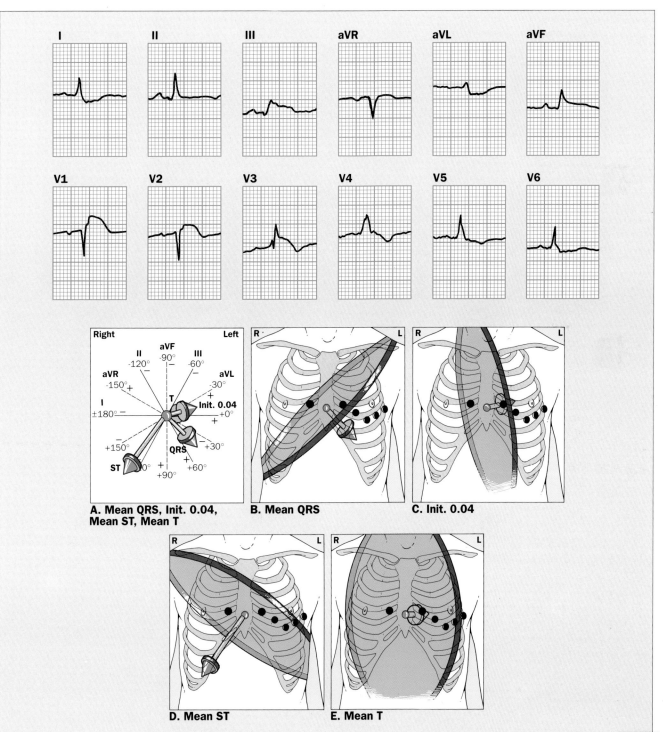

A. Mean QRS, Init. 0.04, Mean ST, Mean T

B. Mean QRS

C. Init. 0.04

D. Mean ST

E. Mean T

(Figure 11.10 continued.)

A. The frontal plane projections of the mean QRS, mean initial 0.04-second QRS, mean ST, and mean T vectors. **B-E.** The spatial orientations of the mean QRS, mean initial 0.04-second QRS, mean ST, and mean T vectors, respectively.

Summary: The unusual electrocardiogram shown in part II exhibits abnormalities characteristic of right ventricular infarction. Tracing I shows an anteroseptal infarction. Tracing II followed coronary angioplasty which was performed to open the right coronary artery which became occluded after coronary artery dissection associated with arteriography. The mean ST segment vector is directed to the right and anteriorly in tracing II. A tracing made from V3R would show an elevated ST segment. The direction of the mean ST segment vector is a better indicator of the culprit artery than that of the mean initial 0.04-second QRS or the mean T vector.

FIGURE 11.11

This electrocardiogram was recorded from a 47-year-old man with anterolateral myocardial infarction. He had a history of angina pectoris at rest. A coronary arteriogram revealed 100 percent obstruction of the left anterior descending coronary artery beyond its first branch, and 75 percent occlusion of the right posterior descending artery. The right ventricular branch of the right coronary artery was missing.

The rhythm is normal and the heart rate is 88 complexes per minute. The PR interval is 0.20 second. The duration of the QRS complex is 0.09 second, and the duration of the QT interval is 0.35 second.

P waves: The P waves are severely notched in leads I and II. The duration of the P wave is 0.14 second. The mean P vector (Pm) is directed at +60° in, and parallel with, the frontal plane. The abnormalities may be due to a localized lesion in the atria, perhaps indicating atrial infarction. The first deflection of what appears to be a P wave could be a U wave, but careful study of several deflections suggests that it is the first part of a notched P wave.

QRS complex: The duration of the QRS complex is 0.09 second. The mean QRS vector is directed about +115 to the right, and about 15° posteriorly. The mean initial 0.04-second QRS vector is directed about +130° to the right, and parallel with the frontal plane. This produces the abnormal Q waves in leads V5 and V6, and is responsible for the rightward deviation of the mean QRS vector. The small R waves seen in leads V2, V3, and V4 are less than 0.04-second in duration, and it is likely that the transitional pathway for the mean initial 0.04-second portion of the QRS complexes is near electrode positions V2, V3 and V4.

ST segment: The mean ST vector is directed -50° to the left, and about 10° anteriorly, toward an area of anterolateral epicardial injury.

T waves: The mean T vector is directed about +45° to the right and 10° anteriorly.

A. The frontal plane projections of the mean P, mean QRS, mean initial 0.04-second QRS, mean ST, and mean T vectors. **B.** The spatial orientation of the mean QRS vector. **C.** The spatial orientation of the mean initial 0.04-second QRS vector. **D.** The spatial orientation of the mean ST vector. **E.** The spatial orientation of the mean T vector.

Summary: This electrocardiogram reveals how anterolateral myocardial infarction can produce right axis deviation of the mean QRS vector. It also exemplifies how P waves may be altered in the setting of infarction. The P wave abnormality may be due to atrial infarction.

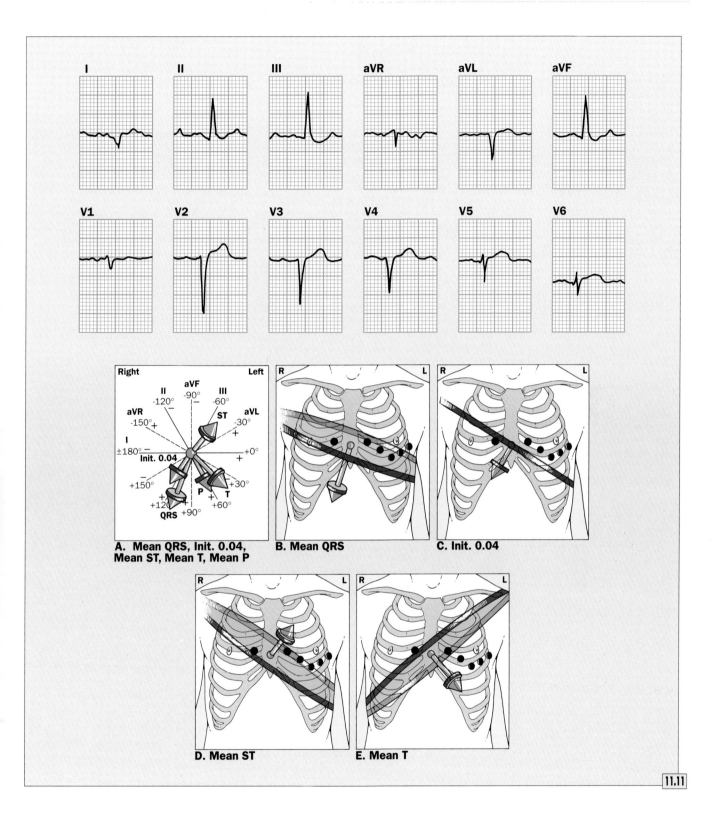

A. Mean QRS, Init. 0.04, Mean ST, Mean T, Mean P

B. Mean QRS

C. Init. 0.04

D. Mean ST

E. Mean T

FIGURE 11.12

This electrocardiogram, showing antero-lateral myocardial infarction, right bundle branch block, and left anterior-superior division block, was recorded from a 48-year-old man with angina pectoris at rest. He gave a history of myocardial infarction. A coronary arteriogram made when the patient was 51 years of age revealed 100 percent obstruction of the proximal portion of the left anterior descending coronary artery. The septum and inferoapical areas of the myocardium were akinetic. The ejection fraction was 20 percent.

The rhythm is normal and the heart rate is 82 complexes per minute. The PR interval is 0.15 second. The duration of the QRS complex is 0.12 second and that of the QT interval is 0.34 second.

P waves: The mean P vector is directed at +30° in the frontal plane. When viewed in space, it is parallel with the frontal plane. P2 is abnormal at -0.06 mm-sec in lead V1, signifying a left atrial abnormality.

QRS complex: The duration of the QRS complex is 0.12 second. The mean QRS vector is directed -75° to the left, and parallel with the frontal plane. The deflections in leads V5 adn V6 are actually negative, whereas the diagram indicates that the deflection recorded at V6 would be positive, and the deflection at V5 would be transitional. The lack of correspondence occurs because the electrodes at V5 and V6 record near the transitional pathway (see previous discussions). The mean terminal 0.04-second QRS vector is directed -100° to the left, and 15° anteriorly. This signifies, when the QRS duration is 0.12 second, the presence of right bundle branch block and left anterior-superior division block, which produces a tall R wave in lead V1, and left axis deviation of the mean QRS vector. The mean initial 0.04-second QRS vector is directed about -60° to the left, and about 80° posteriorly; this signifies an extensive anterior dead zone. The vector produced by left anterior-superior division block shows the direction of depolarization of the myocardium served by the left posterior-inferior division of the conduction system, and retrograde depolarization of that portion of the myocardium served by the left anterior-superior division.

ST segment: The mean ST vector is directed about +75° to the right, and 15° anteriorly, indicating extensive inferior, apical, and perhaps lower septal injury (review the abnormalities in the coronary arteriogram). The mean ST vector of this patient is not parallel with the mean T vector, as it should be when there is uncomplicated bundle branch block. It is directed toward an area of epicardial injury.

T wave: The mean T vector is directed +120° to the right and about 10° posteriorly. This is caused by anterolateral epicardial ischemia.

A. The frontal plane projections of the mean P, mean QRS, mean initial 0.04-second QRS, mean terminal 0.04-second QRS, mean ST, and mean T vectors. **B.** The spatial orientation of the mean QRS vector. **C.** The spatial orientation of the mean initial 0.04-second QRS vector. **D.** The spatial orientation of the terminal 0.04-second QRS vector. **E.** The spatial orientation of the mean ST vector. **F.** The spatial orientation of the mean T vector.

Summary: This electrocardiogram is a good example of the development of right bundle branch block plus left anterior-superior division block due to an anterolateral myocardial infarction. These findings remind us that right bundle branch block does not prevent the identification of abnormal initial QRS forces caused by myocardial infarction. They also reveal how an extensive infarction can produce severe conduction defects. In this tracing, the direction of the initial 0.04-second QRS vector signifies myocardial infarction, as do the directions of the mean ST and T vectors.

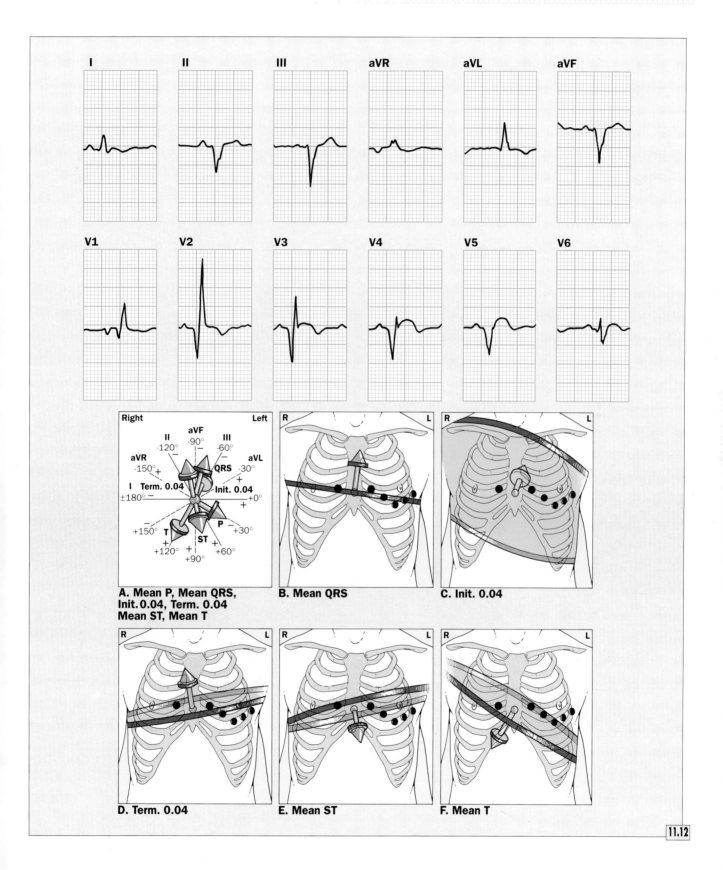

A. Mean P, Mean QRS,
Init. 0.04, Term. 0.04
Mean ST, Mean T

B. Mean QRS

C. Init. 0.04

D. Term. 0.04

E. Mean ST

F. Mean T

11.12

FIGURE 11.13
This electrocardiogram was recorded from a 62-year-old man with an old anteroseptal myocardial infarction.

The rhythm is normal, and the heart rate is 75 complexes per minute. The PR interval is 0.12 second. The duration of the QRS complex is 0.08 second and the QT interval is 0.36 second.

P waves: The P waves are normal.

QRS complex: The mean QRS vector is directed 0° to the left and 20° posteriorly. The mean initial 0.04-second QRS vector

is directed about +30° inferiorly and 30° posteriorly; it is posterior to the mean QRS vector, and signifies an anteroseptal dead zone.

ST segment: The mean ST segment vector is directed +118° to the right and about 40° anteriorly; it signifies anterior epicardial injury.

T waves: The mean T vector is directed about +88° inferiorly and about 30° posteriorly; it signifies anterior epicardial ischemia.

A. The frontal plane projections of the mean QRS, mean initial 0.04-second

QRS, mean ST, and mean T vectors.
B. The spatial orientation of the mean QRS vector. Note that the transitional pathway courses between the electrode sites for V2 and V3. **C.** The spatial orientation of the mean initial 0.04-second QRS vector. Note the transitional pathway which courses between electrode sites V3 and V4. **D.** The spatial orientation of the mean ST vector. **E.** The spatial orientation of the mean T vector.

Summary: This electrocardiogram illustrates the abnormalities associated with

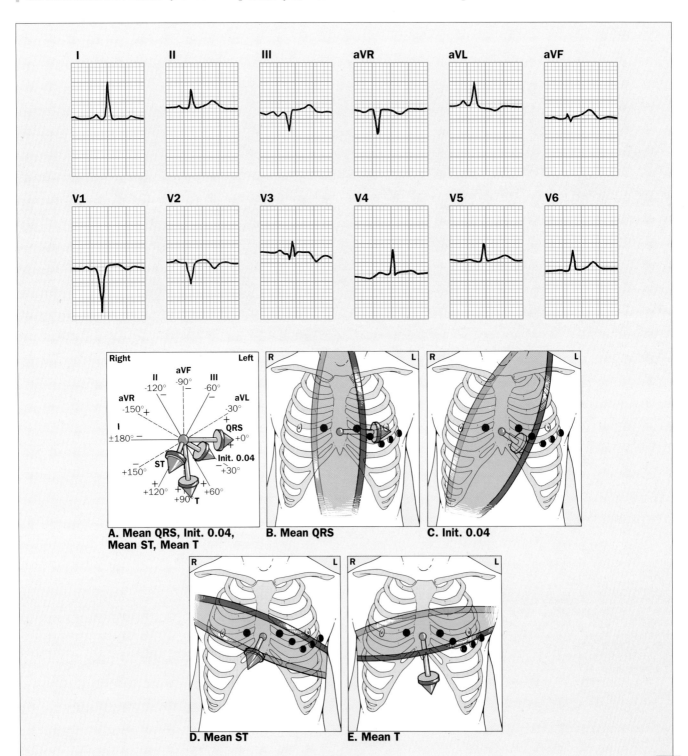

A. Mean QRS, Init. 0.04, Mean ST, Mean T

B. Mean QRS

C. Init. 0.04

D. Mean ST

E. Mean T

(Figure 11.13 continued.)
an anteroseptal myocardial infarction. Note that the mean initial 0.04-second QRS vector is posterior to the mean QRS vector; this arrangement produces the absent R wave in leads V1 and V2, and the Q followed by the R wave in lead V3. (Reproduced with permission from the publisher and author; see Figure Credits.)

FIGURE 11.14

This electrocardiogram, recorded from a hypertensive man, shows complicated left bundle branch block and extensive anterior or epicardial ischemia and injury.

The rhythm is normal, and the heart rate is 70 complexes per minute. The PR interval is 0.16 second. The duration of the QRS complex is 0.16 second, and that of

the QT interval is 0.48 second in lead V2.

P waves: The P waves are abnormal. The mean P vector (Pm) is directed +60° to the right, and 5° posteriorly. P2 is abnormal; the duration-amplitude product of the second half of the P wave is 0.07 mm-sec in lead V1, signifying a left atrial abnormality.

(Figure 11.14 continued on page 11.26.)

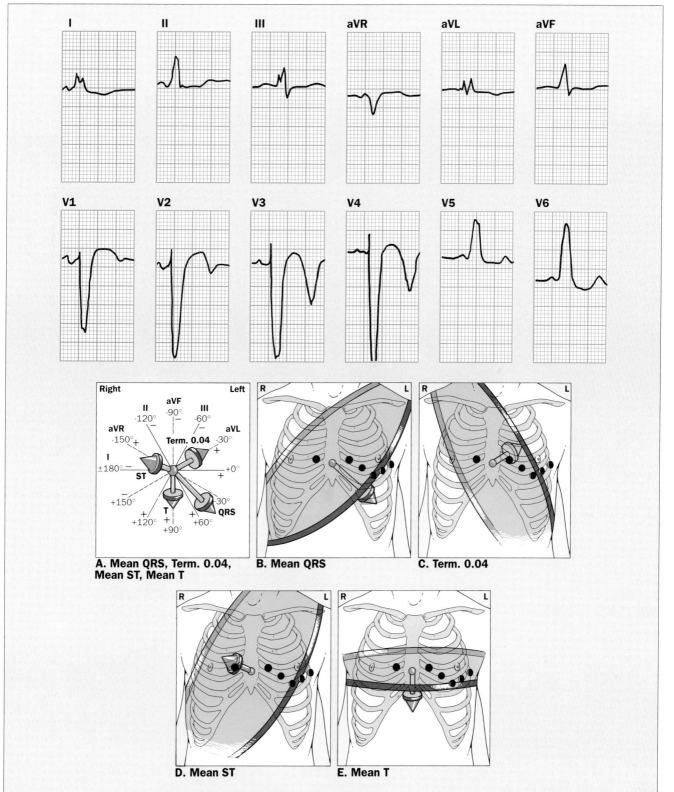

A. Mean QRS, Term. 0.04, Mean ST, Mean T

B. Mean QRS

C. Term. 0.04

D. Mean ST

E. Mean T

(Figure 11.14 continued.)

QRS complex: The duration of the QRS complex is 0.16 second. The mean QRS vector is directed about +45° inferiorly, and about 60° posteriorly. The mean terminal 0.04-second QRS vector is directed about -30° to the left, and about 45° posteriorly, signifying left bundle branch block. Myocyte damage is undoubtedly present in addition to the conduction abnormality.

ST segment: The mean ST segment vector is directed -160° to the left, and about 70° anteriorly; it is not parallel with the mean T vector, as it should be in uncomplicated bundle branch block. It is directed toward an area of anterior epicardial injury.

T waves: The mean T vector is directed +90° to the right, and about 45° posterior-ly. It is directed at least 115° posterior to the mean ST vector, away from an area of epicardial ischemia. It represents a primary T wave abnormality. Note that the T waves are positive (upright) in leads V5 and V6, whereas the diagram indicates that they would be negative (inverted). This lack of correpondence between the actual and predicted T waves arises because the electrodes at positions V4, V5 and V6 record from the area near transitioned pathway of the mean T vector (see previous discussions).

A. The frontal plane projections of the mean QRS, mean terminal 0.04-second QRS, mean ST, and mean T vectors. **B.** The spatial orientation of the mean QRS vector. **C.** The spatial orientation of the mean terminal 0.04-second QRS vector. **D.** The spatial orientation of the mean ST vector. **E.** The spatial orientation of the mean T vector (see previous discussions).

Summary: This electrocardiogram illustrates the presence of epicardial injury and ischemia in a patient with complicated left bundle branch block. Initial QRS abnormalities due to infarction may not be identified when there is left bundle branch block, but the ST and T changes of epicardial injury and ischemia can sometimes be identified in the presence of the block. (Reproduced with permission from the publisher and author; see Figure Credits.)

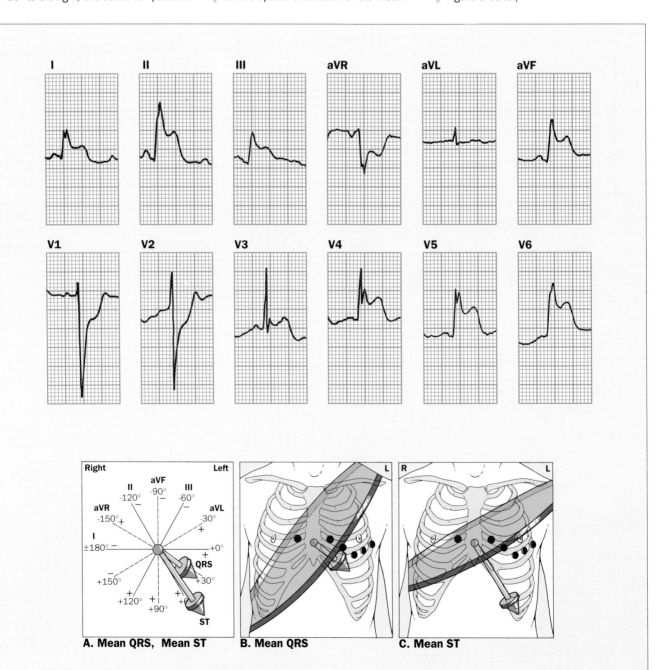

A. Mean QRS, Mean ST　　　B. Mean QRS　　　C. Mean ST

FIGURE 11.15
This electrocardiogram, showing extensive, acute apical epicardial injury associated with myocardial infarction, was recorded from a 52-year-old man. The coronary arteriogram showed 100 percent obstruction of the right coronary artery, 68 percent obstruction of the circumflex coronary artery, 50 percent occlusion of the first marginal coronary artery, and only 25 percent occlusion of the left anterior descending coronary artery, proximal to its left branch. The ejection fraction was 45 percent, and the inferior and posterolateral areas of the left ventricle were hypokinetic.

The rhythm is normal, and the heart rate is 90 complexes per minute. The PR interval is 0.12 second. The duration of the QRS complex is 0.10 second, and that of the QT interval is 0.36 second.

P waves: The P waves are normal.

QRS complex: The mean QRS vector is directed at +35° in the frontal plane and 15° posteriorly.

ST segment: The mean ST vector is huge; it is directed about +60° inferiorly, and 15° posteriorly. The vector is due to extensive epicardial injury associated with myocardial infarction. The frontal plane direction of the mean ST vector could be produced by peri-

carditis. The size of the ST segment vector and its direction both indicate epicardial injury associated with apical myocardial infarction.

T waves: The T waves are difficult to separate from the ST segment.

A. The frontal plane projections of the mean QRS and mean ST vectors. **B.** The spatial orientation of the mean QRS vector. **C.** The spatial orientation of the mean ST vector.

Summary: This electrocardiogram illustrates severe, extensive, epicardial injury associated with acute myocardial infarction. It also illustrates how the ST segment vector reflecting epicardial injury of infarction can, on rare occasions, mimic some of the features of pericarditis. Note that there are no reciprocal changes in the extremity leads in this tracing. An ST segment vector of the magnitude shown here almost never occurs with pericarditis. In this electrocardiogram, the ST segment vector is produced by apical infarction. It is most likely due to epicardial injury produced by occlusion of the circumflex and marginal coronary arteries, because the proximal portion of the left anterior descending artery revealed only 25 percent obstruction. The electrocardiographic

abnormality decreased considerably, as did the patient's chest pain, following the injection of tissue plasminogen activator (tPA).

FIGURE 11.16
This electrocardiogram, showing extensive anterolateral myocardial infarction, was recorded from a 43-year-old man who suffered angina pectoris at rest. He gave a history of previous myocardial infarction. The coronary arteriogram, performed two years later, revealed 100 percent obstruction of the midportion of the left anterior descending coronary artery, 60 percent occlusion of the first diagonal branch, 40 percent obstruction of the first marginal branch and 20 percent occlusion of the distal right coronary artery. The anterior portion of the left ventricular wall was akinetic.

The rhythm is normal, and the heart rate is 56 complexes per minute. The PR interval is 0.12 second. The duration of the QRS complex is 0.08 second, and that of the QT interval is 0.36 second.

P waves: The P waves are normal.

QRS complex: The mean QRS vector is directed about +100° inferiorly, and parallel with the frontal plane. The electrode
(Figure 11.16 continued on page 11.28.)

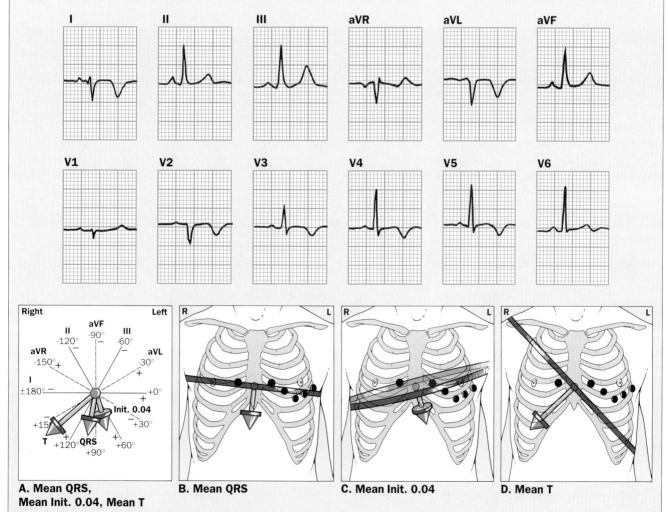

A. Mean QRS,
Mean Init. 0.04, Mean T

B. Mean QRS

C. Mean Init. 0.04

D. Mean T

(Figure 11.16 continued.)
position for lead V6 is near the transitional pathway for the mean QRS vector. Therefore, the QRS complex predicted from the diagram would be resultantly negative whereas it is actually positive in the electrocardiogram. (The cause for this lack of fit is discussed in the section entitled "Comments Regarding the Diagrams Shown in this Chapter.") This abnormal, inferior orientation is the result of an anterolateral dead zone that has removed electrical forces from that region. The mean initial 0.04-second QRS vector is directed inferiorly and posteriorly for the same reason. The mean initial 0.02-second QRS vector is directed about +100° to the right, and the mean initial 0.04-second QRS vector is directed about +80° to the right. The remainder of the QRS complex, represented as mean vector, is directed far to the right. This identifies an abnormality of the early portion of the QRS loop, because this loop is, at first, directed to the right, then less to the right, and finally far to the right.

T waves: The mean T vector is directed +140° to the right and parallel with the frontal plane. It is directed away from an area of extensive anterolateral epicardial ischemia.

A. The frontal plane projections of the mean QRS, mean initial 0.04-second QRS, and mean T vectors. **B.** The spatial orientation of the mean QRS vector. **C.** The spatial orientation of the mean initial 0.04-second QRS vector. **D.** The spatial orientation of the mean T vector.

Summary: This electrocardiogram illustrates how rightward deviation of the mean QRS vector can be produced by myocardial infarction. It also illustrates an abnormally-directed mean initial 0.02-second QRS vector in relation to the mean initial 0.04-second QRS, and the mean QRS vectors. Normally, the initial QRS loop should be directed in a clockwise manner when the mean QRS vector is vertical. Here, it is initially directed to the right (mean 0.02-second vector), then less to the right (mean 0.04-second vector), and then far to the right.

FIGURE 11.17
This electrocardiogram, showing a non-Q wave infarction, was recorded from a 50-year-old woman. The patient had angina pectoris at rest, and gave a history of previous myocardial infarction. The coronary arteriogram revealed 37 percent obstruction of the proximal portion of the left anterior descending artery, and 90 percent obstruction of the left anterior descending coronary artery after its first branch.

The rhythm is normal, and the heart rate is 75 complexes per minute. The duration of the PR interval is 0.20 second. The duration of the QRS complex is 0.07 second, and that of the QT interval is 0.36 second.

P waves: The P waves are normal.

QRS complex: The mean QRS vector is large but normally directed. It is directed +60° inferiorly and 20° posteriorly. The total 12-lead QRS amplitude is 199 mm. This suggests left ventricular hypertrophy, but other methods of examination would be needed to confirm this suspicion. The mean initial 0.04-second QRS vector is normal.

T waves: The mean T vector is directed -95° superiorly and to the left, and 5° posteriorly, away from a large area of inferior, anterior, and lateral ischemia.

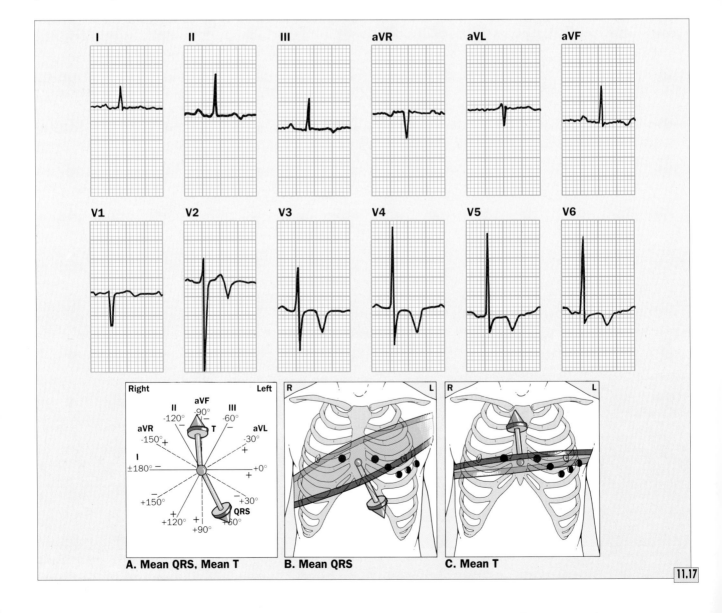

A. Mean QRS, Mean T   **B. Mean QRS**   **C. Mean T**

(Figure 11.17 continued.)
A. The frontal plane projections of the mean QRS and mean T vectors. **B**. The spatial orientation of the mean QRS vector. **C**. The spatial orientation of the mean T vector.

Summary: This electrocardiogram is abnormal owing to extensive inferior, anterior, and lateral epicardial ischemia. It illustrates a non-Q wave infarction. Formerly, some clinicians referred to this as a subendocardial infarction; this terminology is now in disrepute. It must be remembered that some Q wave infarcts are localized to the endocardium while others are actually transmural. Further, some T wave infarcts are actually transmural. It is more scientific to refer to either Q wave or non-Q wave infarcts (1).

FIGURE 11.18
This electrocardiogram, showing anteroseptal infarction and left ventricular hypertrophy, was recorded from an

(Figure 11.18 continued on page 11.30.)

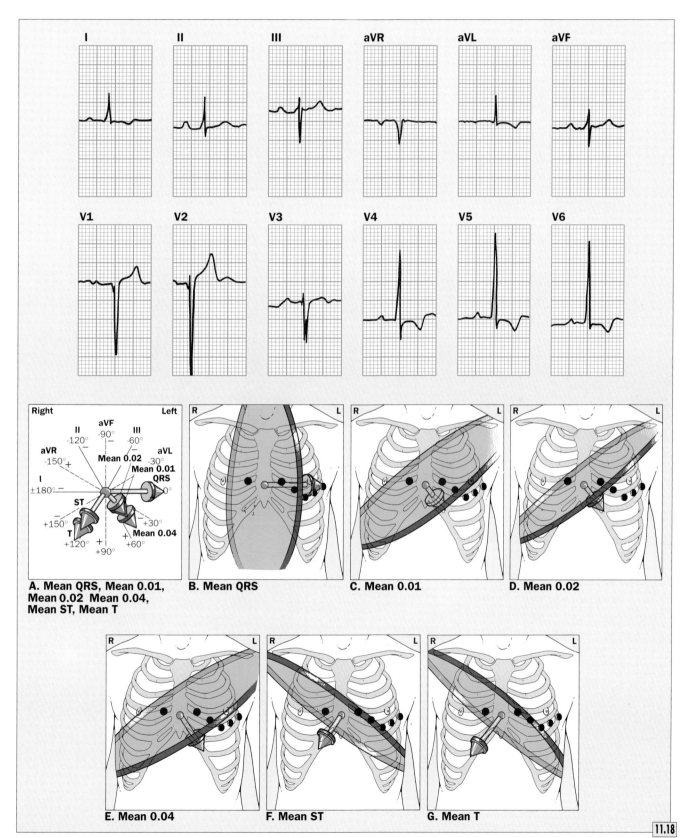

A. Mean QRS, Mean 0.01, Mean 0.02 Mean 0.04, Mean ST, Mean T

B. Mean QRS

C. Mean 0.01

D. Mean 0.02

E. Mean 0.04

F. Mean ST

G. Mean T

11.18

(Figure 11.18 continued.)
80-year-old man. The patient had congestive heart failure and experienced angina pectoris at rest. His systolic blood pressure was 170 mmHg, and his diastolic blood pressure was 60 mmHg. The coronary arteriogram revealed 90 percent obstruction of the left anterior descending coronary artery proximal to its first branch, and three lesions distal to the first branch.

They constituted 50, 40, and 30 percent reductions in luminal diameter, respectively. There was a 40 percent obstruction in the first diagonal branch, a minor lesion in the left circumflex coronary artery, and 70 percent obstruction of the first marginal coronary artery. The left ventricular diastolic pressure was 20 mmHg, and the ejection fraction was 36 percent. The anterior and apical areas of the left ventri-

cle were akinetic and the inferior wall was hypokinetic.

The heart rhythm is normal, and the heart rate is 64 complexes per minute. The duration of the PR interval is 0.20 second. The duration of the QRS complex is 0.08 second, and the duration of the QT interval is 0.35 second.

P waves: The P waves are normal.

QRS complex: The mean QRS vector is

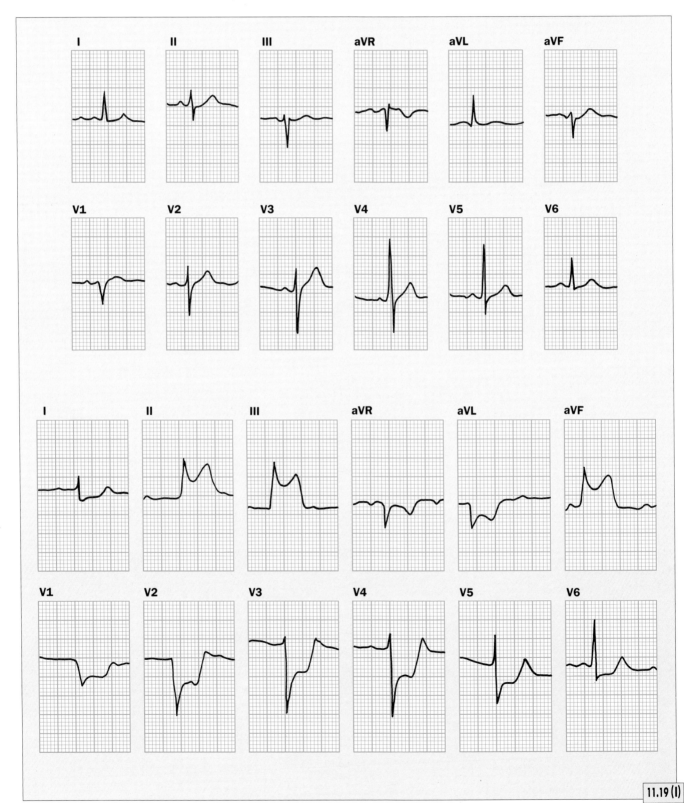

11.19 (I)

(Figure 11.18 continued.)
directed at 0° in the frontal plane and 45° to 60° posteriorly. The mean initial 0.04-second QRS vector is directed about +50° inferiorly and about 45° posteriorly. The mean initial 0.01-second QRS vector is directed about +50° inferiorly and about 45° posteriorly, but the mean initial 0.02-second vector is directed about +50° inferiorly and about 30° posteriorly. This produces a notch on the S wave in lead V1, and a small Q wave followed by an R and then an S wave in leads V2 and V3. It identifies an initial abnormality of the QRS loop, and serves to emphasize that a Q wave need not be 0.04-second wide to signify infarction. The 12-lead QRS amplitude is greater than 180 mm, suggesting the presence of left ventricular hypertrophy.

ST segment: The mean ST vector is directed +120° inferiorly and about 20° anteriorly. It is relatively parallel with the mean T vector.

T waves: The mean T vector is directed +120° inferiorly and about 20° anteriorly. The vector could be abnormal because of

systolic pressure overload of the left ventricle.

A. The frontal plane projections of the mean QRS, mean 0.01-second QRS, mean 0.02-second QRS, mean 0.04-second QRS, mean ST, and mean T vectors.
B. The spatial orientation of the mean QRS vector. **C.** The spatial orientation of the mean initial 0.01-second QRS vector. Note that it is posterior to the 0.02-second vector. **D.** The spatial orientation of the mean initial 0.02-second QRS vector; note that it is anterior to the 0.01-second vector. **E.** The spatial orientation of the mean initial 0.04-second QRS vector; note that it is posterior to the 0.02-second vector. **F.** The spatial orientation of the mean ST vector; note that it parallels the mean T vector. **G.** The spatial orientation of the mean T vector.

Summary: This electrocardiogram illustrates an anteroseptal myocardial infarction associated with left ventricular hypertrophy due to systolic pressure overload of the left ventricle secondary to hypertension. The direction of the initial 0.01-sec-

ond QRS vector and its relationship to the mean initial 0.02-second and mean initial 0.04-second QRS vectors signify anteroseptal infarction. This creates the slur in the initial part of the S wave in lead V1, and the small Q wave followed by an R wave in leads V2 and V3. The directions of the mean ST and T vectors indicate left ventricular hypertrophy, but epicardial ischemia may play a role. First degree atrioventricular block is present.

FIGURE 11.19 (I AND II)
These electrocardiograms were recorded from a 59-year-old male with Prinzmetal angina pectoris, who was experiencing repeated anterior chest discomfort at rest.

I. The top electrocardiogram was recorded at 10 am; the patient was having no chest pain at the time. The bottom electrocardiogram was recorded at 5 pm during an episode of chest pain. Note the high degree of atrioventricular block, and marked ST segment displacement.

(Figure 11.19 continued on page 11.32.)

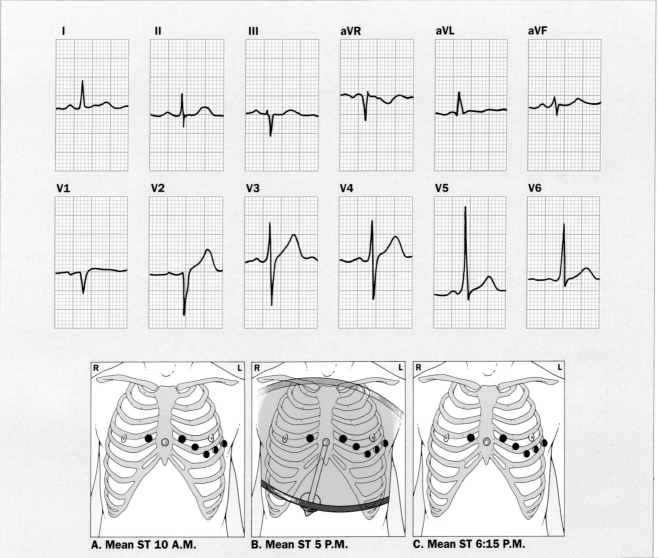

A. Mean ST 10 A.M.   B. Mean ST 5 P.M.   C. Mean ST 6:15 P.M.

(Figure 11.19 continued.)
The mean ST vector is directed inferiorly and posteriorly.

II.This electrocardiogram was recorded at 6:15 pm the same day. It is similar to the one recorded at 9 am.

Parts **A-C** illustrate the appearance (or absence) of the mean ST vector at 10 am, 5 pm, and 6:15 pm. Note that no ST vector was present at 10 am and 6:15.

Summary: Coronary arteriography revealed a discrete lesion (95 percent obstruction) in the right coronary artery. This series of electrocardiograms illustrate a patient with obstructive coronary disease who also had coronary artery spasm. (Reproduced with permission from the publisher and author; See Figure Credits).

FIGURE 11.20
This electrocardiogram, illustrating an example of pseudoinfarction, was recorded from a 31-year-old man with Friedreich's ataxia.

An atrial ectopic rhythm is present; the atrial rate is about 210 depolarizations per minute, and 2:1 atrioventricular block is also present. The ventricular rate is 105 depolarizations per minute, the duration of the QRS complex is 0.08 second, and the duration of the QT interval is 0.34 second.

TABLE 11.3 ELECTROCARDIOGRAPHIC ABNORMALITIES OF PSEUDOINFARCTION THAT MUST BE DIFFERENTIATED FROM THOSE OF MYOCARDIAL ISCHEMIA, INJURY, AND DEAD ZONE

The electrocardiographic abnormalities associated with the conditions listed below cannot always be distinguished from those of true infarction. The entire clinical picture may enable the physician to identify pseudoinfarction, but patients with electrocardiographic signs of pseudoinfarction may also have true infarctions. For example, a patient with the Wolff-Parkinson-White syndrome, a condition in which the electrocardiographic abnormalities mimic those of infarction, may actually have a myocardial infarction.

T wave abnormalities:

- T wave abnormalities due to pericarditis may simulate those of epicardial myocardial ischemia. However, the mean T vector of pericarditis points away from the centroid of epicardial damage, whereas the mean T vector of epicardial myocardial ischemia is directed away from a localized area of ischemia (see Chapter 10).
- Subarachnoid hemorrhage or brain tumor may produce large, broad T waves which, when represented as a mean vector, are directed away from the mean QRS vector. There is no way to distinguish this abnormality from myocardial ischemia other than to recognize its possibility in the appropriate clinical setting.
- In cases of pulmonary embolism, the mean T vector may be directed posteriorly. In such cases, there is no way to distinguish the electrocardiographic abnormality from that of a non-Q wave anterior infarction. The mean T vector may shift to the left in patients with acute pulmonary embolism; this produces an inverted T wave in leads II, III, and aVF, suggesting inferior infarction. The clinical setting may or may not help, and other techniques are often needed to establish the diagnosis.
- The T wave abnormality associated with hypertrophic cardiomyopathy may simulate the mean T vector of epicardial ischemia due to hypoxia. The T wave abnormalities of hypertrophic cardiomyopathy do not change over time, as they frequently do in cases of *acute* myocardial ischemia. The T wave abnormality caused by *chronic* ischemia may not change. Accordingly, there may be no specific way to distinguish the T wave abnormalities of hypertrophic cardiomyopathy from those of chronic myocardial ischemia.

ST segment abnormalities:

- Pericarditis may simulate epicardial myocardial injury electrocardiographically. However, the ST segment vector of pericarditis is directed toward the cardiac apex, whereas the ST segment vector of epicardial injury is usually directed toward a localized segment of the left ventricular wall (see Chapter 10).
- The abnormal ST segment vector associated with hypertrophic cardiomyopathy may simulate the ST segment vector of epicar-

dial injury due to hypoxia. However, the abnormal ST segment vector of the former is persistent, whereas in the latter, except when the abnormality is due to a ventricular aneurysm, it usually evolves toward normal (see Chapter 9).

The mean initial 0.04-second QRS abnormalities of pseudoinfarction may be caused by several different conditions including:

- Systolic pressure overload of the left ventricle, which may produce a posterior rotation of the QRS loop resulting in the absence of R waves in leads V1, V2, and V3. This abnormality cannot always be distinguished from septal infarction.
- Diastolic pressure overload of the left ventricle, which may produce large Q waves in leads I, aVL, V4, V5, and V6. Without the use of other procedures, these abnormalities cannot be consistently distinguished from those due to lateral myocardial infarction.
- Acute myocarditis, in which abnormal Q waves may occur.
- Dilated cardiomyopathy in which Q wave abnormalities suggesting myocardial infarction can occur. Without using other procedures, there is no way to consistently distinguish these Q waves from those due to myocardial infarction.
- Hypertrophic cardiomyopathy, in which abnormal Q waves commonly occur. Without the use of other procedures, there is no way to consistently distinguish the abnormal Q waves associated with this condition from those of infarction.
- Restrictive cardiomyopathy. Abnormal Q waves are especially likely when the cardiomyopathy is due to amyloid. Without using other procedures, there is no way for a clinician to consistently distinguish these abnormal Q waves from those associated with myocardial infarction.
- Pre-excitation of the ventricles, as in the Wolff-Parkinson-White syndrome, may produce abnormal Q waves. Other electrocardiographic features of this condition, such as the short PR interval and the delta wave, serve to alert the clinician to the true diagnosis. Remember, however that such patients may also have myocardial infarction.
- Neoplastic disease, sarcoid, and other conditions all of which can produce abnormal Q waves that mimic those associated with myocardial infarction.
- Acute pulmonary embolism, which may produce abnormal Q waves. This condition may produce initial QRS forces that are shifted to the left, generating new Q waves in leads II, III, and aVF, and terminal QRS forces that are shifted to the right. Only by assessing the total clinical picture is it possible to distinguish these abnormal Q waves from those due to myocardial infarction.
- Complex congenital heart disease, in which abnormal Q waves may simulate those of myocardial infarction.

Note: All of the QRS complex, ST segment, and T wave abnormalities described above may occur in the same patient, producing the electrocardiographic condition known as pseudoinfarction.

(Figure 11.20 continued.)

P waves: The shape of the P waves is abnormal; note the tall, narrow, sharp P waves in lead V1. This is probably due to an unusual atrial conduction defect.

QRS complex: Although the QRS duration is only 0.08 second, there is evidence of a peculiar conduction defect within the ventricles. The mean QRS vector is directed -120° superiorly, and parallel with the frontal plane. The mean initial 0.04-second QRS vector is directed so that Q waves are recorded in leads I, II, III, and aVF. This could lead an observer to consider an inferior and lateral infarction. The mean terminal 0.04-second QRS vector is also directed about -120° superiorly, and more than 15° to 20° posteriorly.

The exact type of conduction defect in this case cannot be determined. It is likely that the left anterior-superior division is involved, but diseases of the heart muscle responsible for the initial 0.04 second of the QRS complex may play a role. The 12-lead QRS amplitude is 69 mm, indicating a low QRS voltage.

T waves: It is difficult to determine the direction of the mean T vector because the P waves interrupt them. The vector seems to be directed slightly anteriorly.

A. The frontal plane projections of the *(Figure 11.20 continued on page 11.34.)*

TABLE 11.4 CAUSES OF PSEUDOINFARCTION OF THE MYOCARDIUM

- Pericarditis
- Myocarditis
- Subarachnoid hemorrhage (and other acute cerebral diseases)
- Left ventricular hypertrophy (diastolic and systolic pressure overload).
- Dilated cardiomyopathy
- Hypertrophic cardiomyopathy

- Restrictive cardiomyopathy (such as from amyloid)
- Pre-excitation of the ventricles
- Pulmonary embolism
- Neoplastic disease of the ventricles
- Sarcoid of the left ventricle
- Complex congenital heart diseases

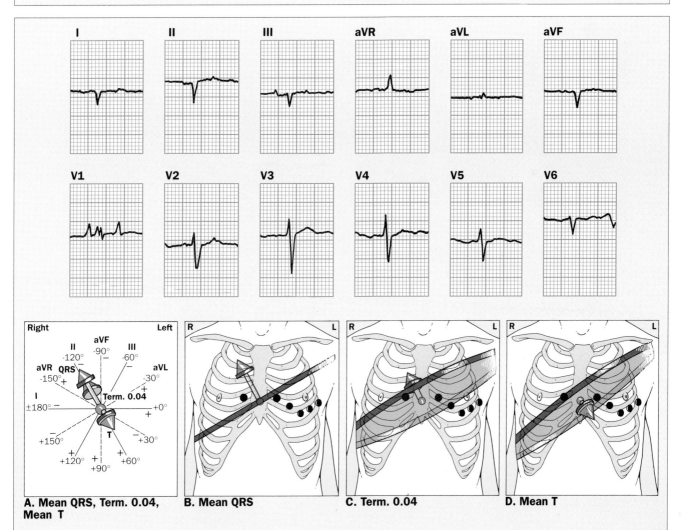

A. Mean QRS, Term. 0.04, Mean T

B. Mean QRS

C. Term. 0.04

D. Mean T

11.20

(Figure 11.20 continued.)
mean QRS, mean terminal 0.04-second QRS, and mean T vectors. **B**. The spatial orientation of the mean QRS vector. **C**. The spatial orientation of the mean terminal 0.04-second QRS vector. **D**. The spatial orientation of the mean T vector.

Summary: This electrocardiogram exhibits peculiar P waves and peculiar QRS complexes due to the cardiomyopathy associated with Friedreich's ataxia. In this condition, the cardiac conduction system and myocytes are involved; note the extremely low QRS voltage. These ventricular abnormalities can produce an electrocardiogram that mimics that of myocardial infarction; hence the term "pseudoinfarction." Patients with dilated, hypertrophic, or restrictive cardiomyopathy may have electrocardiograms that exhibit pseudoinfarction.

FIGURE 11.21

This electrocardiogram, recorded from a 43-year-old man, illustrates a pseudoinfarction due to sarcoid of the heart. The patient had recurrent episodes of refractory ventricular tachycardia for which an internal defibrillator was installed.

The heart rhythm is normal and the heart rate is 63 complexes per minute. The PR interval is 0.16 second. The duration of the QRS complex is 0.11 second, and that of the QT interval is 0.40 second.

P waves: The P waves are abnormal. In lead I, they are notched, and their duration is 0.12 second. The second half of the P wave vector (P2),representing left atrial depolarization, is directed about +30° inferiorly and about 30° posteriorly. Note that the second half of the P wave is isoelectric in lead III. The amplitude-duration product of last half of the P wave in V1 is greater than -0.03 mm-sec. These abnormalities suggest a left atrial abnormality.

QRS complex: The mean QRS vector is directed about +20° to 30° inferiorly, and about 40° posteriorly. The mean initial 0.02-second QRS vector is directed +180° to the right, and 30° anteriorly. The mean initial 0.03-second QRS vector is directed about +130° to the right, and about 40° anteriorly. The "Q waves" seen in leads I, II, aVL, V4, V5, and V6 suggest lateral myocardial infarction.

T waves: The mean T vector is directed -115° to -120° superiorly, and about 20° anteriorly. The vector is abnormal, suggesting lateral or generalized epicardial ischemia.

A. The frontal plane projections of the mean QRS, mean 0.02-second QRS, mean 0.03-second QRS, and mean T vectors. **B**. The spatial orientation of the mean QRS vector. **C**. The spatial orientation of the mean initial 0.03-second QRS vector. **D**. The spatial orientation of the mean T vector.

Summary: This tracing shows a pseudoinfarction due to sarcoid involving the myocardium. Certain neoplastic diseases, amyloid deposits, and many of the connective tissue diseases that involve the heart may produce abnormalities of pseudoinfarction in the electrocardiogram. Some of these diseases, such as amyloid and collagen diseases, may also involve the coronary arteries, and when they do, they may cause obstructive coronary disease and atrial myocardial infarction.

FIGURE 11.22

This tracing, showing the electrocardiographic abnormalities of the Wolff-Parkinson-White syndrome and atrial fibrillation (see diagram F), was recorded from a 35-year-old man. The abnormalities

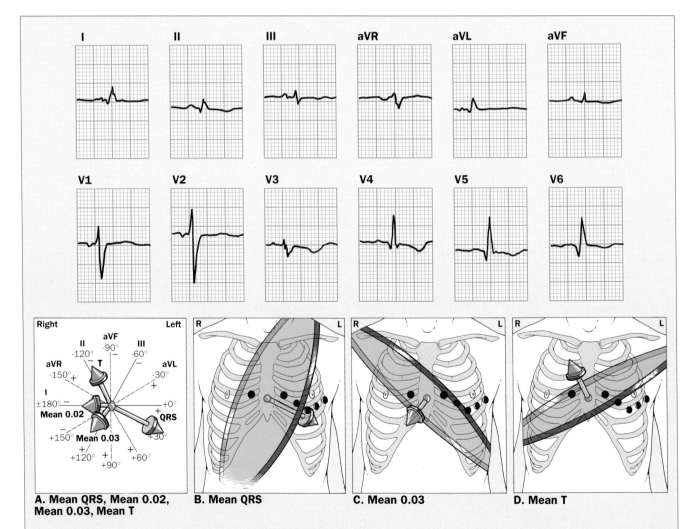

A. Mean QRS, Mean 0.02, Mean 0.03, Mean T   **B. Mean QRS**   **C. Mean 0.03**   **D. Mean T**

(Figure 11.22 continued.)
simulate myocardial infarction, and represent another common cause of pseudoinfarction.

The rhythm is normal in the 12-lead tracing, and the heart rate is 60 complexes per minute. The PR interval is about 0.12 second. The duration of the PR interval appears to be 0.16 second in some leads, but this is an illusion, because the the electrical forces seen during the early part of the QRS complex are isoelectric in those leads. Note that the QRS complex appears to be about 0.10 second in lead II. However, when simultaneous leads are studied, it is apparent that the early QRS forces are perpendicular to lead axis II, producing a PR interval that falsely appears to be at least 0.16 second. The duration of the QRS complex is 0.14

(Figure 11.22 continued on page 11.36.)

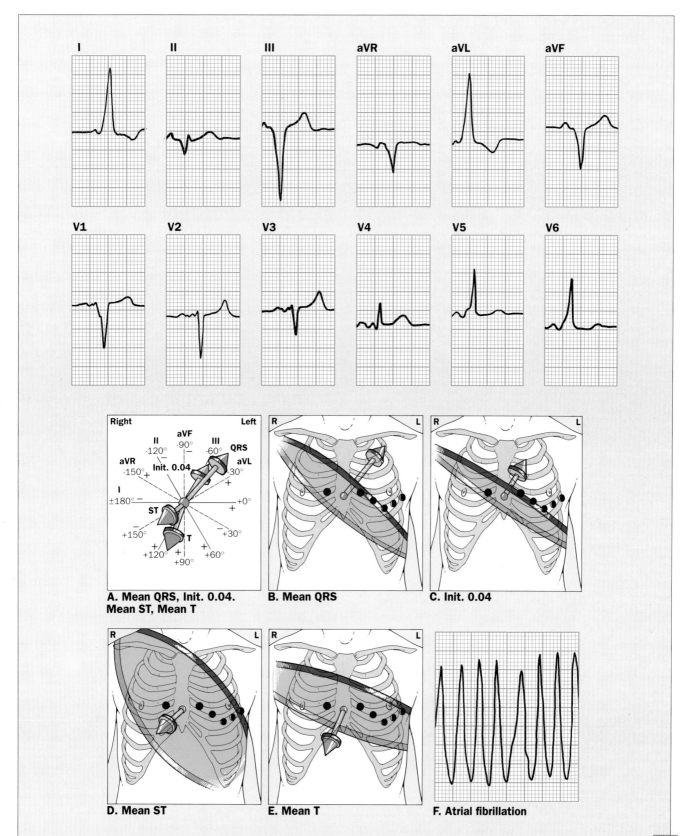

A. Mean QRS, Init. 0.04.
Mean ST, Mean T

B. Mean QRS

C. Init. 0.04

D. Mean ST

E. Mean T

F. Atrial fibrillation

11.22

(Figure 11.22 continued.)
second, and that of the QT interval is 0.48 second.

P waves: The P waves are normal, and the PR interval is short. Atrial fibrillation with a rapid ventricular rate is shown in diagram F.

QRS complex: The mean QRS vector is directed about -50° to the left, and about 20° posteriorly. The mean initial 0.04-second QRS vector is directed -60° to the left and about 10° posteriorly, simulating the abnormality due to inferior infarction. Note the slurring of the initial portion of the QRS complexes; this is a classic delta wave. The delta wave is best seen in leads V1, V5, and V6.

ST segment: The direction of the mean ST segment vector is about +145° inferiorly, and about 80° anteriorly.

T waves: The direction of the mean T vector is about +110° inferiorly and about 60° anteriorly.

A. The frontal plane projections of the mean QRS, mean initial 0.04-second QRS, mean ST, and mean T vectors. **B.** The spatial orientation of the mean QRS vector. **C.** The spatial orientation of the mean initial 0.04-second QRS vector. **D.** The spatial orientation of the mean ST vector. **E.** The spatial orientation of the mean T vector. **F.** This electrocardiogram was recorded during an episode of tachycardia. It shows atrial fibrillation with a high ventricular rate.

Summary: The short PR interval (0.12 second) and the delta waves are characteristic of pre-excitation of the ventricles in a patient with the Wolff-Parkinson-White syndrome. The duration of the QRS complex in this patient is 0.14 second and also simulates left bundle branch block. However, the short PR interval and delta wave distinguish this type of electrocardiogram from one showing true left bundle branch block.

The QRS duration may be as short as 0.10 second or as long as 0.18 second in patients with pre-excitation of the ventricles. In these cases, electrocardiograms may simulate anterior or inferior

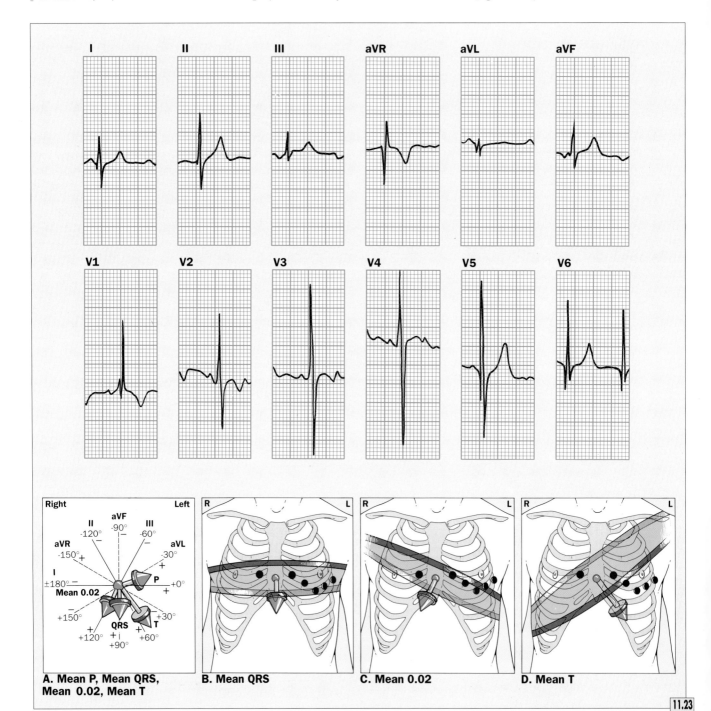

A. Mean P, Mean QRS, Mean 0.02, Mean T   **B. Mean QRS**   **C. Mean 0.02**   **D. Mean T**

11.23

(Figure 11.22 continued.)
infarction. There is usually no other evidence of heart disease in patients with the Wolff-Parkinson-White syndrome, but the clinician is obligated to search for idiopathic ventricular hypertrophy, Ebstein's anomaly, and atrial septal defect, since these conditions occur with greater than average frequency in such patients.

When atrial fibrillation occurs in a patient with a bypass tract, the ventricular rate may reach 220-280 complexes per minute.

FIGURE 11.23

This electrocardiogram shows a pseudoinfarction as well as right and left ventricular hypertrophy. The tracing was recorded from a 7-year-old boy with a large aortic septal defect.

The rhythm is abnormal owing to lower atrial rhythm. Note that the mean P vector is directed -20° to the left and about 30° anteriorly. The heart rate is 110 complexes per minute. The PR interval is 0.12 second. The duration of the QRS complex is 0.08 second, and the duration of the QT interval is 0.36 second.

P waves: The mean P vector (Pm) is directed -20° to the left, and 30° anteriorly. The depolarization of the atria is abnormal because of an ectopic atrial rhythm.

QRS complex: The mean QRS vector is directed about +90° inferiorly, and about 30° anteriorly. The QRS complexes recorded from leads V5 and V6 are from the area near the transitional pathway in this seven-year-old child (see previous discussions). The QRS amplitude is large; the QRS complexes are almost off the electrocardiographic paper in leads V3 and V4. Their direction and magnitude suggest right and left ventricular hypertrophy. The initial 0.02-second vector is large; it is directed about +120° inferiorly in the frontal plane, and 20° anteriorly. The size of this vector might be interpreted as being due to myocardial infarction.

T waves: The mean T vector is directed +50° inferiorly, and about 15° posteriorly.

A. The frontal plane projections of the mean P, mean QRS, mean initial 0.02-second QRS, and mean T vectors.
B. The spatial orientation of the mean QRS vector. **C.** The spatial orientation of the mean initial 0.02-second QRS vector. **D.** The spatial orientation of the mean T vector.

Summary: This patient with congenital heart disease had a large left-to-right shunt through an aortic septal defect. Diastolic pressure overload of both the left and right ventricles was undoubtedly present. The tracing shows an atrial ectopic rhythm and suggests left and right ventricular hypertrophy and lateral infarction (thought this is not present). This is a good example of the many types of congenital heart disease that exhibit pseudoinfarction on the electrocardiogram. (Reproduced with permission from the publisher and author; see Figure Credits.)

REFERENCES

1. Antaloczy Z, Barcsak J, Magyar E: Correlation of electrocardiologic and pathologic findings in 100 cases of Q wave and non-Q wave myocardial infarction. *J Electrocardiol* 1988; 21(4):331.
2. Hurst JW: Coronary spasm as viewed by Wilson and Johnston in 1941. *Am J Cardiol* 1988; 57:1000.
3. Prinzmetal M, Kennamer R, Merlis R, et al: Angina pectoris. I. A variant form of angina pectoris. *Am J Med* 1959; 27:375.
4. Hurst JW, Pollak SJ, Brown CL, Lutz JF: Electrocardiographic signs suggesting inferior infarction associated with angiographic evidence of obstruction of the left anterior descending coronary artery or its branches. *Emory Univ J Med* 1988; 2(3):170.

FIGURE CREDITS

Figure 11.1 From Hurst JW, Woodson GC Jr: *Atlas of Spatial Vector Electrocardiography*. New York: Blakiston, 1952, p. 123.

Figure 11.13 From Hurst JW, Woodson GC Jr: *Atlas of Spatial Vector Electrocardiography*. New York: Blakiston, 1952, p. 149.

Figure 11.14 From Hurst JW, Woodson GC Jr: *Atlas of Spatial Vector Electrocardiography*. New York: Blakiston, 1952, p. 181.

Figure 11.19 I and II From Hurst JW, King III SB, Walter PF, Friesinger GC, Edwards JE: Atherosclerotic coronary heart disease: angina pectoris, myocardial infarction, and other manifestations of myocardial ischemia, in Hurst JW (ed): *The Heart* Ed. 5. New York: McGraw-Hill, 1982, p. 1090. The electrocardiogram was originally provided by Dr. Joel Felner.

Figure 11.23 From Cabrera E, Estes EH, Hellerstein HK: Case 40 in Hurst JW, Wenger NK (eds.): *Electrocardiographic Interpretation*. New York: McGraw-Hill., 1963, p. 217.

CHAPTER TWELVE

The Effects of Digitalis and Other Drugs

THE EFFECTS OF DIGITALIS

Digitalis medication may produce prolongation of the PR interval, atrial arrhythmias, ventricular arrhythmias, and higher grades of atrioventricular block. Hypokalemia and hypomagnesemia may precipitate the arrhythmias, especially atrial tachycardia with a 2:1 atrioventricular block, when digitalis blood levels are within an acceptable range. This chapter emphasizes the effect of digitalis on the ventricular electrocardiogram. The mechanisms responsible for the rather unique electrocardiographic abnormalities seen with digitalis medication is discussed in Chapter 6.

The electrocardiographic characteristics of the effects of digitalis medication are listed in Table 12.1. The electrocardiographic abnormalities that must be differentiated from these are listed in Table 12.2. Examples of its effects on the electrocardiogram are shown in Figures 12.1 through 12.4.

THE EFFECTS OF OTHER DRUGS

Certain antidepressant drugs, most antiarrhythmic drugs, the beta blockers, and calcium antagonists are known to alter the electrocardiogram. The alteration is not specific, but can often be recognized if the clinician correlates the electrocardiographic features present prior to giving the drug with those that develop after the drug has been administered.

TRICYCLIC ANTIDEPRESSANTS AND PHENOTHIAZINE

The abnormalities produced by tricyclic antidepressant and phenothiazine medications are: rhythm disturbances including sinus bradycardia, sinus arrest, sinoatrial block, ventricular tachycardia, ventricular fibrillation, atrioventricular block, prolongation of the QT interval, prolongation of the QRS complex, bundle branch block, ST segment displacement, primary T wave abnormalities, and a prominent U wave.

ANTIARRHYTHMIC DRUGS

Almost all antiarrhythmic drugs are potentially proarrhythmic; many produce serious conduction disturbances and T wave abnormalities.

QUINIDINE: The electrocardiographic abnormalities produced by quinidine are: rhythm disturbances, including sinus arrest, atrioventricular block, and ventricular arrhythmias; prolongation of the QT interval; ventricular conduction defects; primary T wave abnormalities; and prominent U waves. These abnormalities are more likely to occur with large or toxic doses of the drug.

PROCAINAMIDE AND DISOPYRAMIDE: The electrocardiographic abnormalities produced by procainamide are similar to those produced by quinidine.

Disopyramide also produces most of electrocardiographic changes that occur with quinidine.

LIDOCAINE: Lidocaine may produce sinus arrest and atrioventricular block. As a rule, however, average doses produce no electrocardiographic abnormalities.

TOCAINIDE: This drug usually has little effect on the electrocardiogram, but primary T wave abnormalities can occur. As with many antiarrhythmic drugs, ventricular arrhythmia may develop.

MEXELETINE: Mexeletine may produce sinus arrest, junctional rhythm, and atrioventricular block. Theoretically, ventricular arrhythmia can occur.

AMIODARONE: Amiodarone may increase the length of the QT interval.

BETA-BLOCKING DRUGS: The beta-blocking drugs produce sinus bradycardia and atrioventricular block. The latter is more likely to occur when the patient is also receiving digitalis or verapamil. The "brady-tachy" syndrome may especially be precipitated in elderly patients, who may already have a "sick sinus" or "sick atrioventricular node."

CALCIUM ANTAGONISTS: Nifedipine does not produce electrocardiographic abnormalities. Diltiazem may produce slight bradycardia and may have a minor effect on atrioventricular conduction. Verapamil, however, may have considerable effect on the sinus node, producing sinus bradycardia. The drug also slows conduction in the atrioventricular node, producing a long PR interval and higher grades of atrioventricular block. These electrocardiographic abnormalities are more likely to occur when the patient is receiving digitalis or a beta-blocking drug.

TABLE 12.1 EFFECTS OF DIGITALIS ON THE ELECTROCARDIOGRAM

- Occasionally increases the length of the PR interval.
- Can produce atrial arrhythmias, ventricular arrhythmias, and higher grades of atrioventricular block.
- Does not alter the magnitude or direction of the mean QRS vector.
- May decrease the magnitude of the mean T vector without changing its direction or altering the PR or QT intervals.
- Commonly shortens the QT interval to 0.32—0.36 second. This is associated with an early T vector (seen during the ST segment), referred to in practice as an ST segment vector. This is usually directed opposite the mean QRS vector. There is, at the same time, a decrease in the magnitude, but no change in the direction of the late T vector.
- The U wave may become larger while the late T wave is becoming smaller.
- May be responsible for a false-positive exercise test for myocardial ischemia.
- May increase the ST-T abnormality of left ventricular hypertrophy.

F I G U R E   1 2 . 1
This normal electrocardiogram was recorded from a 29-year-old subject before digitalis was administered. The PR interval is 0.16 second and the QT interval is 0.36 second. **A.** The frontal plane projections of the mean QRS and T vectors. **B.** The spatial orientation of the mean QRS vector. This vector is almost parallel with lead II, but slightly positive in lead III. The transitional pathway on the chest courses between leads V3 and V4. **C.** The spatial orientation of the mean T vector. The T wave is isoelectric to lead aVF, and the mean T vector is perpendicular to this lead. The transitional pathway passes through lead V1 because the T wave is slightly positive in this lead. (Reproduced with permission from the publisher and author; see Figure Credits.)

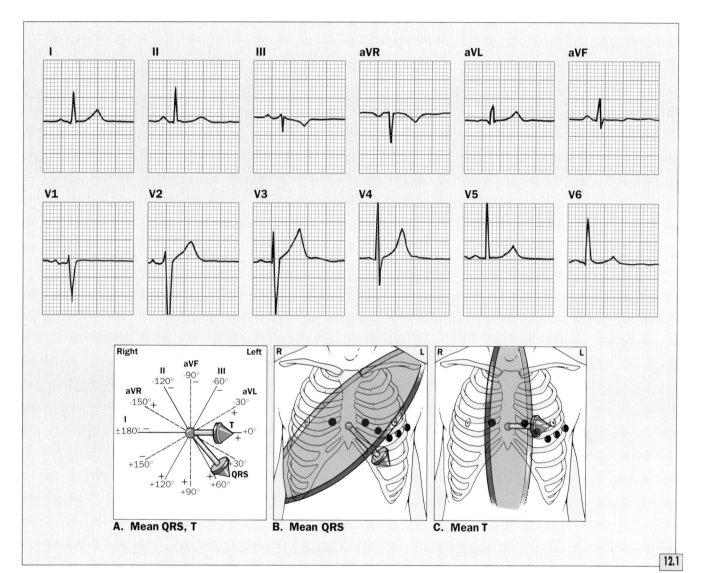

A. Mean QRS, T   B. Mean QRS   C. Mean T

12.1

TABLE 12.2 ELECTROCARDIOGRAPHIC ABNORMALITIES THAT MUST BE DIFFERENTIATED FROM THOSE DUE TO DIGITALIS MEDICATION

Subendocardial injury due to hypoxia may produce ST-T abnormalities similar to those of digitalis medication. Useful clues that assist in the separation of the two conditions are listed below:

- If the ST-T wave abnormalities as described in Table 12.1 are associated with a short QT interval (0.32 to 0.34 second), and the heart rate is within the normal range, the electrocardiographic abnormalities are probably due to digitalis.

- If ST-T abnormalities are present but the QT interval is normal, a digitalis effect could be considered as a possible cause, but is less likely than when the QT interval is short.

- If the heart rate is rapid and the QT interval is normal or short, the ST-T abnormalites may be due to digitalis, subendocardial injury, or both.

- When the heart rate is rapid, ST-T abnormalities are present, and the QT interval is long, subendocardial injury is likely.

- If an ST segment vector is directed opposite the mean QRS vector but the mean T vector is large and the QT interval is normal, the abnormality is most likely due to subendocardial injury rather than digitalis medication.

FIGURE 12.2

This electrocardiogram was recorded from the same subject described in Fig. 12.1, after he was given 2 mg of digoxin over a period of 24 hours. The PR interval is 0.16 second and the QT interval is 0.35 second. **A.** The frontal plane projections of the mean QRS and mean T vectors. Note that the mean QRS vector has not changed in direction or magnitude. The direction of the late T vector has not changed significantly, but its magnitude has decreased considerably. Note that the U wave is a little more prominent in lead V4 than in the previous electrocardiogram. **B.** The spatial orientation of the mean QRS vector. **C.** The spatial orientation of the new ST vector. Owing to early repolarization, it is actually occurring immediately after depolarization is complete. **D.** The spatial orientation of the mean late T vector. Note that it has decreased in size, but its direction has not changed significantly from that shown in Fig. 12.1. (Reproduced with permission from the publisher and author; see Figure Credits.)

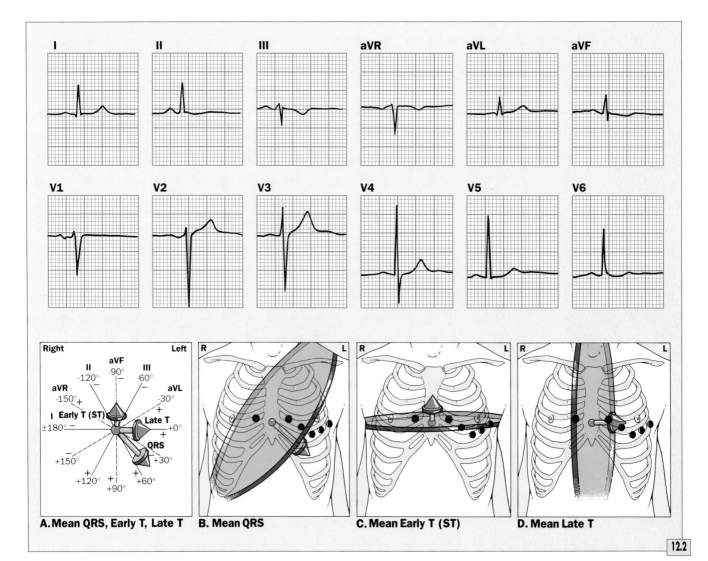

A. Mean QRS, Early T, Late T   B. Mean QRS   C. Mean Early T (ST)   D. Mean Late T

12.2

FIGURE 12.3

This electrocardiogram was recorded from a 72-year-old man with hypertension. It was made prior to the administration of digitalis. The PR interval is 0.16 second and the QT interval is 0.40 second. Note the presence of U waves. **A**. The frontal plane projections of the mean QRS and T vectors. The QRS complex is slightly positive in lead aVF.

Accordingly, the mean QRS vector is almost perpendicular to lead aVF. The direction and magnitude of the QRS vector is normal. The mean T vector is barely visible in lead aVL; it is almost perpendicular to this lead. **B.** The spatial orientation of the mean QRS vector. The transitional pathway courses between leads V3 and V4. **C.** The spatial orientation of the mean T vector.

The transitional pathway is not apparent because all of the T waves are upright in the precordial leads. The larger T wave in lead V6 as compared to lead V1 suggests that the mean T vector is directed anteriorly by less than 45°. This electrocardiogram shows no definite abnormality. (Reproduced with permission from the publisher and author; see Figure Credits.)

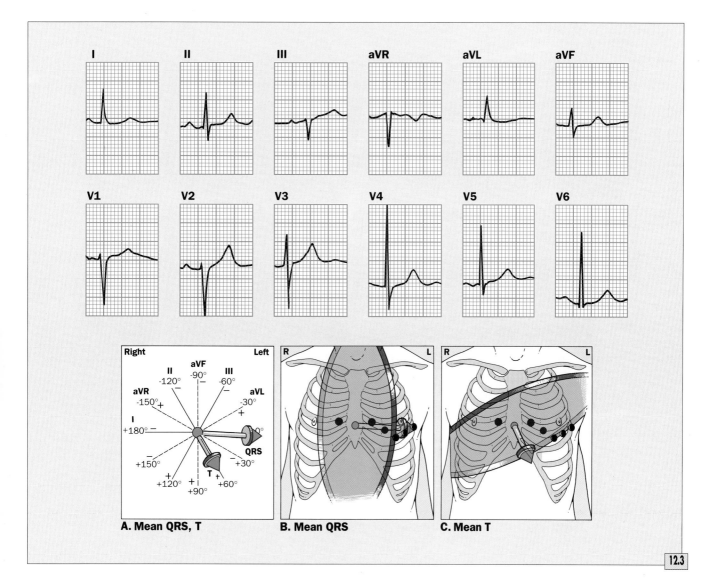

A. Mean QRS, T   B. Mean QRS   C. Mean T

12.3

FIGURE 12.4

This electrocardiogram was recorded from the same 72-year-old patient in Fig. 12.3. The tracing shown here was recorded after digitalis was administered. The PR interval is 0.20 second and the QT interval is about 0.28 second. Note the difference in these measurements as compared to those in Fig. 12.3. **A.** The frontal plane projections of the mean QRS and the early T (ST) vector. The mean QRS vector is slightly negative in lead aVF. Accordingly, the mean QRS vector is amost perpendicular to this lead. The early T vector (seen during the ST segment) is large, isoelectric in lead aVF and negative in lead I. Accordingly, it is directed to the right and is perpendicular to lead aVF. The late T vector is difficult to plot because the T wave is small. It is not possible to determine when it begins and ends. **B.** The spatial orientation of the mean QRS vector. The transitional pathway courses between leads V3 and V4. Note that the size and direction of the vector have not changed significantly from those shown in Fig. 12.3B. **C.** The early ST segment change. In reality, this is due to repolarization and should be referred to as an early T change. The transitional pathway courses through lead V2. The mean ST vector is in an opposite direction from the mean QRS vector.

The spatial orientation of the late T vector cannot be calculated because it cannot be identified.

Summary: This electrocardiogram shows the expected changes in the PR interval, QT interval, early T (ST) vector, and late T vector due to digitalis medication. When these potential changes are remembered, it is often possible to anticipate what will occur when digitalis is given to a patient. It may require less digitalis to alter the ST-T segments of a patient with a condition such as hypertension or aortic valve disease than in an individual with a normal left ventricle. (Reproduced with permission from the publisher and author; see Figure Credits.)

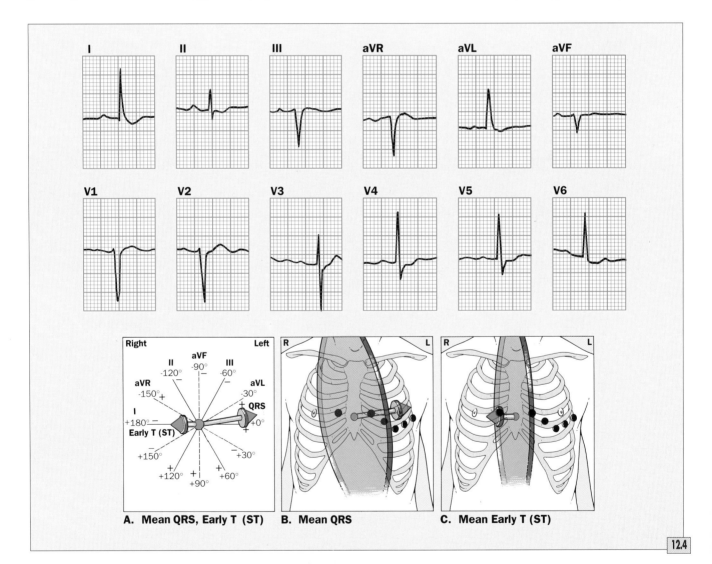

A. Mean QRS, Early T (ST)   B. Mean QRS   C. Mean Early T (ST)

12.4

FIGURE CREDITS

Figure 12.1 From Hurst JW, Woodson GC Jr: *Atlas of Spatial Vector Electrocardiography*. New York, Blakiston Co., 1952, p 189.

Figure 12.2 From Hurst JW, Woodson GC Jr: *Atlas of Spatial Vector Electrocardiography*. New York, Blakiston Co., 1952, p 191.

Figure 12.3 From Hurst JW, Woodson GC Jr: *Atlas of Spatial Vector Electrocardiography*. New York, Blakiston Co., 1952, p 193.

Figure 12.4 From Hurst JW, Woodson GC Jr: *Atlas of Spatial Vector Electrocardiography*. New York, Blakiston Co., 1952, p 195.

CHAPTER THIRTEEN

OTHER IMPORTANT CONDITIONS

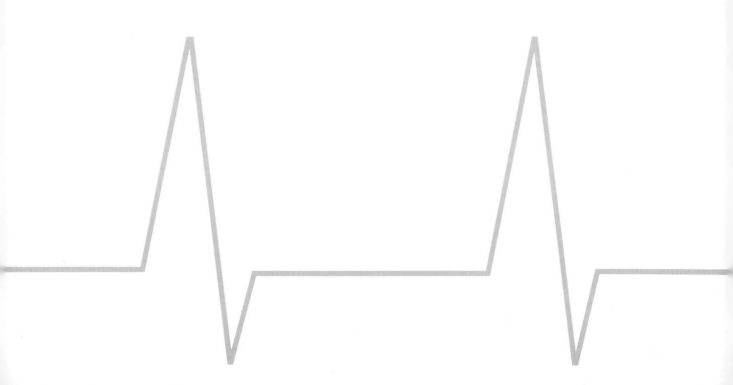

COR PULMONALE WITH EMPHYSEMA

Cor pulmonale with pulmonary emphysema is a common problem. When the electrocardiogram shows the characteristic features of this condition, one can usually deduce that the arterial PO_2 is lower than normal, and that pulmonary hypertension and heart failure are present.

The electrocardiographic abnormalities due to cor pulmonale and pulmonary emphysema are listed in Table 13.1. Fowler et al(1) studied 15 patients with cor pulmonale and pulmonary emphysema proven by autopsy (Table 13.2). An example of an electrocardiogram made from one of their patients is shown in Figure 13.1.

PULMONARY EMBOLI

ACUTE COR PULMONALE DUE TO ACUTE PULMONARY EMBOLISM

McGinn and White(2) described the electrocardiographic characteristics of acute pulmonary embolism in 1935. Their observations were made prior to the use of angiography as a diagnostic tool. Stein et al(3) summarized the electrocardiographic abnormalities produced by acute pulmonary embolism proven by pulmonary angiography. These abnormalities can be produced by sudden dilatation of the right atrium and ventricle, pressure overload of the right ventricle, hypoxia, and right ventricular ischemia.

The electrocardiographic characteristics of acute pulmonary embolism are listed in Table 13.3. Table 13.4, from a report by Stein et al(3), indicates the abnormalities they observed in 90 patients with massive or submassive pulmonary embolism in whom the catastrophic condition was proven by pulmonary angiography. The differentiation of acute pulmonary embolism from other conditions producing similar electrocardiographic abnormalities is described in Table 13.5. Examples of the electrocardiogram in acute pulmonary embolism are shown in Figures 13.2 and 13.3.

REPEATED PULMONARY EMBOLI WITH CHRONIC PULMONARY HYPERTENSION

Repeated pulmonary emboli may produce chronic pulmonary hypertension and systolic pressure overload of the right ventricle. The electrocardiographic characteristics of this condition are listed in Table 13.6. Other diseases may produce similar abnormalities, and the differentiation between them is described in Table 13.7. An example of an electrocardiogram recorded from a patient with repeated pulmonary emboli and chronic pulmonary hypertension is shown in Figure 13.4.

ELECTROCARDIOGRAPHIC ABNORMALITIES DUE TO NEUROMUSCULAR DISEASE, HEAD TRAUMA, CENTRAL NERVOUS SYSTEM AND CEREBROVASCULAR LESIONS

Almost all of the *neuromuscular diseases* may be associated with intraventricular conduction abnormalities and cardiomyopathy. An exception to this may be myasthenia gravis.

CENTRAL NERVOUS SYSTEM LESIONS

Millar and Abildskov(7) described the electrocardiographic abnormalities of 89 young individuals with central nervous system lesions stemming from subarachnoid hemorrhage, internal carotid occlusion, intracerebral hematoma, brain tumors, and an array of cerebral diseases. They reported the development of ST and T wave abnormalities of a nonspecific type, as well as severely notched T waves. They believe that the abnormal notching of the T waves might have been caused by the "asymmetrical alteration" in the "tone" of the sympathetic nervous system as it influences the ventricles. The true cause of the abnormality remained unknown.

HEAD TRAUMA

Hersch(8) studied the electrocardiograms of 164 patients with *head trauma.* He found "inverted T waves" in leads V4, V5, and V6, U waves greater than 1 mm in height, and sinus arrhythmia. He further reported that the "frequency of electrocardiographic abnormalities increased as (the) level of consciousness deteriorated."

Burch, Meyers, and Abildskov(9) called attention to a new abnormality associated with cerebrovascular accidents: the development of huge, inverted T waves and a long QT interval (Fig. 13.5). Their patients had cerebral hemorrhage, subarachnoid hemorrhage, and cerebral arterial thrombosis. Whereas some investigators have attributed the electrocardiographic abnormalities resulting from central nervous system damage to an alteration in ventricular sympathetic tone, Connor(10), a pathologist, reported focal myocytosis, "a form of myocardial damage," in eight percent of patients dying of intracranial lesions.

The clinician should remember that notched T waves often occur in normal children, and that deeply inverted, broad T waves may occur in patients with apical hypertrophic cardiomyopathy.

Note: As stated in several places in this book, the model presented here is a clinically useful approximation of the real situation within the heart. At times, the explanation moves beyond the known evidence. When this occurs, every effort has been made to extend the facts in a logical manner.

ATHLETE'S HEART

The changes in the heart produced by long-term, intense training have been the subject of clinical research for a long time. As new techniques were developed, the research methods came to include physical examination, chest radiography and electrocardiography, as well as Holter monitoring, cardiac catheterization, and echocardiography. However, even with all of these techniques, there remain unanswered questions and problems related to the electrocardiograms recorded from athletes.

Zeppilli(11,12) has divided the electrocardiographic abnormalities of athletes into three categories: *physiologic changes,* which are clearly due to the effects of training; *borderline abnormalities,* which may be due to training but cannot be distinguished from abnormalities due to heart disease; and *abnormalities not due to training,* which can nevertheless be observed in athletes.

The electrocardiographic abnormalities observed in athletes are listed in Table 13.8. The differentiation of training-related electrocardiographic abnormalities from those due to other causes is described in Table 13.9. An example of an electrocardiogram of a trained athlete is shown in Figure 13.6, and electrocardiograms of athletes with two types of hypertrophic cardiomyopathy are shown in Figures 13.7 and 13.8.

In athletes, it is not always possible to distinguish the features of hypertrophic cardiomyopathy from the changes produced by long-term training. At present, asymmetric septal hypertrophy and apical hypertrophy identified by echocardiography are not considered to be consequences of exercise. Generalized left ventricular hypertrophy is more likely to be exercise-related.

ENDOCRINE DISEASE AND THE ELECTROCARDIOGRAM

HYPOTHYROIDISM

Hypothyroidism produces bradycardia and low voltages of the QRS complexes and T waves (Figure 13.9). The P wave voltages are less likely to be reduced than are the voltages of the QRS complexes and T waves. The decreased QRS complex and T wave voltages are the result of three factors: pericardial effusion, which may accompany hypothyroidism; increased skin resistance, which may also occur in hypothyroidism; and changes in the ventricular myocardium. The P wave amplitude is less affected by pericardial effusion than

are the amplitudes of the QRS complexes and T waves. Further, the change in the atrial myocardium may have less effect on the P waves than the change in the ventricular myocardium has on the QRS complexes and T waves.

ADDISON'S DISEASE

The electrocardiogram in patients with Addison's disease varies according to the stage of the disease, the associated electrolyte abnormality, and the stage of treatment. The QRS voltage may be diminished. There may be signs of hyperkalemia and a short QT interval or, during treatment with desoxycorticosterone acetate and cortisone, signs of hypokalemia and, and under certain circumstances, hypocalcemia with a prolonged QT interval (see Figs. 13.10 and 13.11).

HYPERTHYROIDISM

Hyperthyroidism usually produces no abnormalities in the ventricular electrocardiogram. However, when atrial fibrillation is uncontrolled, the ST segments and T waves may become abnormal. Sinus tachycardia or atrial fibrillation with a ventricular rate of 180 to 220 depolarizations per minute is usually present. When atrial fibrillation occurs in the absence of thyrotoxicosis, the ventricular rate is usually less than 180 depolarizations per minute. Therefore, with ventricular rates higher than this, it is wise to consider the presence of thyrotoxicosis or some other factor, such as pre-excitation of the ventricles.

HYPOPARATHYROIDISM

Hypoparathyroidism may produce hypocalcemia, which in turn produces a long QT interval in the electrocardiogram; the mean T vector remains normal. The QT interval is long because the ST segment is abnormally long (Fig 13.12).

ECTROLYTE ABNORMALITIES AND THE ELECTROCARDIOGRAM

HYPOKALEMIA

Hypokalemia may contribute to the development of atrial and ventricular arrhythmias, especially in patients receiving digitalis. Prolongation of the PR interval and of the QRS complex can occur on rare occasions. Hypokalemia increases the size of the U wave and decreases the size of the T wave. The U wave tends to "join" the T wave, producing a long QU interval that is often erroneously designated as a long QT interval. The direction of the mean T vector may change. The electrocardiographic changes occur when the plasma concentration of potassium is about 2.3 mEq/L. An example of the electrocardiographic effects of hypokalemia is shown in Figure 13.13.

HYPERKALEMIA

Hyperkalemia may lead to sinoatrial exit block, in which case no P waves may be visible. It may also produce an increase in the duration of the P wave, PR interval, and QRS complex. The T wave assumes a characteristic shape, as discussed below. Every conceivable type of intraventricular conduction defect can occur in hyperkalemia, including right bundle branch block, left bundle branch block, left anterior-superior division block, left posterior-inferior division block, left bundle branch block plus left anterior-superior division block, right bundle branch block plus left anterior-superior division block, or right bundle branch block plus left posterior-inferior division block. As a rule, both the initial and terminal portions of the QRS complexes become abnormal, providing a clue to possible hyperkalemia.

The T waves in hyperkalemia become tall and tent-shaped (Fig. 13.14). The ascending limb of a normal T wave has a more gradual slope than its descending limb, whereas in hyperkalemia, both the ascending and descending limbs are equally slanted. The base of the wave in these cases becomes narrow, and the direction of the mean T wave vector may also be altered.

In normal dogs, there is a close relationship between the level of plasma potassium and the changes in the electrocardiogram when potassium is administered. The correlation is less definite in human patients with other electrolyte abnormalities in addition to hyperkalemia. Figure 13.15 shows an example of an electrocardiogram with the abnormalities caused by hyperkalemia.

OTHER ELECTROLYTE ABNORMALITIES

HYPERCALCEMIA: Hypercalcemia, as occurs in hyperparathyroidism, produces a shortening of the QT interval. This is caused by a decrease in duration of the ST segment. Hypercalcemia may produce ST and T wave abnormalities that resemble those associated with digitalis.

HYPOCALCEMIA: Hypocalcemia produces prolongation of the QT interval by prolonging the ST segment (see Fig. 13.12).

HYPOCALCEMIA AND HYPERKALEMIA: Hypocalcemia and hyperkalemia may occur at the same time in patients with renal failure. The electrocardiogram may reveal prolongation of the ST segment and tented T waves.

HYPOCALCEMIA AND HYPOKALEMIA: Hypocalcemia and hypokalemia may produce a long ST segment and prominent U waves.

EXERCISE ELECTROCARDIOGRAPHY: The reader is referred to Chapter 107 in the 7th edition of *The Heart* for a complete discussion of this subject(13).

PSEUDOINFARCTION

This important subject is discussed in Chapter 11. Examples of electrocardiograms showing pseudoinfarction are shown in Figures 11.20 through 11.23.

ELECTROCARDIOGRAPHIC ABNORMALITIES DUE TO ACCIDENTAL COOLING

Cooling of the body may cause atrial fibrillation, bradycardia, and alteration of the QRS complexes of the electrocardiogram. The QRS duration becomes prolonged, and an Osborn wave develops. This subject is discussed in Chapter 8, with Figure 8.22 providing an example of an electrocardiogram showing an Osborn wave.

RESIDUAL ABNORMALITIES IN THE ELECTROCARDIOGRAM FOLLOWING CARDIAC SURGERY

The electrocardiographic abnormalities that follow cardiac surgery may be similar to those observed prior to surgery; alternatively, previous abnormalities may be altered, taking on more normal characteristics. Postoperative abnormalities may, at times, represent a combination of preoperative abnormalities and new ones caused by the surgery itself.

The electrocardiographic evidence of ventricular hypertrophy may gradually diminish, but only rarely does it disappear completely following an operation that eliminates the cause of the hypertrophy. Conduction disturbances reflected in the QRS complex, such as right ventricular delay or right or left bundle branch block, are less likely to disappear following surgery. This would imply that damage to the conduction system is more likely to be permanent, while hypertrophy *per se* is more likely to be reversible. These observations are personal; to my knowledge, this issue has not been studied scientifically.

Certain surgical procedures are more likely than others to produce atrioventricular block, new left or right bundle branch block, or some other QRS conduction abnormality. This is the case with surgery involving replacement of the mitral valve, replacement of the aortic valve, closure of an interventricular septal defect, coronary artery bypass, or removal of a ventricular aneurysm.

Figure 13.16 shows an example of right ventricular conduction delay that persisted after surgical closure of a high-flow ostium secundum atrial septal defect.

LEFT PLEURAL EFFUSION

The electrocardiograms of patients with normal or abnormal hearts who have substantial left pleural effusion may show decreased QRS-T amplitudes in leads V5 and V6 (see Fig. 13.17).

TWO HEARTS IN THE SAME PATIENT

Cardiac transplantation has created new electrocardiographic abnormalities. In these cases, the heart of the recipient is removed except for a rim of the atria. The rim of the new heart is sutured to the rim of the old heart, and two different P waves may be seen in the electrocardiogram.

Occasionally, the entire diseased heart is left in place and a new heart is attached to it; two ventricular electrocardiograms are produced by this arrangement (Fig. 13.18 (I) and (II)), which is known as a "piggyback" (PB) heart.

GENETICS AND THE HEART

Genetic abnormalities may be responsible for certain types of heart disease. Genetically determined heart disease, for example, may be responsible for the electrocardiographic abnormalities associated with neuromuscular diseases. Some types of congenital heart disease are genetically determined; a good example is hereditary pulmonary valve stenosis. One variety of hypertrophic cardiomyopathy is also genetically determined, as may be defects of the ventricular conduction system. Finally, there are times when the clinician may suspect, but cannot prove the presence of genetically determined heart disease.

Examples of left bundle branch block occurring in two sisters, suggesting a possible genetic determination, are shown in Figures 13.19 and 13.20. These sisters were discovered to have conduction defects of the left bundle branch system while in their early forties. One had left bundle branch block plus left anterior-superior division block, while the other had left bundle branch block alone. They exhibited no other evidence of heart disease. There was a family history of atherosclerotic coronary heart disease occurring at a relatively early age in their father, uncles, brother, and a cousin. The question is whether the sisters' conduction system disease is an isolated condition or whether they have atherosclerotic coronary heart disease. If the conduction system disease is isolated, it is more likely to be genetically determined than to have occurred independently in both of them at the same age. If they have atherosclerotic coronary disease, the only indication of it is disease in the left bundle branch system, which would suggest the possibility of an inherent, perhaps genetically detemined vulnerability of the conduction system. In fact, however, there is no definite explanation for the unusual appearance of this condition in the two sisters.

EFFECTS OF PHYSIOLOGIC PHENOMENA ON THE ELECTROCARDIOGRAM

The deflections in the electrocardiogram may be altered by physiologic phenomena. Four examples will be discussed here.

RESPIRATION

The effects of full inspiration, full expiration, and quiet breathing on the deflections of the electrocardiogram are shown in Figure 13.21A-C. These changes are due to the changes in position of the diaphragm plus the change in blood volume within the ventricles during the different phases of respiration. Some years ago, it was believed that a Q wave in lead III that disappeared with inspiration was not due to inferior infarction. Whereas this is often true, the predictive value of this response is not adequate for clinical use.

HYPERVENTILATION

Patients with anxiety who hyperventilate to the extent that their blood PCO_2 becomes lower than normal may exhibit electrocardiographic abnormalities (Fig. 13.22A and B). It is likely that alkalosis of any cause will have the same effect.

SUDDEN CATECHOLAMINE RELEASE

The changes in the electrocardiogram produced by the startle reaction precipitated by a pistol shot are shown in Figure 13.23. Whereas catecholamine release must play a role in this condition, other factors not yet identified may also be operative.

THE INFLUENCE OF BODY POSITION ON THE ELECTROCARDIOGRAM

In the era of Waller and Einthoven, it was necessary to record leads I, II, and III with the patient seated because contact between the patient and the galvanometer was achieved by placing the hands and feet into buckets of saline (see Fig. 4.15). Consequently, early descriptions of electrocardiograms were of tracings recorded from seated subjects. As improved electrodes were developed, it became possible to create precordial leads, and to routinely record tracings with the patient in the recumbent position.

Figure 13.24A and B shows the effect of body position on the electrocardiogram. The mean QRS vector may be directed more vertically when the patient is seated than when supine. This is because the diaphragm is lower when the patient is in a seated position. Additionally, the mean T vector is directed more to the left and superiorly when the patient is seated than when supine, because the ventricular volume and heart size are slightly smaller when the patient is seated. This alters the repolarization process and shifts the mean T vector.

Whereas electrocardiograms are routinely made with the patient in the supine position, there are times when seriously ill patients may not be able to assume this position; this often occurs in intensive care units.

Although there are no studies regarding the effect of body position on the electrocardiogram in the intensive care unit, it is wise to recall that a change in position may produce changes in the electrocardiogram.

SITUS INVERSUS

Situs inversus, a condition in which the positions of all of the body's organs are reversed, produces a characteristic electrocardiogram (see Fig.13.25). The deflections recorded by the extremity leads resemble those created when the left arm electrode is placed on the right arm and the right arm electrode is placed on the left arm. The difference between the electrocardiogram achieved by switching the arm electrodes and that of a patient with situs inversus can be detected in the precordial leads. Reversal of the left and right arm electrodes will not influence the precordial lead deflections. In a patient with situs inversus, the precordial lead deflections will resemble those recorded from the usual electrode positions for leads V1 and V2, but the deflections will become progressively smaller as one records from positions V3, V4, V5, and V6. If situs inversus is suspected, it is proper to place the precordial electrodes on the right side of the chest rather than the left, using the same anatomic guidelines as are used on the left side of the chest.

MISPLACED ELECTRODES

MISPLACED PRECORDIAL ELECTRODES

Misplacement of the precordial electrodes is undoubtedly a frequent occurrence. Under certain circumstances, a misplacement of a centimeter or two for a precordial electrode will not alter the tracing significantly.

However, in other circumstances, a one-centimeter misplacement can produce major changes. When the mean QRS vector, mean initial 0.04-second QRS vector, mean terminal

0.04-second QRS vector, mean ST vector, or mean T vector is directed between 0° and +90°, or between -90° and ±180°, misplacement of the precordial electrode will not make a major difference in the recording of serial electrocardiograms. On the other hand, when electrical forces represented as vectors are directed about halfway between 0° and -90°, or between +90° and ±180°, a slight change in electrode position can substantially alter the precordial deflections. This occurs because the transitional pathways of electrical forces that are directed between 0° and -90°, or between +90° and ±180° are more likely to pass near all of the precordial electrode position sites than when these forces are directed between 0 and +90°, or between -90° and ±180° (Fig. 13.26). Whenever this occurs, an electrode misplacement of one to two centimeters may change the direction of a deflection from negative to positive or vice versa. This must be kept in mind, or the clinician interpreting the electrocardiogram will believe that a significant change has occurred from one recording to the next.

MISPLACED EXTREMITY LEADS

The most common error in recording an electrocardiogram is to place the left arm electrode on the right arm and vice versa ("switched arm leads"). An example of this mistake is shown in Figure 13.27(I) and (II). In such a case, the deflection recorded in lead I is an upside-down mirror image of the correct deflection; the deflection recorded by lead II is actually the deflection recorded by lead III; the deflection recorded by lead III is actually the deflection recorded by lead II; and the deflections recorded by leads aVR and aVL are actually those recorded by leads aVL and aVR, respectively. The deflection recorded in lead aVF is the true deflection recorded by this lead.

Whereas the deflections recorded by extremity leads are altered as described above, the deflection from the chest leads are recorded properly. How does this occur? Remember, the chest leads are part of the Wilson unipolar lead system, in which the negative pole of the electrocardiograph machine is attached to a central terminal, created by attaching wires to both arms and a leg, and connecting them at a common point. The exploring electrode (chest lead) is then attached to the positive pole of the electrocardiograph machine. The central terminal will record almost zero potential regardless of where on the extremities the electrodes are placed, so long as an electrode is placed on each of the arms and one leg. Accordingly, when the exploring electrode records from the usual precordial electrode sites, it records properly because the precordial electrode measures the difference between the electrical potential recorded at the precordial sites and that recorded by the central terminal. Because the central terminal records almost zero potential, the potentials recorded at the standard precordial electrode sites are uninfluenced by what is recorded by the central terminal. Accordingly, a switching of the extremity leads will not alter the precordial electrode deflections.

TABLE 13.1 THE ELECTROCARDIOGRAPHIC FEATURES OF COR PULMONALE WITH PULMONARY EMPHYSEMA

- Atrial arrhythmia may be present.

- A right atrial abnormality may be present. The mean P vector shifts to the right and anteriorly; it may be directed as much as +90° vertically. The P wave amplitude may be increased.

- The mean QRS vector tends to shift to the right and anteriorly.

- There may be low voltage of the QRS complex. The P and T waves may also exhibit low voltage.

- Right ventricular conduction delay may be present.

- Right bundle branch block may be present.

- The R/S ratio may be more than 1 in lead V1.

TABLE 13.2 ELECTROCARDIOGRAPHIC CHANGES IN COR PULMONALE WITH EMPHYSEMA

Case	Age and Sex	P Wave Axis 90°		Low Voltage QRS Limb Leads		R<5 mm in V5 or V6		QRS<5 mm in V5 or V6	
		Final	Any	Final	Any	Final	Any	Final	Any
1	77M	0	0	+	...	+	...	0	0
2	72M	+	...	+	...	+	...	0	+
3	68M	+	...	0	+	+	...	+	...
4	67M	+	...	0	0	0	+	0	+
5	67M	0	0	0	0	0	+	0	0
6	67M	+	...	+	...	+	...	0	0
7	65M	0	0	0	0	0	0	0	0
8	65M	+	...	+	...	0	0	0	0
9	62M	0	0	0	0	+	...	+	...
10	60M	0	+	+	...	+	...	+	...
11	58M	+	...	0	0	+	...	+	...
12	56M	+	...	+	...	+	...	+	...
13	55F	+	...	0	0	0	0	0	0
14	48M	0	0	0	0	0	+	0	+
15	44M	0	0	0	0	0	0	0	0

Reproduced with permission from the publisher and author(1); see Figure Credits.

FIGURE 13.1

Characteristic rsR' pattern of right ventricular hypertrophy in lead V1 of a patient with emphysema and cor pulmonale. The P waves are large in lead II. The mean P vector is directed +90° in the frontal plane; a right atrial abnormality is present.

There is an abnormal right axis deviation of the mean QRS complex. The voltage of the QRS complexes is low. The initial R wave is small in all precordial leads.

A. Frontal plane projection of the mean P, mean QRS, terminal 0.04–second QRS and mean T vectors. **B**. Spatial orienta-

tion of the mean P vector. **C.** Spatial orientation of mean QRS vector. **D** Spatial orientation of the terminal 0.04–second QRS vector. **E.** Spatial orientation of the mean T vector. (Reproduced with permission from the publisher and author (1); see Figure Credits.)

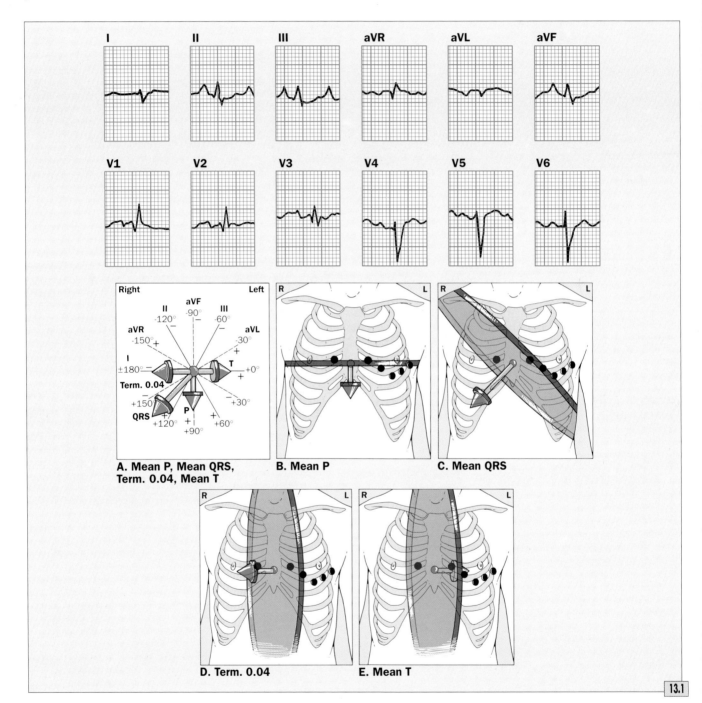

A. Mean P, Mean QRS, Term. 0.04, Mean T

B. Mean P

C. Mean QRS

D. Term. 0.04

E. Mean T

TABLE 13.3 ELECTROCARDIOGRAPHIC CHARACTERISTICS OF ACUTE PULMONARY EMBOLISM

- A right atrial abnormality may develop.

- Cardiac arrhythmia may develop.

- Sinus tachycardia may occur.

- Atrial fibrillation or atrial tachycardia may occur, especially in patients with pre-existing heart disease.

- Right ventricular conduction delay may develop; the QRS duration may remain normal.

- The early and late QRS forces may be altered. Early QRS changes may simulate inferior infarction because they shift to the left, producing new Q waves in lead III and occasionally in leads II and aVF.

The late QRS forces shift to the right and anteriorly, producing S waves in leads I and V6, and terminal R waves in lead V1.

- The mean T vector may shift to the left, suggesting inferior ischemia or inferior myocardial infarction.

- The mean T vector may be directed to the left and posteriorly, suggesting the ischemia of acute anterior infarction.

- Abnormalities are often transient, lasting less than 24 to 48 hours. At times, however, the abnormalities may last for weeks.

- Acute right bundle branch block may develop.

- A mean ST vector of subendocardial injury may develop.

- The mean QRS vector may, on rare occasions, shift to the left.

TABLE 13.4 ELECTROCARDIOGRAPHIC MANIFESTATIONS OF PULMONARY EMBOLISM: PATIENTS WITHOUT PRIOR CARDIAC OR PULMONARY DISEASE*

Electrocardiogram	Massive Pulmonary Embolism: 50 Pts. (%)	Submassive Pulmonary Embolism: 40 Pts. (%)	Massive or Submassive Pulmonary Embolism: 90 Pts.
Normal	6	23	13
Rhythm disturbances:			
• Premature atrial beats	2	3	2
• Premature ventricular beats	4	3	3
Atrioventricular conduction disturbances:			
• First-degree A-V block	0	3	1
• P pulmonale	6	5	6
QRS abnormalities:			
• Right axis deviation	8	5	7
• Left axis deviation	4	10	7
• Clockwise rotation (V5)	10	3	7
• Incomplete right bundle branch block	8	3	6
• Complete right bundle branch block	8	10	9
• Right ventricular hypertrophy	6	5	6
• S1, S2, S3 Pattern	6	8	7
• S1, Q3, T3 Pattern	18	5	12
• Pseudoinfarction	16	5	11
• Low voltage (frontal plane)	8	3	6
Primary RST segment and T wave abnormalities:			
• RST segment depression (not reciprocal)	28	23	26
• RST segment elevation (not reciprocal)	18	13	16
• T wave inversion	46	38	42

*Some patients had more than one abnormality.
The prevalence of the various electrocardiographic abnormalities did not differ significantly between patients with massive and submassive pulmonary embolism (chi-square >0.05).

F I G U R E   1 3 . 2

A. Leads I, II, III recorded two hours after pulmonary embolism. **B.** Same leads recorded four weeks after pulmonary embolism. These electrocardiograms have been reproduced from McGinn and White's original article published in 1935(2). Note the change in direction of the mean QRS, mean T, mean initial 0.04–second, and mean terminal 0.04–second vectors. No chest leads were recorded. Accordingly, the spatial orientation of the vectors cannot be determined. (Reproduced with permission from the American Medical Association(2); see Figure Credits.)

F I G U R E   1 3 . 3

The electrocardiogram of a 54-year-old patient made shortly after pulmonary embolism. The direction of the mean terminal 0.04–second QRS vector indicates right ventricular conduction delay, and that of the mean T vector indicates right ventricular ischemia. Note that as the QRS vector influences the electrode at V5 and V6, negative deflections should be recorded whereas resultantly positive deflections are actually recorded. This discrepancy occurs either because electrode sites for V4 and V5 are too high or because the transitional pathway undulates. (Reproduced with permission from the publisher and author; see Figure Credits)

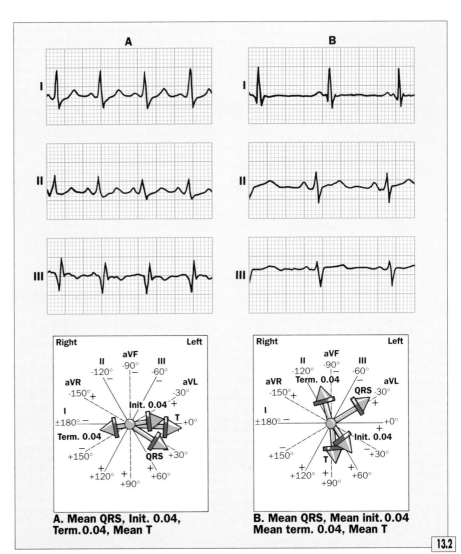

A. Mean QRS, Init. 0.04, Term. 0.04, Mean T

B. Mean QRS, Mean init. 0.04 Mean term. 0.04, Mean T

13.2

TABLE 13.5 DIFFERENTIATION OF THE ELECTROCARDIOGRAPHIC ABNORMALITIES OF ACUTE PULMONARY EMBOLISM FROM THOSE OF OTHER CONDITIONS

- Pulmonary embolism must be differentiated from acute inferior or anterior myocardial infarction. It may not be possible to accomplish this by examining the electrocardiogram alone. Accordingly, the clinical setting, symptoms, and at times, other diagnostic procedures such as determination of blood gases, pulmonary scan, right ventricular echocardiography, and pulmonary angiography are needed to make the diagnosis.

- Epicardial injury, recognized by a new ST segment vector, is less likely with pulmonary embolism than with myocardial infarction.

- The abnormalities usually associated with extensive anterior myocardial infarct are less likely as a result of pulmonary embolism than of infarct itself, but both conditions may be present in the same patient.

- Deep vein thrombosis of the legs must be excluded in patients with pulmonary embolism. There may be no signs of the disease; non-invasive studies and, at times, venography may be indicated.

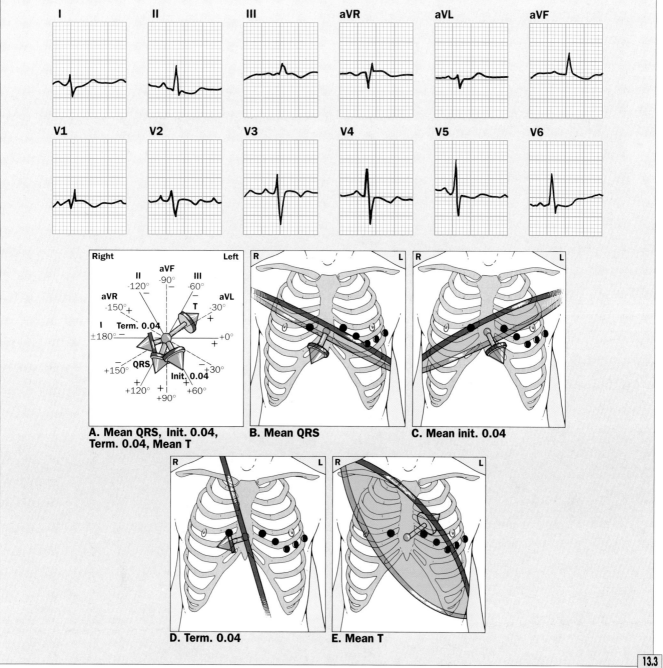

A. Mean QRS, Init. 0.04, Term. 0.04, Mean T
B. Mean QRS
C. Mean init. 0.04
D. Term. 0.04
E. Mean T

13.3

TABLE 13.6 ELECTROCARDIOGRAPHIC CHARACTERISTICS OF REPEATED PULMONARY EMBOLI AND CHRONIC PULMONARY HYPERTENSION

- A right atrial abnormality may be present.

- There may be a gradual shift of the mean QRS vector from its normal leftward, inferior, and posterior position toward a right-ward, inferior, and anterior orientation; the QRS duration may remain less than 0.10 second. The QRS shift results from the shift of the initial and mid-QRS forces.

- The electrocardiographic abnormalities indicate right ventricular hypertrophy due to systolic pressure overload of the right ventricle.

- The mean T vector tends to be directed opposite the mean QRS vector.

- The mean ST vector is relatively parallel with the mean QRS vector.

- Right bundle branch block may develop.

TABLE 13.7 ELECTROCARDIOGRAPHIC DIFFERENTIATION OF REPEATED PULMONARY EMBOLI AND CHRONIC PULMONARY HYPERTENSION FROM OTHER CONDITIONS

- The electrocardiographic abnormalities of repeated pulmonary emboli and chronic pulmonary hypertension are similar to those produced by primary pulmonary hypertension and Eisenmenger's syndrome.

- Systolic overload of the right ventricle produced by mitral stenosis may be suspected when a left atrial abnormality is definitely present.

- When the usual screening examination, including the history, physical examination, and chest x-ray film does not identify the abnormalities that are known to cause acquired systolic pressure overload of the right ventricle, it is usually necessary to use other procedures, including cardiac catheterization and angiography, to make the differentiation.

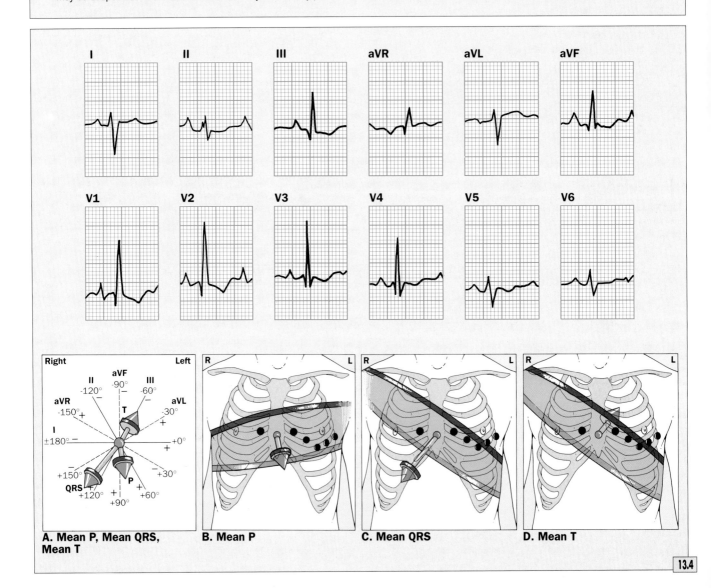

A. Mean P, Mean QRS, Mean T

B. Mean P

C. Mean QRS

D. Mean T

13.4

FIGURE 13.4

This electrocardiogram was recorded from a patient with repeated pulmonary emboli. (**A–D**) Frontal plane projections and spatial orientation of the mean P, mean QRS, and mean T vectors, respectively. Part B shows the right atrial abnormality. Part C illustates the mean QRS vector which is directed to the right and anteriorly, signifying right ventricular hypertrophy. The T wave vector shown in part D, which is directed opposite the mean QRS vector, also signifies right ventricular hypertrophy.

Summary: These electrocardiographic abnormalities cannot be differentiated from those of the right ventricular hypertrophy produced by Eisenmenger's physiology or primary pulmonary hypertension. Other diagnostic methods are needed to make the differentiation. (Reproduced with permission from the publisher and author(6); see Figure Credits.)

FIGURE 13.5

Abnormal T waves sometimes associated with cerebral vascular accidents (subarachnoid hemorrhage, cerebral hemorrhage, or cerebral thrombosis). (Reproduced with permission from the American Heart Association and the author(9); see Figure Credits.)

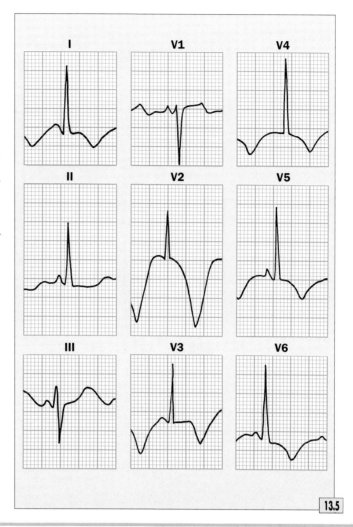

13.5

TABLE 13.8 ELECTROCARDIOGRAPHIC ABNORMALITIES OBSERVED IN ATHLETES

Physiologic changes clearly due to training:

- Increase in P wave amplitude.

- Sinus bradycardia (nocturnal rates may be as low as 30 depolarizations per minute or less).

- Premature atrial, junctional, or ventricular depolarizations.

- First-degree atrioventricular block, second-degree atrioventricular block, and Mobitz type I block.

- Increased amplitude of the mean QRS vector, possibly indicating left ventricular hypertrophy; there may be clues to biventricular hypertrophy.

- The preceding abnormalities are reversible, usually disappearing after exercise is eliminated. The atrioventricular block can produce syncope, and this may occasionally persist after dynamic exercise training is discontinued. A pacemaker is occasionally needed.

Borderline abnormalities that may be due to training but cannot be distinguished from those due to heart disease:

- Large ST segment vector due to early repolarization; this disappears when the training is discontinued

- The mean T vector may be changed considerably; it may be directed to the right and anteriorly, due to left ventricular hypertrophy, or it can be directed posteriorly. These abnormalities cannot always be differentiated from the T wave abnormalities of mitral valve prolapse or hypertrophic cardiomyopathy.

Abnormalites not due to training but that can be identified in athletes:

- Atrial and ventricular tachycardia.

- Initial mean 0.04–second QRS complex abnormalities simulating the abnormal Q waves of myocardial infarction. These abnormalities may be seen in patients with hypertrophic cardiomyopathy.

- QRS conduction defects.

Reproduced with permission from the publisher and author(11); see Figure Credits.

TABLE 13.9 DIFFERENTIATION OF THE ELECTROCARDIOGRAPHIC ABNORMALITIES OF THE TRAINED ATHLETE FROM THOSE DUE TO OTHER CAUSES

Physiologic changes clearly due to training:

- It may not be possible to differentiate the increased QRS amplitude seen in the trained athlete from left ventricular hypertrophy due to heart diseases such as hypertrophic cardiomyopathy.

Borderline abnormalities that may be due to either training or heart disease:

- An unusual ST segment vector that must be differentiated from the ST segment abnormality of epicardial injury due to percarditis. The clinical setting assists in distinguishing these two problems.

- An ST segment abnormality simulating that seen in epicardial injury due to myocardial infarction. The direction of the means T vector in an athlete is toward the apex; the mean ST vector is not usually directed toward a localized area of myocardium as it is in myocardial infarction.

- A T wave abnormality that may not be distinguished from that associated with mitral valve prolapse or hypertrophic cardiomyopathy, even if the T waves become more normal after the exercise is dicontinued. Other clinical data and echocardiographic examinations needed.

Abnormalities that are not due to training but may be observed in athletes:

- QRS duration of 0.12 second or greater.

- Abnormalities of the initial QRS forces, including those suggesting myocardial infarction. This should stimulate the clinician to consider the presence of hypertrophic cardiomyopathy. A conduction defect of the Wolff-Parkinson-White type may be noted, but this abnormality is not due to exercise.

Reproduced with permission from the publisher and author (11); See Figure Credits.

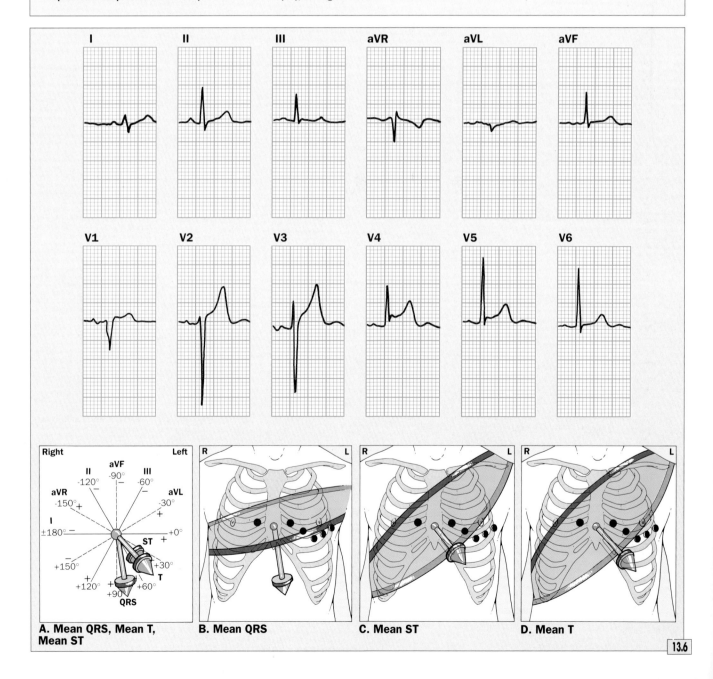

A. Mean QRS, Mean T, Mean ST

B. Mean QRS

C. Mean ST

D. Mean T

FIGURE 13.6

This electrocardiogram, showing a large ST segment vector, was recorded from a normal 27-year-old athlete. An electrophysiologic study was normal.

(A–D) Frontal plane projection and spatial orientations of the mean QRS, mean ST and mean T vectors, respectively.

Summary: Sinus bradycardia is present; there are 46 complexes per minute. Note that the direction of the large mean ST vector parallels that of the mean T vector. This finding, if stable, distinguishes the mean T vector seen here from that associated with pericarditis or infarction. Note also that the ascending limb of the T wave is more slanted than the descending limb; this distinguishes the mean ST vector from the ST vector due to hyperkalemia.

FIGURE 13.7

This electrocardiogram, showing left anterior-superior division block and terminal T wave inversion in leads V1 and V2, was recorded from a 16-year-old canoeist. An echocardiogram showed an asymmetric thickening of the interventricular septum considered characteristic of hypertrophic cardiomyopathy.

(A–D) Frontal plane projection and spatial orientations of the mean QRS, mean ST and mean T vectors, respectively.

QRS complex: The mean QRS vector is directed –60° to the left and 30° posteriorly; when the QRS duration is 0.10 second or less, this degree of left axis deviation indicates the presence of left anterior-superior division block.

Summary: This young athlete apparently had hypertrophic cardiomyopathy unrelated to his athletic exercise. This case illustrates the problem of distinguishing the hypertrophy of exercise from hypertrophic cardiomyopathy. (Reproduced with permission from the publisher and author (11); see Figure Credits.)

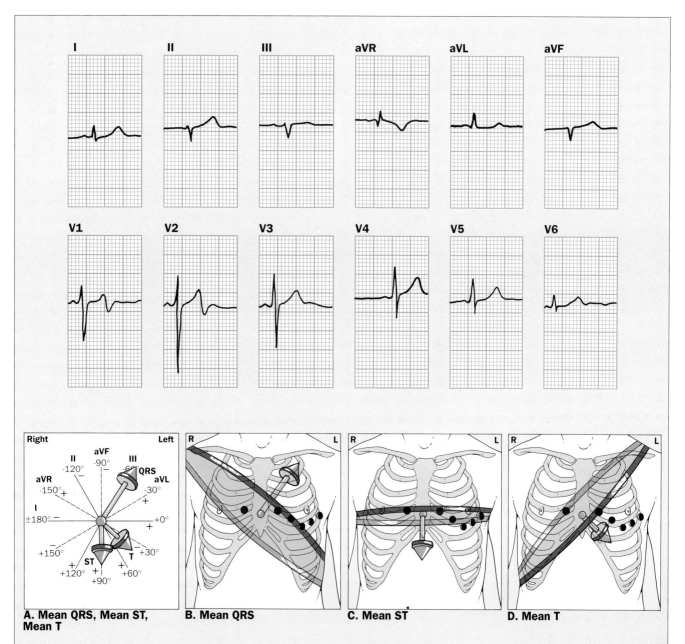

A. Mean QRS, Mean ST, Mean T

B. Mean QRS

C. Mean ST

D. Mean T

FIGURE 13.8

This electrocardiogram, showing left ventricular hypertrophy and left ventricular conduction delay, was recorded from an asymptomatic 31-year-old sprinter.

(**A–D**) Frontal plane projection and spatial orientations of the mean QRS, mean ST and mean T vectors, respectively.

QRS Complex: The QRS voltage is enormous. The mean QRS vector is directed +70° inferiorly, and 15° to 20° posteriorly. The patient shows left ventricular hypertrophy, and the absence of a Q wave in leads I and V6 suggests the presence of left ventricular conduction delay.

ST segment: The mean ST vector is directed about +110° superiorly and parallel with the frontal plane. The mean ST vector is parallel with the mean T vector.

T waves: The mean T vector is directed +115° superiorly and parallel with the

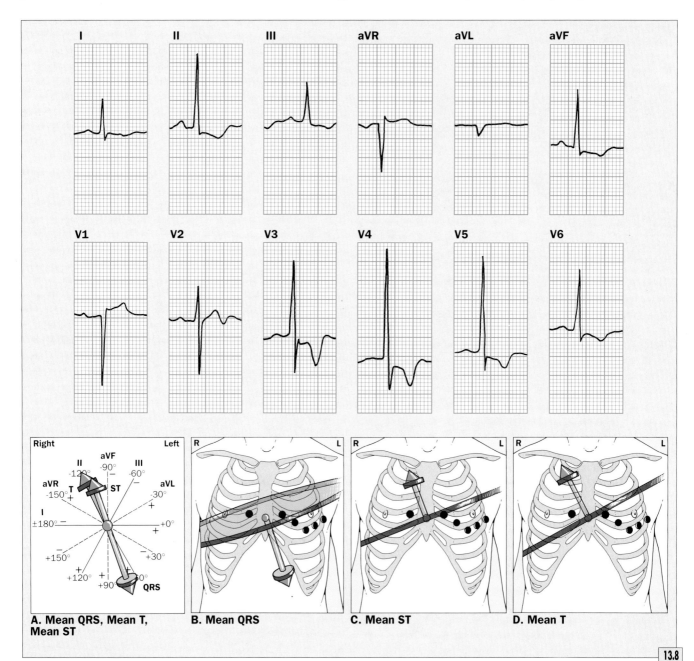

A. Mean QRS, Mean T, Mean ST

B. Mean QRS

C. Mean ST

D. Mean T

13.8

(Figure 13.8 continued.)
frontal plane. The T wave abnormality is due to left ventricular hypertrophy.

Summary: An echocardiogram taken from this patient showed apical hypertrophic cardiomyopathy, unrelated to his exercise. (Reproduced with permission from the publisher and author(11); see Figure Credits.)

FIGURE 13.9
This electrocardiogram was recorded from a 67-year-old woman with hypothyroidism. Sinus bradycardia is present. The heart rate is 48 complexes per minute. The total 12-lead QRS voltage is decidedly low at 88 mm. (**A–C**) Frontal plane projection and spatial orientations of the mean QRS and mean T vectors, respectively. Bradycardia and low QRS and T voltages are clues to hypothyroidism.

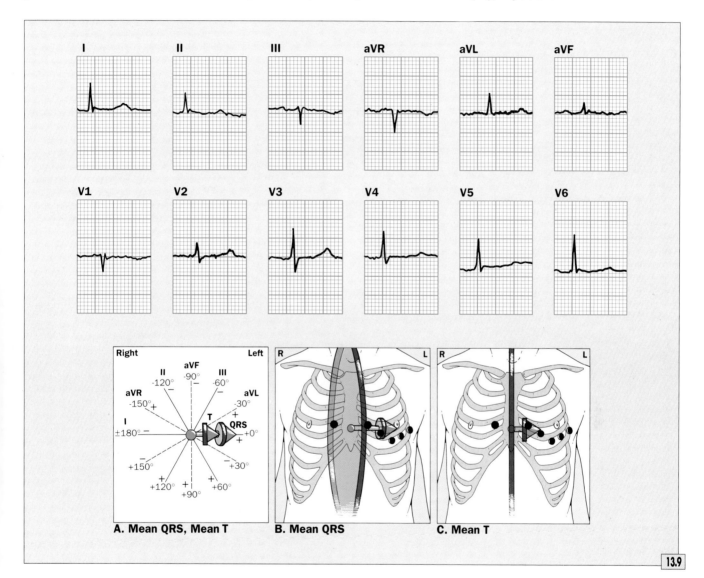

A. Mean QRS, Mean T   B. Mean QRS   C. Mean T

13.9

FIGURE 13.10

Addison's disease was diagnosed in this woman at age 52. Her symptoms included vomiting, weight loss, and progressive weakness. She was malnourished, and her systolic blood pressure was 98 mm Hg, with a diastolic pressure of 70 mm Hg. There was considerable brownish pigmentation of the skin, especially marked in the creases and over the elbows and knuckles. She responded very well to treatment with desoxycorticosterone acetate (DOCA), and was discharged one month later. She was then maintained with implantation of DOCA pellets and testosterone therapy.

Three and one-half years later she was readmitted because of psychotic behavior, but was discharged after unsuccessful attempts to alter the psychosis by hormone and electrolyte manipulation.

A. The electrocardiogram shows a normal sinus rhythm at a rate of 100 complexes per minute; low T waves in leads I and II and in precordial leads V2 through V6; and a QT duration of 0.36 second (the upper limit of normal for this heart rate is 0.35 second). The QRS complexes are rather low in amplitude. **B.** The electrocardiogram taken nine days after the one reproduced in part A shows a normal sinus rhythm at a rate of 75 complexes per minute. The T waves are sharp and peaked, and the QRS complexes are rather low in amplitude. The duration of the QT interval measures 0.32 second (the upper limit of normal is 0.39 second for this heart rate).

Summary: The tracing in A, which was taken 17 days after admission, following a long period of treatment with DOCA and testosterone, is consistent with, but not diagnostic of a low-potassium effect. The serum sodium level on that date was 130.3 mEq/L, and the serum potassium level was 3.7 mEq/L. The latter was initially questioned because the patient had been taking potassium chloride by mouth for 10 days. It was later thought to represent a true value.

The tracing in B shows the changes of early hyperkalemia. The serum potassium level two days prior to this recording was 5.7 mEq/L. This series of changes is strongly suggestive of what might be expected with the emergence of the patient from a low or low-normal potassium state to one above normal. The evidence is not conclusive, and it should be remembered that serum levels are only rough indicators of potassium distribution through the body. Thus, it is perfectly possible that the patient was in low potassium balance at the time of tracing A. The changes seen in B indicate that the serum potassium levels were rising above normal, suggesting caution in the further administration of potassium. It should also be remembered that other factors may have been important in producing the pattern seen in A. These tracings illustrate the limitations as well as the usefulness of the electrocardiogram in the treatment of Addison's disease. (This figure and most of the legend are

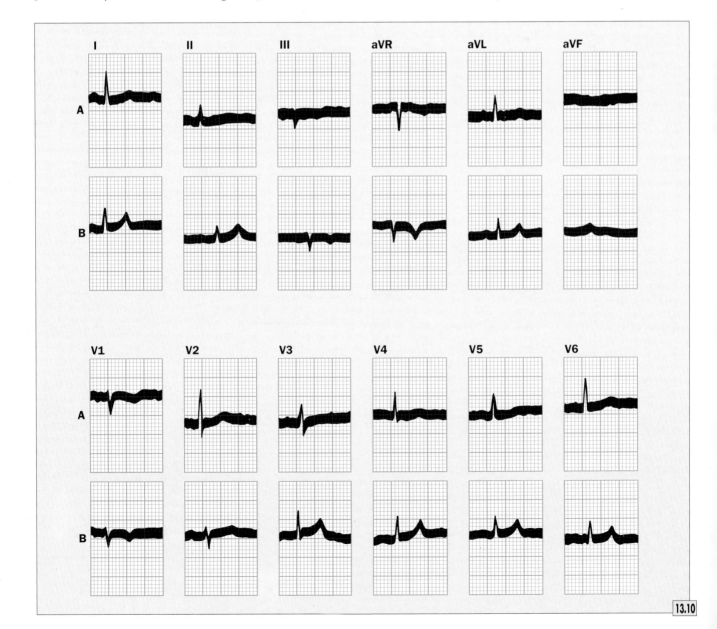

(Figure 13.10 continued.) reproduced with permission from the publisher and author(6); see Figure Credits.)

FIGURE 13.11

Hypocalcemia of obscure endocrine origin in a nine-year-old schoolgirl who was hospitalized at the age of seven with classical symptoms and findings of Addison's disease. She responded well to treatment with desoxycorticosterone acetate (DOCA) and cortical extract. Physical examination revealed extensive skin pigmentation in this patient. The serum sodium was 143 mEq/L, the serum chloride was 99.2 mEq/L, and the sugar, 45 mg %. A low level of serum calcium was first suspected on the basis of an electrocardiogram.

The electrocardiogram shown here was recorded when the serum calcium was 7.9 mg % and the serum phosphorus was 11 mg %. Several potassium determinations were within the normal range.

This tracing shows sinus arrhythmia at a rate averaging 70 complexes per minute, a PR interval of 0.15 second, normal QRS complexes, upright T waves, and long ST segments. The QT duration is prolonged, and measures 0.42 second (the upper limit of normal is 0.39 second for this heart rate).

Summary: This tracing shows a long QT

interval with T waves of normal appearance. Prolongation of the ST segment with little shift from the baseline is a distinguishing feature of hypocalcemia. In this case, the electrocardiographic patterns led to a diagnosis. However the exact cause of the low calcium levels in this patient with Addison's disease was never discovered. (This figure and much

of the legend are reproduced with permission from the publisher and author(6); see Figure Credits.)

FIGURE 13.12

This tracing was recorded from a 44-year-old woman with advanced renal failure. The duration of the QT interval
(Figure 13.12 continued on page 13.20.)

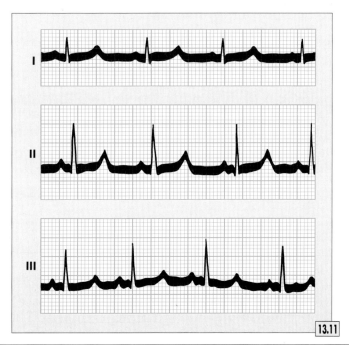

13.11

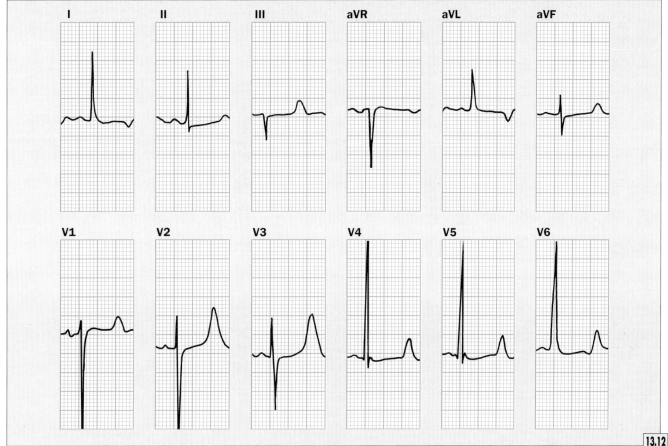

13.12

(Figure 13.12 continued.)
is 0.56 second. This prolongation is due to hypocalcemia (a serum calcium of 1.8 mg %). The tent-shaped T waves are the result of hyperkalemia (6.7 mEq/L). The tracing also shows left ventricular hypertrophy. (Reproduced with permission from the publisher and author; see Figure Credits.)

FIGURE 13.13
Both of the tracings (lead V3) in this figure were recorded from a patient with hypokalemia. Note the tall U waves partially fused with diphasic T waves in the upper tracing. The lower strip, taken one hour later, shows further elevation of the U wave, with coupled ventricular extrasystoles originat-

ing from the ascending branch of the U wave. (Reproduced with permission from the publisher and author; see Figure Credits.)

FIGURE 13.14
This figure shows the relationship of the serum potassium concentration to abnormalities in the electrocardiogram.

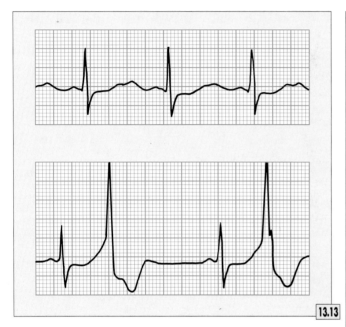

13.13

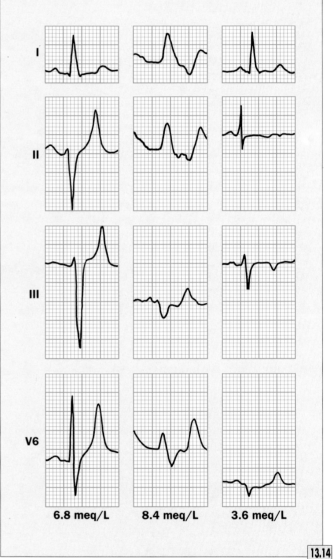

| 6.8 meq/L | 8.4 meq/L | 3.6 meq/L |

13.14

(Figure 13.14 continued.)
After treatment, and at a potassium level of 3.6 mEq/L, the PR intervals and the durations of the QRS complexes are normal (the shapes of the T waves are normal, although the direction of the mean T vector and the baseline QRS complex durations are abnormal). At 6.8 mEq/L, the PR intervals and QRS complexes are prolonged, with a shift of the QRS vector to the left. The T waves are symmetrical, narrow-based, and tall--the so-called "tented" T waves. At a potassium concentration of 8.4 mEq/L there is further prolongation of the PR interval, the P wave becoming difficult to identify. The means QRS vector is shifted to the right, and the QRS duration is prolonged to 0.20 second. The characteristic prolongation of both the initial and terminal portions of the QRS is best illustrated in V6. (The figure and most of the legend are reproduced with permission from the publisher and author; see Figure Credits.)

FIGURE 13.15
This electrocardiogram was recorded from a 26-year-old man with severe renal failure. His serum potassium was 8.7 mEq/L. Note the severe intraventricular conduction defect and peaked T waves. (The figure and much of the legend are reproduced with permission from the publisher and author; see Figure Credits.)

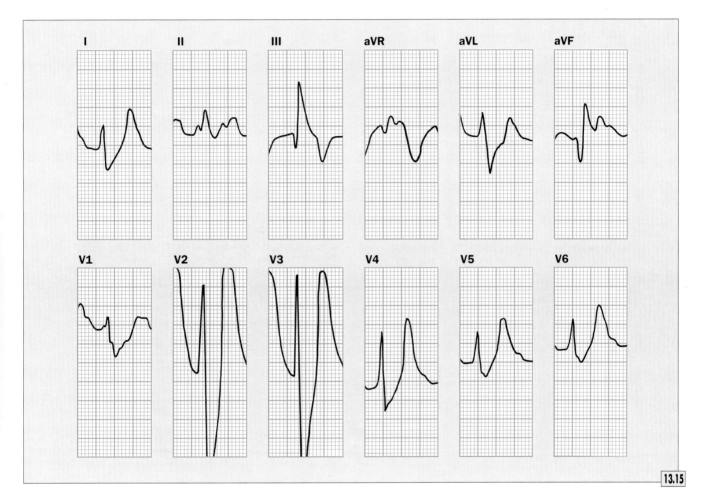

13.15

FIGURE 13.16
This electrocardiogram, showing a slight right ventricular conduction delay, was recorded from a 56-year-old woman several years after the surgical closure of a secundum type atrial septal defect.

The rhythm is normal and the heart rate is 80 complexes per minute. The duration of the PR interval is 0.17 second. The duration of the QRS complex is 0.08 second, and the duration of the QT interval is 0.36 second. The P waves

are pointed, and the first half of the P wave is prominent in lead V1. Whereas these P waves suggest a right atrial abnormality, they do not fit the established criteria for its identification.

A. Frontal plane projection of the mean P, mean QRS, mean terminal 0.04-second QRS, and mean T vectors. (**B-E**) Spatial orientations of the mean P, mean QRS, mean terminal 0.04-second QRS and mean T vectors, respectively.

Summary: Right ventricular conduction delay, an abnormality of repolarization in the anterior portion of the heart (in this case, the right ventricle), and a possible right atrial abnormality have persisted following the surgical closure of a secundum atrial septal defect.

FIGURE 13.17
This electrocardiogram, showing an anteroseptal myocardial infarction and left pleural fluid effusion, was recorded

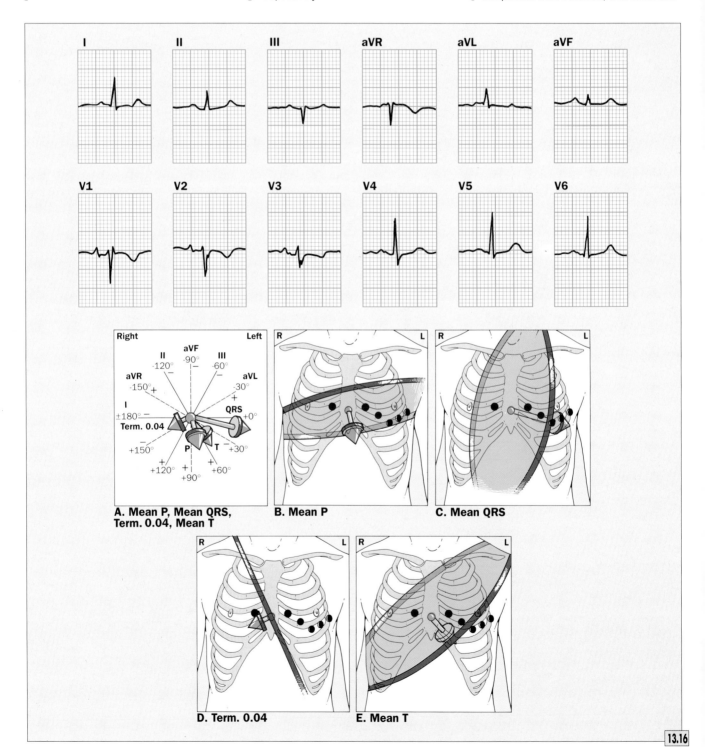

A. Mean P, Mean QRS, Term. 0.04, Mean T

B. Mean P

C. Mean QRS

D. Term. 0.04

E. Mean T

13.16

(Figure 13.17 continued.)
from a 59-year-old man with severe atherosclerotic coronary heart disease. An echo-Doppler study showed a severely dilated left ventricle, and a moderate mitral and tricuspid valve regurgitation.

Sinus tachycardia is present, and the heart rate is 104 complexes per minute. The duration of the PR interval is 0.14 second, that of the QRS complex is 0.08 second and that of the QT

interval is 0.29 second.

A. Frontal plane projection of the mean QRS, mean 0.02-second QRS, mean ST, and mean T vectors. (**B-E**) Spatial orientations of the vector shown in A.

Summary: The initial 0.02-second QRS vector is abnormal. It is posterior to the subsequent QRS force (notice the lack of R waves in leads V1, V2, and V3, and the small Q waves fol-

lowed by R and then S waves in leads V4, V5, and V6.) This abnormality is caused by the anteroseptal myocardial infarction. The mean ST vector is difficult to plot, but it is directed toward a large area of anterolateral epicardial injury. The mean T vector is directed away from this ischemic area. The amplitude of the complexes decreases considerably in leads V5 and V6; this is caused by the left pleural effusion.

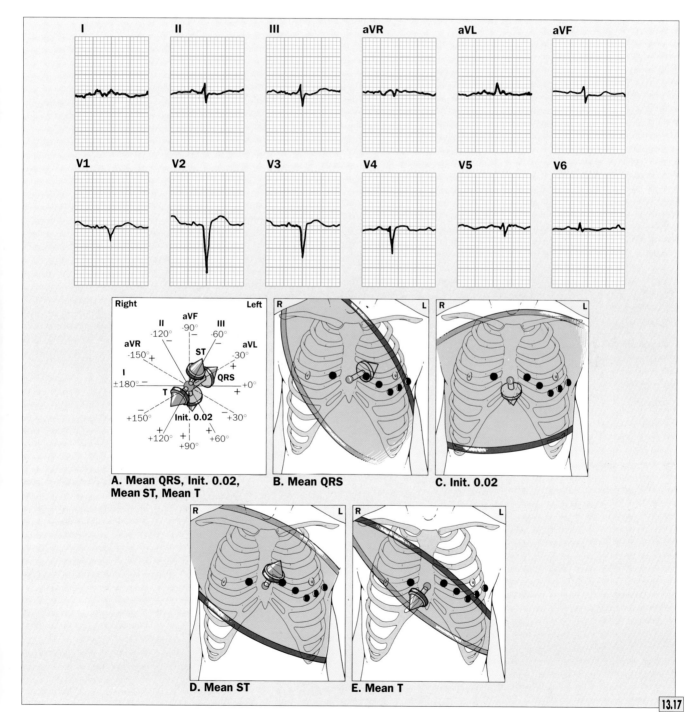

A. Mean QRS, Init. 0.02, Mean ST, Mean T

B. Mean QRS

C. Init. 0.02

D. Mean ST

E. Mean T

13.17

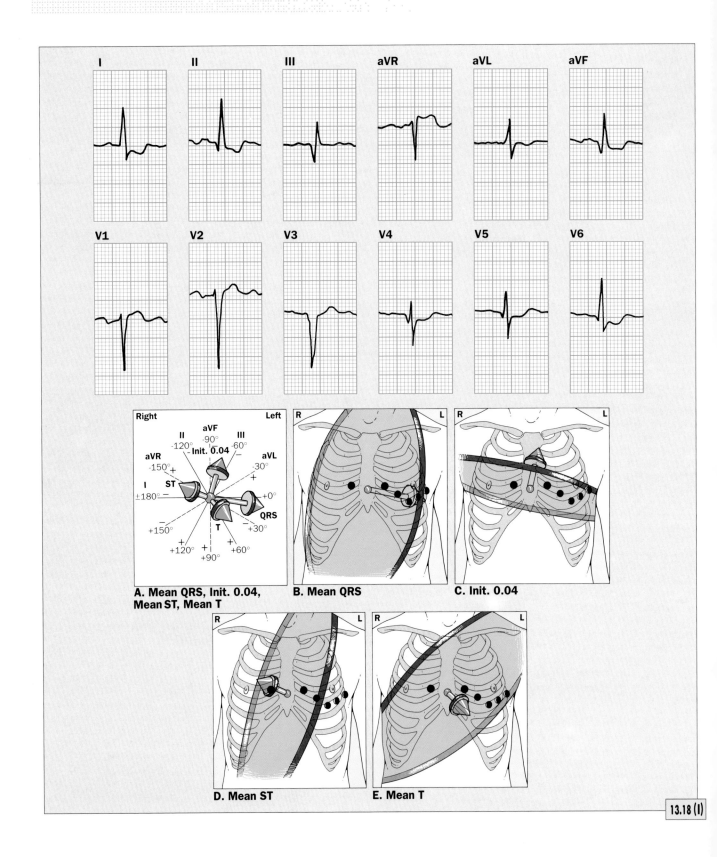

A. Mean QRS, Init. 0.04, Mean ST, Mean T

B. Mean QRS

C. Init. 0.04

D. Mean ST

E. Mean T

13.18 (I)

FIGURE 13.18
(I AND II)

These electrocardiograms, created by two hearts in the same patient, were recorded from a 50-year-old man with advanced ischemic cardiomyopathy. He had a heart transplant in which the donor's heart was attached to his own heart ("piggyback heart").

I. Tracings made prior to cardiac transplantation. (**A-D**) Frontal plane projection and spatial orientations of the mean QRS, mean initial 0.04-second QRS, mean ST, and mean T vectors, respectively. The tracing shows extensive inferior and lateral infarctions.

II. Tracings recorded after a new heart (the piggyback heart) was attached to the patient's old heart. The QRS complexes of the transplanted heart are identified by the symbol (PB).

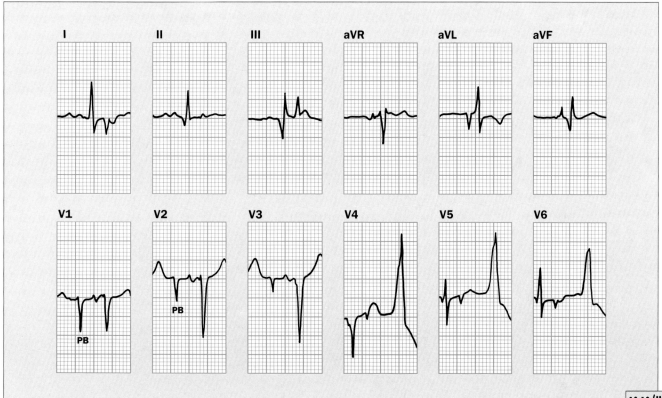

13.18 (II)

FIGURE 13.19

This electrocardiogram, showing left bundle branch block plus left anterior-superior division block, was recorded from a woman in her early forties with no other evidence of heart disease. Her sister, who also showed no other evidence of heart disease, developed left bundle branch block while also in her early forties (see Figure 13.20). There was a family history of atherosclerotic coronary heart disease occurring at a relatively early age.

The duration of the QRS complex is 0.12 second, and the mean QRS vector is directed about -45° to the left and 60°posteriorly. The mean terminal 0.04-second QRS vector is directed about -55° to the left and 40° posteriorly. The mean T vector is directed 50° inferiorly and about 30° anteriorly. The ventricular gradient is borderline.

(A-D) Frontal plane projection and spatial orientation of the mean QRS, mean terminal 0.04-second QRS, and mean T vectors, respectively.

Summary: The mean QRS vector is directed too far leftward for uncomplicated left bundle branch block; left anterior-superior division block is also present.

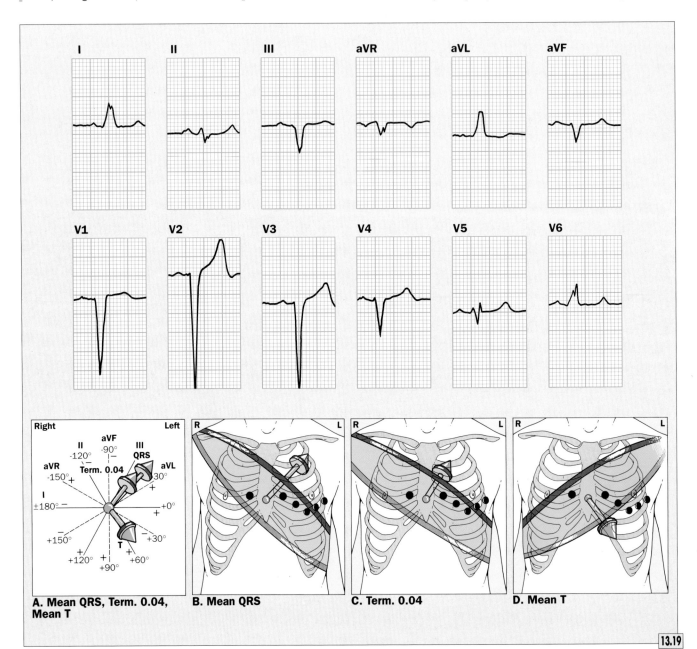

A. Mean QRS, Term. 0.04, Mean T

B. Mean QRS

C. Term. 0.04

D. Mean T

13.19

FIGURE 13.20

This electrocardiogram, showing left bundle branch block, was recorded from the sister of the patient whose electrocardiogram is reproduced in Figure 13.19. Left bundle branch block is present without evidence of other abnormalities.

The duration of the QRS complex is 0.12 second, and the mean QRS vector is directed about +70° inferiorly and 40° posteriorly. The mean terminal 0.04-second QRS vector is directed about –42° to the left and about 30° posteriorly. The mean T vector is directed +70° inferiorly and an undetermined number of degrees anteriorly. The ventricular gradient is normal.

(A-D) Frontal plane projection and spatial orientations of the mean QRS, mean terminal 0.04-second QRS, and mean T vectors, respectively. (Electro-cardiogram reproduced with the permission of Dr. John T. Cardone, Hartford, Conn.)

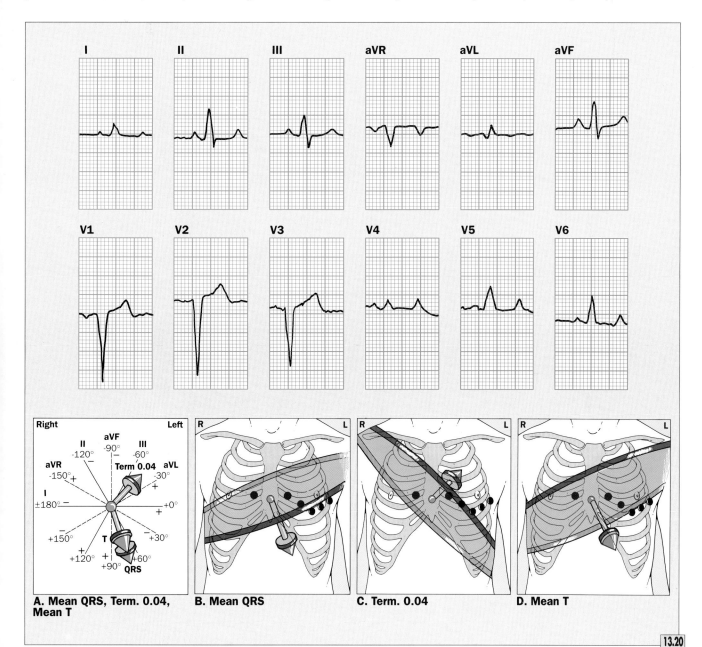

A. Mean QRS, Term. 0.04, Mean T

B. Mean QRS

C. Term. 0.04

D. Mean T

13.20

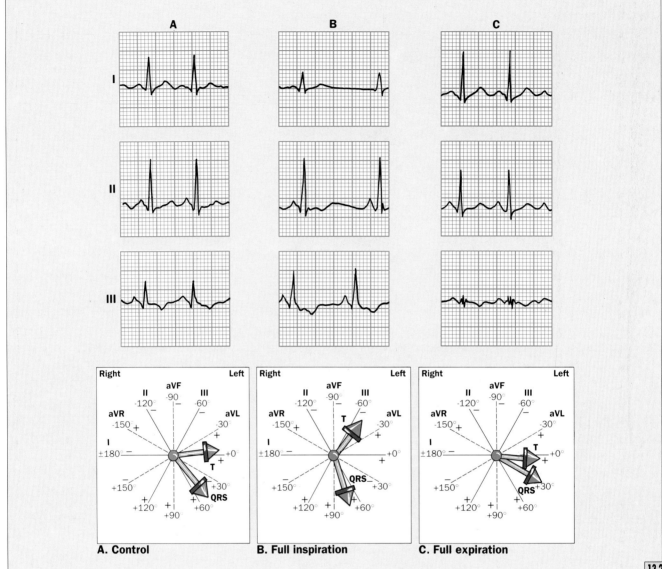

A. Control

B. Full inspiration

C. Full expiration

13.21

FIGURE 13.21
Alterations in the electrocardiogram and the directions of the mean QRS and T vectors associated with changes in respiration: **A.** control; **B.** full inspiration; **C.** full expiration. (Reproduced with permission from the publisher and author(6); see Figure Credits.)

FIGURE 13.22
The effect of hyperventilation in a patient with neurocirculatory asthenia: **A.** control; **B.** overventilation. (Reproduced with permission from the publisher and author (6); see Figure Credits.)

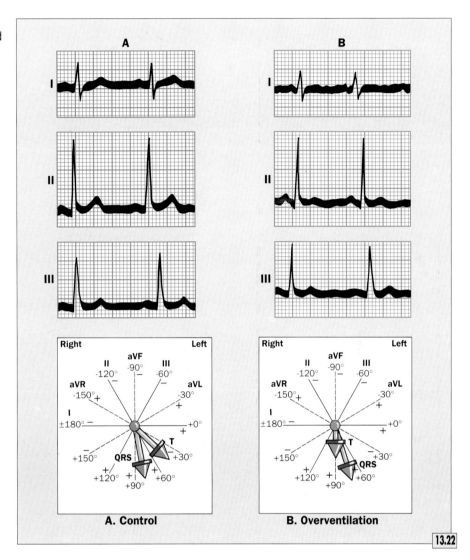

FIGURE 13.23
Startle reaction as the result of a pistol shot producing bundle branch block:
A. control; **B.** reaction. (Reproduced with permission from the publisher and author(6); see Figure Credits.)

FIGURE 13.24
This electrocardiogram and frontal plane vector projections are from a 14-year-old.

A. Note the wide QRS-T angle, with the T wave directed leftward and supe-

riorly when the patient is seated.
B. When the patient is supine, the direction of the mean QRS vector has changed very little. It should be pointed out that a vertically-directed mean QRS vector identified in the supine tracing

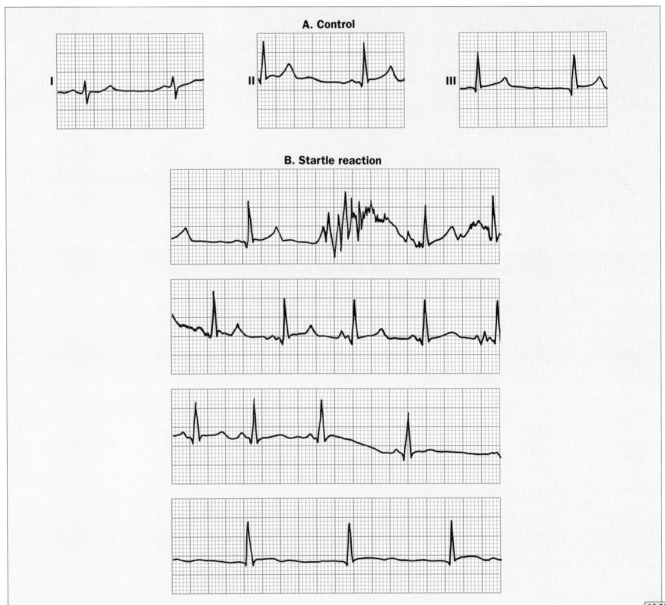

A. Control

I   II   III

B. Startle reaction

13.23

(Figure 13.24 continued.)
will change very little in direction when the patient assumes the seated or upright position. This is in contrast with a horizontal mean QRS vector recorded in the supine position, which shifts toward a more vertical position when the patient assumes an upright or seated position.

In this tracing, there is a shift of the mean T vector to the left and superiorly when the patient sits upright. This is due to a change in ventricular volume and heart size and the influence of these two factors on repolarization. (Reproduced with permission from the publisher and author(6); see Figure Credits.)

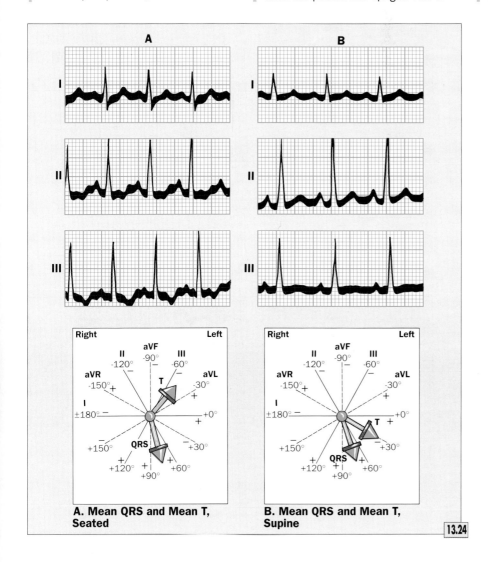

A. Mean QRS and Mean T, Seated

B. Mean QRS and Mean T, Supine

13.24

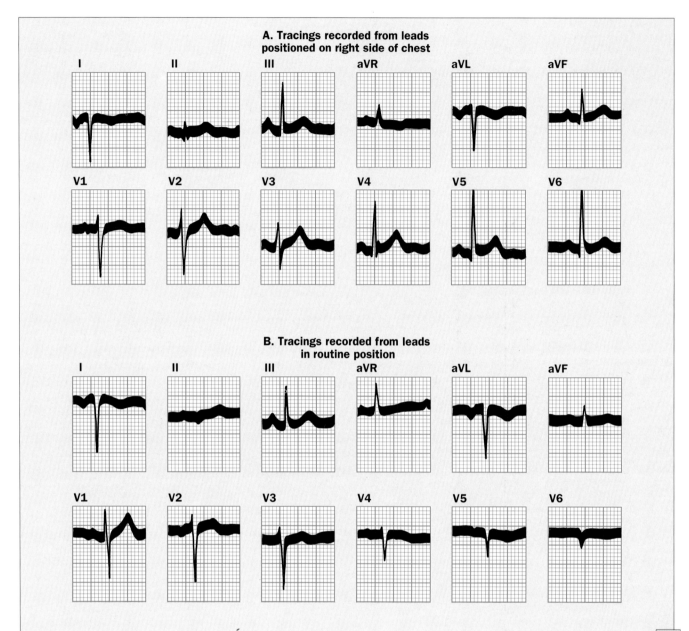

A. Tracings recorded from leads positioned on right side of chest

B. Tracings recorded from leads in routine position

13.25

FIGURE 13.25

This electrocardiogram was recorded from a 52-year-old man with situs inversus.

A. The P, QRS, and T waves are inverted in lead I. The precordial leads were recorded from the right side, and the deflections are normal. **B.** When the precordial leads were recorded from their routine positions, the deflections become progressively smaller from lead V1 to lead V6. In addition, all of the QRS complexes are negative.

Summary: When the P wave, QRS complex, and T wave are negative in lead I, and the QRS complexes are negative in the precordial leads (but are smaller in V6 than in V1, V2, and V3), it is highly likely that situs inversus is present. (Reproduced with permission from the publisher and author(6); see Figure Credits.)

FIGURE 13.26

The influence of precordial electrode misplacement on the precordial electro-cardiogram. When an electrical force, represented as a vector, is directed between 0° and +90°, the transitional pathway of the vector will be located between two of the chest lead deflections, or it will pass through one of the chest lead deflections. This makes it quite easy to identify which complexes are resultantly negative, which are resultantly positive, and which are resultantly zero.

A. In this figure, the deflections recorded at electrode positions V1, V2, and V3 would be negative, and those recorded at electrode positions V4, V5 and V6 would be positive. This occurs because the transitional pathway is *perpendicular* to a line connecting the V2, V3, and V4 positions.

When an electrical force, represented as a vector, is directed between 0° and -90° or between +90° and ±180°, the transitional pathway may be oriented in a way that makes it difficult to identify which complexes are resultantly nega-tive, which complexes are resultantly positive, and which are resultantly zero.

B. In this figure, the deflection recorded at electrode position V1 would be resultantly negative, those recorded at electrode positions V5 and V6 would be resultantly positive, and those recorded at the electrode positions for leads V2, V3, and V4 would all be resultantly 0° (or nearly so). This is because a line connecting electrode positions V2, V3, and V4 is parallel with the transitional pathway of the vector in question. Note that if, on a repeat electrocardiogram, the V2 electrode position were placed one centimeter higher than is shown here, a positive deflection would be recorded, whereas a the misplacement of lead V2 by several centimeters in part A would not change the positivity or negativity of the deflection, with the exception of those deflections recorded near the transitional pathway. This would not change the spatial orientation of the vector very much.

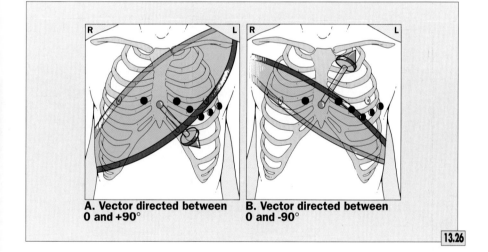

A. Vector directed between 0 and +90°

B. Vector directed between 0 and -90°

13.26

FIGURE 13.27 (I AND II)

The influence of switched arm leads on the electrocardiogram of a young adult male.

I. This electrocardiogram was recorded from a normal, young adult male physician. **A.** Frontal plane projection of the mean P, mean QRS, and mean T vectors. (**B-D**) Spatial orientations of the mean P, mean QRS, and mean T vectors, respectively.

II. This electrocardiogram was recorded from the same subject as above. In this recording, the electrode that should have been placed on the right arm was placed on the left arm, and vice versa. Note that the deflection in lead II in this tracing looks like the deflection recorded in lead III in the tracing labeled(I); the deflection in lead III in this tracing looks like the deflection in lead II in part I; and lead I in this tracing is the upside-down mirror image

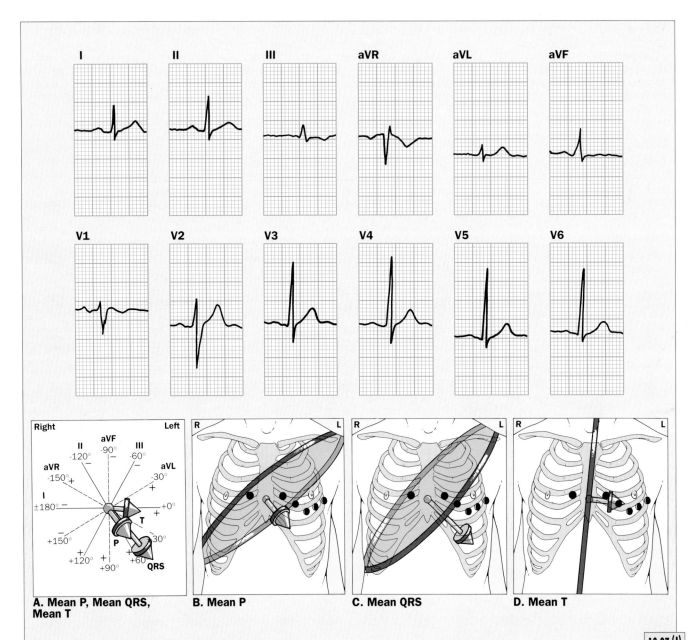

A. Mean P, Mean QRS, Mean T

B. Mean P

C. Mean QRS

D. Mean T

13.27 (I)

of lead I in the tracing shown in part I. The deflection in lead aVL in this tracing looks like that recorded in lead aVR in the first tracing; the deflection in aVR looks like the one recorded in lead aVL; and the deflection in lead aVF matches the one in lead aVF in the first tracing.

(**A-B**) It is not possible to construct the spatial orientation of the mean P vector, mean QRS vector or mean T vector in a case such as this: no arrangement will fit.

One can deduce that the arm leads have been reversed because the precor-

dial deflections appear normal while the frontal plane projections of the mean P, mean QRS and mean T vector are highly abnormal, and because the deflections in leads V3, V4, V5, and V6 are positive. (I wish to thank Dr. Henry Sadlo for providing both of these electrocardiograms.)

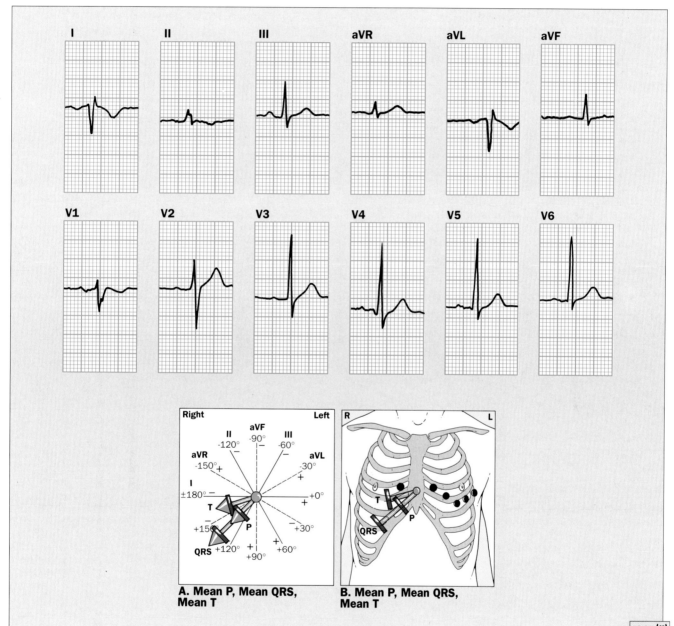

A. Mean P, Mean QRS, Mean T

B. Mean P, Mean QRS, Mean T

13.27 (II)

REFERENCES

1. Fowler NO, Daniels C, Scott RC, et al: The electrocardiogram in cor pulmonale with and without emphysema. *Am J Cardiol* 1965;16:500.
2. McGinn S, White PD: Acute cor pulmonale resulting from pulmonary embolism. its clinical recognition. *JAMA* 1935;104(17):1473.
3. Stein PD, Dalen JE, McIntyre KM, Sasahara AA, Wenger NK, Willis PW III:The electrocardiogram in acute pulmonary embolism. *Prog Cardiovasc Dis* 1975;27(4):247.
4. Hurst JW, Woodson GC Jr: *Atlas of Spatial Vector Electrocardiography*. New York and Toronto, Blakiston, 1952, p 203.
5. Castleman B, Bland EF: Organized emboli of the tertiary pulmonary arteries. *Arch Pathol* 1947;42:581.
6. Graybiel A, White PD, Wheeler L, Williams C: *Electrocardiography in Practice*, Ed 3. Philadelphia, WB Saunders, 1952, p 186.
7. Millar K, Abildskov JA: Notched T waves in young persons with central nervous system lesions. *Circulation* 1968;37:597.
8. Hersch C: Electrocardiographic changes in head injuries. *Circulation* 1961;23:853.
9. Burch GE, Meyers R, Abildskov JA: A new electrocardiographic pattern observed in cerebrovascular accidents. *Circulation* 1954;9:719.
10. Connor RCR: Heart damage associated with intracranial lesions. *Br Med J* 1968;3:29.
11. Zeppilli P: The athlete's heart: differentiation of training effects from organic heart disease. *Pract Cardiol* 1988;14(8):61.
12. Zeppilli P, Venerando A: Sudden death and physical exertion. *J Sports Med Phys Fitness* 1981;21:299.
13. DeBusk RF: Techniques of exercise testing. In Hurst JW (ed): The Heart, Ed 7. New York, McGraw-Hill, 1990, p 1825.

FIGURE CREDITS

Table 13.2 From Fowler NO, Daniels C, Scott RC, et al: The electrocardiogram in cor pulmonale with and without emphysema. *Am J Cardiol* 1965; 16:501.

Table 13.4 From Stein PD, Dalen JE, McIntyre KM, Sasahara AA, Wenger NK, Willis PW III: The electrocardiogram in acute pulmonary embolism. *Prog Cardiovasc Dis* 1975; 27(4)247.

Table 13.8 From Zeppilli P: The athlete's heart: differentiation of training effects from organic heart disease. *Prac Cardiol* 1988; 14(8):61.

Table 13.9 From Zeppilli P: The athlete's heart: differentiation of training effects from organic heart disease. *Prac Cardiol* 1988; 14(8):61.

Figure 13.1 From Fowler NO, Daniels C, Scott RC, et al: The electrocardiogram in cor pulmonale with and without emphysema. *Am J Cardiol* 1965; 16:503.

Figure 13.2 From McGinn S, White PD: Acute cor pulmonale resulting from pulmonary embolism: its clinical recognition. *JAMA* 1935; 104(17):1475.

Figure 13.3 From Hurst JW, Woodson GC Jr: Atlas of Spatial Vector Electrocardiography. New York and Toronto, Blakiston, 1952, p 203.

Figure 13.4 From Graybiel A, White PD, Wheeler L, Williams C: Electrocardiography in Practice, Ed 3. Philadelphia, WB Saunders, 1952, p 186.

Figure 13.5 From Burch GE, Meyers R, Abildskov JA: A new electrocardiographic pattern observed in cerebrovascular accidents. *Circulation* 1954; 9:720.

Figure 13.7 From Zeppilli P: The athlete's heart: differentiation of training effects from organic disease. *Pract Cardiol* 1988; 14:61.

Figure 13.8 From Zeppilli P: The athlete's heart: differentiation of training effects from organic disease. *Pract Cardiol* 1988; 14:61.

Figure 13.10 From Graybiel A, White PD, Wheeler L, Williams C: *Electrocardiography in Practice*, Ed 3. Philadelphia, WB Saunders, 1952, p 247.

Figure 13.11 From Graybiel A, White PD, Wheeler L, Williams C: *Electrocardiography in Practice*, Ed 3. Philadelphia, WB Saunders, 1952, p 248.

Figure 13.12 From Chung EK: *Cardiac Arrhythmias: Self-Assessment*. Baltimore, Williams and Wilkins, 1977, p 435.

Figure 13.13 From Lepeschkin E: Physiologic basis of the U wave. In Schlant RC, Hurst JW (eds): *Advances in Electrocardiography*. New York, Grune & Stratton, 1976, p 369.

Figure 13.14 From Fisch C: Electrolytes and the heart. In Hurst JW (ed): *The Heart*, Ed 6. New York, McGraw-Hill, 1986, p 1473.

Figure 13.15 From Chung EK: *Cardiac Arrhythmias: Self-Assessment*. Baltimore, Williams and Wilkins, 1977, p 277.

Figure 13.21 From Graybiel A, White PD, Wheeler L, Williams C: *Electrocardiography in Practice*, Ed 3. Philadelphia, WB Saunders, 1952, p 69.

Figure 13.22 From Graybiel A, White PD, Wheeler L, Williams C: *Electrocardiography in Practice*, Ed 3. Philadelphia, WB Saunders, 1952, p 71.

Figure 13.23 From Graybiel A, White PD, Wheeler L, Williams C: *Electrocardiography in Practice*, Ed 3. Philadelphia, WB Saunders, 1952, p 71.

Figure 13.24 From Graybiel A, White PD, Wheeler L, Williams C: *Electrocardiography in Practice*, Ed 3. Philadelphia, WB Saunders, 1952, p 70.

Figure 13.25 From Graybiel A, White PD, Wheeler L, Williams C: *Electrocardiography in Practice*, Ed 3. Philadelphia, WB Saunders, 1952, p 219.

APPENDIX

T A B L E 1 :

DATA FOR COMPUTATION OF HEART RATE AND VALUES FOR THE MAXIMUM NORMAL QT INTERVALS AT VARIOUS RATES IN ADULTS*

Cycle Time (0.04-sec intervals)	Rate	Max. QT (sec) Male	Max. QT (sec) Female	Cycle Time (0.04-sec intervals)	Rate	Max. QT (sec) Male	Max. QT (sec) Female
5	300	.19	.20	28	52	.42	.47
6	250	.20	.22	29	51	.43	.47
7	214	.21	.23	30	50	.44	.48
8	187	.23	.25	31	48	.45	.49
9	166	.24	.26	32	46	.45	.50
10	150	.25	.28	33	45	.46	.51
11	136	.26	.29	34	43	.47	.51
12	125	.28	.30	35	42	.47	.52
13	115	.29	.32	36	41	.48	.53
14	107	.30	.33	37	40	.49	.54
15	100	.31	.34	38	39	.49	.54
16	93	.32	.35	39	38	.50	.55
17	88	.33	.36	40	37	.51	.56
18	83	.34	.37	41	36	.51	.56
19	78	.35	.38	42	35	.52	.57
20	75	.36	.39	43	35	.52	.58
21	71	.37	.40	44	34	.53	.58
22	68	.38	.41	45	33	.54	.59
23	65	.38	.42	46	32	.54	.60
24	62	.39	.43	47	32	.55	.60
25	60	.40	.44	48	31	.56	.61
26	57	.41	.45	49	30	.56	.62
27	55	.42	.46	50	30	.57	.62

* Rate computation for regular rhythms only.
Reprinted by permission from Ferrer MI: *Electrocardiographic Notebook* (4th ed.). Futura, Mt. Kisco, N.Y., 1973.

T A B L E 2 :

NORMAL VALUES FOR PR INTERVALS

Upper Limits of the Normal PR Interval (Corrected for rate)*

Rate	Below 70	71-90	91-110	111-130	Above 130
LARGE ADULTS	0.21	0.20	0.19	0.18	0.17
SMALL ADULTS	0.20	0.19	0.18	0.17	0.16
CHILDREN, AGES 14 TO 17	0.19	0.18	0.17	0.16	0.15
CHILDREN, AGES 7 TO 13	0.18	0.17	0.16	0.15	0.14
CHILDREN, AGES 11/2 TO 6	0.17	0.165	0.155	0.145	0.135
CHILDREN, AGES 0 TO 11/2	0.16	0.15	0.145	0.135	0.125

Range of the Normal PR Interval and P Wave Duration (Uncorrected for rate)†

Age	PR Interval(sec) Range	P Wave Duration(sec) Range
0-1 WEEK	0.08-0.15	0.04-0.08
1 WEEK-1 MONTH	0.08-0.14	0.03-0.08
1 MONTH-3 MONTHS	0.08-0.14	0.04-0.08
3 MONTH-6 MONTHS	0.08-0.14	0.04-0.08
6 MONTH-1 YEAR	0.08-0.15	0.04-0.08
1 YEAR-3 YEARS	0.08-0.15	0.06-0.09
3 YEARS-5 YEARS	0.10-0.17	0.05-0.11
5 YEARS-16 YEARS	0.10-0.20	0.05-0.12
16 YEARS-20 YEARS	0.12-0.20	0.08-0.12

* Reprinted by permission from Ferrer, MI: *Electrocardiographic Notebook (4th ed.)*. Futura, Mt. Kisco, N.Y., 1973.
† Adapted by permission from Burch GE, DePasquale NP: *Electrocardiography in the Diagnosis of Congenital Heart Disease*. Lea & Febiger, Philadelphia, 1967.

T A B L E   3 :

NORMAL VALUES FOR ECG WAVES IN AV AND V LEADS IN ADULTS

Criteria for Normal Deflections (mm) in Adults in Augmented Extremity Leads aVR, aVL, aVF
(with normal instrument sensitivity)

	P		Q		R*		S		S-T†		T‡	
	Min.	Max.	Min.	Max.	Min.	Max.	Min.	Max	Min.	Max.	Min.	Max.
aVR	-1.5	-08	0	12.0	0	4.5	0	16.0	0	0	-6.0	-1.0
aVL	-1.0	1.0	0	2.0	0	8.0	0	10.0	0	0	-1.5	2.0
aVF	0	3.0	0	2.5	1.5	20.0	0	7.0	0	0	0.2	5.0

Criteria for Normal Deflections (mm) in Adults in Precordial Leads V1 to V6. (With instrument sensitivity at half normal
[1 mv = 0.5 cm]. Values must be doubled if records are made at normal sensitivity [1 mv = 1cm]).

	P		Q		R*		S		S-T†		T‡	
	Min.	Max.	Min.	Max.	Min.	Max	Min.	Max.	Min.	Max.	Min.	Max.
V1	0	1.0	0	0	0.5	5.0	2.0	12.5	0	0.5	-1.5	2.5
V2	-0.3	1.0	0	0	1.5	10.0	2.0	20.0	0	0.5	1.0	6.0
V3	0.3	1.0	0	0.5	3.0	20.0	0	12.0	0	1.0	1.0	8.0
V4	0	1.0	0	2.0	4.0	22.0	0	8.0	0	0.5	0.8	7.0
V5	0	0.5	0	1.5	4.0	17.0	0	4.0	0	0	0.5	5.0
V6	0	0.5	0	1.5	3.5	110	0	1.5	0	0	0.5	3.0

* Includes value of R′ if present.
† ST junction with reference to PR segment.
‡ T with reference to isoelectric line.
Reprinted by permission from Ferrer to MI: *Electrocardiographic Notebook (4th ed.)*. Futura, Mt. Kisco, N.Y., 1973.

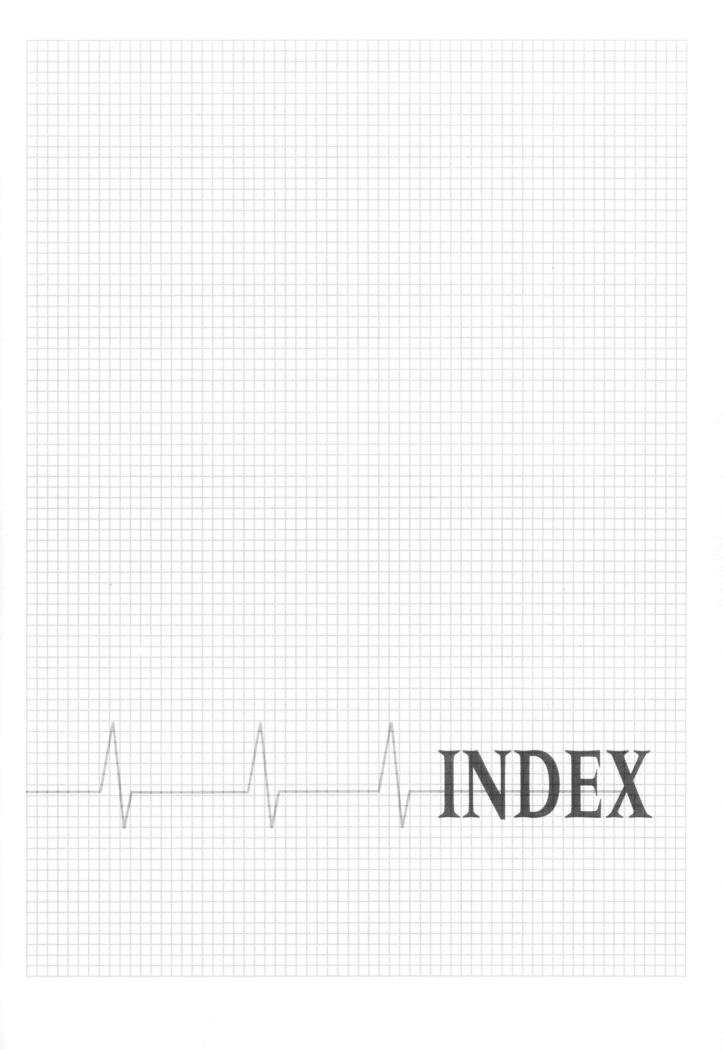

INDEX